Current Research in Chiropractic and Rehabilitation Medicine

Edited by **Esther Henson**

SYRAWOOD
PUBLISHING HOUSE
New York

Published by Syrawood Publishing House,
750 Third Avenue, 9th Floor,
New York, NY 10017, USA
www.syrawoodpublishinghouse.com

Current Research in Chiropractic and Rehabilitation Medicine
Edited by Esther Henson

International Standard Book Number: 978-1-68286-239-1 (Hardback)

Printed in China.

Contents

Preface

Chiropractic is rapidly becoming a prominent field of alternative medicine for treatment of musculoskeletal disorders. The researches based on chiropractic and rehabilitation medicine focus on musculoskeletal, social, emotional and neurological health and treatment. Some of the topics that are included in this book are postoperative rehabilitation and assessment, clinical studies on patient life style and dietary habits, risks associated with rehabilitation medicine and chiropractic, etc. It strives to provide a fair idea about this discipline and to help develop a better understanding of the latest advances within this field. This book is a resource guide for experts as well as students.

The information contained in this book is the result of intensive hard work done by researchers in this field. All due efforts have been made to make this book serve as a complete guiding source for students and researchers. The topics in this book have been comprehensively explained to help readers understand the growing trends in the field.

I would like to thank the entire group of writers who made sincere efforts in this book and my family who supported me in my efforts of working on this book. I take this opportunity to thank all those who have been a guiding force throughout my life.

Editor

Chiropractic wellness on the web: the content and quality of information related to wellness and primary prevention on the Internet

Marion Willard Evans Jr[1*], Stephen M Perle[2], Harrison Ndetan[3]

Abstract

Background: The Internet has become a common source of information for patients wishing to learn about health information. Previous studies found information related to back pain poor and often contradictory to current guidelines. Wellness has become a common topic in the field of chiropractic and accrediting agencies have standards on delivery of wellness-based content in college curricula as well as directives for clinical applications. The purpose of this study was to evaluate the quality of the information on the Internet using the terms "chiropractic wellness," or "wellness chiropractic".

Methods: Five commonly used search engines were selected and the first 10 sites found using the strategy above were evaluated by two raters. Demographic assessments of the sites were made along with whether they were Health on the Net Foundation (HON) certified, contained standard wellness content, mentioned any Healthy People Focus Areas, and other chiropractic topics. Kappa statistics compared inter-rater agreement.

Results: Potential patients appeared to be the audience 87% of the time and a private doctor of chiropractic appeared to be the typical site owner. The sites usually promoted the provider. No sites displayed HON certification logo nor did any appear to meet the HON certification criteria. Twenty-six sites (55%) promoted regular physical activity in some manner and 18 (38%) had information on health risks of tobacco. Four (9%) had mental health or stress-reduction content but none had information supportive of vaccination. Some had information contradictory to common public health measures.

Conclusions: Patients searching the Internet for chiropractic wellness information will often find useless information that will not help them maintain health or become well. Most simply market the chiropractic practice or allow for a patients to provide personal information in exchange for more 'wellness' information. More research should be done on how providers determine site content, pay any attention to the details on their sites, or agree with content as some appear to be prefabricated sites. Website content could be enhanced by sharing of information from reputable sources like US Centers for Disease Control, the National Institutes of Health and other authoritative sources. HON certification should also be sought.

Background

The Internet has become a common source of information for patients wishing to learn about health and medical information [1-4]. Internet sites can now be set up by virtually anyone and may contain information simply chosen at will by the site developers. Butler and Foster found information related to back pain on the Internet to be of poor quality with information often contradictory to current guidelines for management of back pain [5]. Studies on home management of childhood fever and depression on the Internet were also rated poorly in separate studies [6,7].

Specific evaluations of Internet-based information have been performed for back and spinal pain, scoliosis and spine-related education [8-10]. Li and colleagues searched the Internet for information on back pain using a search strategy of what a typical patient might utilize and found a lack of quality control, problems

* Correspondence: wevans@txchiro.edu
[1]Texas Chiropractic College, Pasadena, TX, USA
Full list of author information is available at the end of the article

with credibility of information on the sites, and a minority of sites containing evidence-based information related to back pain [8]. Mathur and associates investigated the quality of information related to management of scoliosis on Internet sites and stated that the information was typically of limited quality and of poor information value [9]. They suggested that physicians assume more responsibility for the content of information on their sites. In a review of readability of sites related to spine-related educational information on websites reading levels were typically way above recommended levels averaging over the 10th grade reading level [10].

Wellness has become a common topic in the field of chiropractic and the accrediting agency for chiropractic degree programs has standards on delivery of wellness-based content in college curricula as well as directives for practical application at the clinical level [11]. In addition, the United States (US) has established goals for the nation through the ***Healthy People*** (HP) initiatives that should guide content provided by all health care providers and community health programs related to wellness and primary prevention [12]. The Association of Chiropractic Colleges and the American Chiropractic Association, the largest trade group in the US for the chiropractic profession have mission statements supportive of these efforts [13,14]. The Chiropractic and Osteopathic College of Australasia has within its objectives to; "promote the integration of chiropractors and osteopaths into the broader community health team" and; to, "participate in activities related to public health" [15]. Wellness content then should be content that is congruent with the recommendations of such documents mentioned above, not in opposition to accepted public or community health measures, and not simply advertisement for services in a provider's office. The purpose of this study was to specifically evaluate the quality of the information patients searching the Internet with the terms "chiropractic wellness," or "wellness chiropractic" would find based on whether the information is in line with current, accepted health promoting measures related to general health and wellness described above. Further, sites were evaluated to see if they followed the criteria called for by Health on the Net Foundation (HON) http://www.hon.ch/ which provides guidelines for responsible health and medical information sites on the Internet. Sites were also assessed as to whether they contained typical chiropractic terms such as subluxation, innate intelligence, or spinal care and whether the presence of these terms would predict more or less health promotion and wellness advice available on the site.

Methods

The search terms selected were "chiropractic wellness," and "wellness chiropractic." These terms are commonly used in signage on chiropractic offices in marketing materials so the rationale or aim of the investigators was to see what content this would net on the World Wide Web and evaluate that content. Five search engines commonly used by laypersons were selected. These were Google.com, Yahoo.com, Microsoft Bing.com, Ask.com, and AOL.com. These were selected because of their rankings as the most used websites from http://www.comscore.com. The first 10 sites found anywhere on the web by using the strategy above on each search engine were selected for evaluation.

Demographic assessments of the sites were made such as determining the audience they were aimed at, the source of the website, the purpose, whether they were Health on the Net Foundation (HON) certified http://www.hon.ch/, whether they contained standard wellness content, mentioned any HP Focus Areas, HP Ten Leading Health Indicators, and typical chiropractic topics. The typical chiropractic topics determined if the site mentioned subluxation, prevention of spinal pain, innate or presented anti-vaccination, anti-drug or anti-medical viewpoints. The site was judged using the 8 principles defined by HON:

1–Information must be authoritative giving qualifications of authors

2–Purpose of the website should be apparent

3–Confidentiality that respects the privacy site users

4–Information must be documented: citing sources and dates of medical information

5–Justification of claims

6–Website contact details should be apparent

7–Disclosure of funding sources

8–Advertising policy stated that clearly distinguishes advertising from editorial content

Data about websites were placed in an Excel spreadsheet with assessment of each of the criteria described. Assessment was made separately by two researchers (Rater1 and Rater2). Data was reviewed and converted into SPSS version 16 (SPSS Inc, Chicago, IL) for analysis. Primarily, frequencies were generated on the web content of each site as reviewed by Rater1 and Rater2. Kappa statistics was used to assess agreement beyond chance between the two reviewers. Kappa value is reported as a percent and commonly interpreted as follows: <20% negligible improvement over chance agreement alone, 21-40% minimal improvement, 41-60% fair, 61-80% good improvement, 81-92% very good, and 93-100% excellent [16]. The main chiropractic topic assessed was whether or not a webpage specifically mentioned subluxation, innate and/or spinal pain. Odds ratios (OR) and 95% confidence intervals (CI) were computed from binary cross-tabulations that assessed whether or not sites that mentioned each of those chiropractic topics (such as 'subluxation', 'innate', or management of spinal conditions) were also likely to mention anti-vaccination, anti-drug, or anti-medical information. It should be stated that the term 'subluxation' is a chiropractic term suggestive of nerve interference occurring when spinal alignment or function is altered by such events as trauma and that innate refers to the body having an innate or inborn ability to heal itself if spinal nerve interference is not present. These terms are unique to chiropractic in a historical sense and are commonly used by some practitioners adhering to a traditional belief that spinal conditions are a source of other diseases; hence, the interest in the evaluators as to presence or non-presence of these terms and their potential for effect modification of any analysis.

Results

General purpose and content of the site

A total of 47 unique websites were obtained from the 5 search engines for testing. All of the sites appear to be sites in North America. Nineteen sites were captured under the term 'chiropractic wellness,' and 18 with the term 'wellness chiropractic' and 10 of these were found with both search phrases. The results reported below are mainly based on one reviewer (Rater2), however, details on both reviewers as well as percent agreement between them are present in the tables.

Potential patients appeared to be the audience the websites were aiming at 87% of the time and a private doctor of chiropractic appeared to be the site owner 87% of the time. The purpose of the site was typically to promote the provider (87% of sites). None of the web sites displayed HON certification logo nor did any appear to meet the HON certification criteria. One site appeared to offer authoritative information and 1 stated the purpose of the site. Thirteen had statements related to confidentiality of the site. Only 2 had referenced and dated content and 2 had justification of claims. Contact details were unavailable on >90% of sites. Demographics of websites and Rater1 and 2 responses with kappa statistics appear in table 1.

Table 1 General website demographic information and rater responses

Variable	Rater1 n (%)	Rater2 n (%)	Kappa (%)
Audience			
Patient	44(94)	41(87)	100
Chiropractor	3(6)	3(7)	
Gen public	0(0)	2(4)	
Missing	0(0)	1(2)	
Owner			
Chiropractor	43(92)	41(87)	100
Non-profit	2(4)	3(7)	
Commercial	2(4)	2(4)	
Missing	0(0)	1(2)	
HON certified			
Yes	0(0)	0(0)	100
No	47(100)	47(100)	
Info is authoritative			
Yes	0(0)	1(2)	100
No	47(100)	46(98)	
Purpose defined			
Product	3(6)	1(2)	98
Service	0(0)	2(4)	
Provider	44(94)	41(88)	
Profession	0(0)	2(4)	
Missing	0(0)	1(2)	
Confidentiality			
Yes	0(0)	13(28)	72
No	47(100)	34(72)	
Info documented, referenced, dated			
Yes	0(0)	2(4)	96
No	47(100)	45(96)	
Justification of claims			
Yes	0(0)	2(4)	96
No	47(100)	45(96)	
Website contact details			
Yes	0(0)	2(6)	94
No	47(100)	44(94)	
Discloses funding			
Yes	0(0)	0(0)	100
No	47(100)	47(100)	
Advertising policy			
Yes	0(0)	1(2)	98
No	47(100)	46(98)	

General health-related content on the site

Twenty-six sites (53%) promoted regular physical activity in some manner and 18 (38%) had information on tobacco or health risks of smoking. Four (9%) had mental health or stress-reduction content but none had information supportive of vaccination. Other data on general health information is noted in table 2 along with both raters' assessments and kappa statistics.

Healthy People content areas

No website specifically mentioned the topic of HP 2010 but 25 (53%) had some content that fell loosely under one of the HP headings. For example, one site had some content related to cancer prevention and one had information on prevention of stroke or heart disease but none had information specific to prevention of kidney disease, disability, secondary conditions, or family planning. Content related to prevention falling under HP Focus areas was rare on all of the websites reviewed. Table 3 lists content-specific information related to HP Focus areas.

Table 2 General health and wellness topics mentioned on websites

Variable	Rater1 n (%)	Rater2 n (%)	Kappa (%)
Site promotes physical activity			
Yes	17(36)	26(53)	83
No	30(64)	22(47)	
Smoking cessation information			
Yes	2(4)	18(38)	66
No	45(96)	29(62)	
Mental health and stress reduction			
Yes	9(19)	4(9)	89
No	38(81)	43(91)	
Safety (helmet, seatbelt use)			
Yes	1(2)	0(0)	98
No	46(98)	47(100)	
Healthy diet			
Yes	15(32)	27(57)	74
No	32(68)	20(43)	
Alcohol use in moderation			
Yes	0(0)	0(0)	100
No	47(100)	47(100)	
Safe sex practices			
Yes	0(0)	0(0)	100
No	47(100)	47(100)	
Substance abuse			
Yes	0(0)	0(0)	100
No	47(100)	47(100)	
Supportive of vaccines			
Yes	0(0)	0(0)	100
No	47(100)	47(100)	

Among the HP Leading Health Indicators, 25 (53%) sites specifically mentioned a topic that would fall under one of them. Some mention of physical activity (PA) was noted on 26 (53%) of sites and 21 (45%) mentioned issues related to overweight and obesity. As stated, 18 (38%) had some information related to the health issues associated with tobacco use. Only 1 site contained any information on injury and violence prevention and no site had information on the benefits of immunization, responsible sexual behavior, vision and hearing problems, or substance abuse.

Chiropractic topic information

Thirty-six (77% of sites) contained information on chiropractic 'subluxation' and 28 (60%) had information on 'innate.' Thirty-one (66%) sites had information related to prevention of spinal pain. Regarding information expressing negative aspects of medical interventions or vaccines, 16 (34%) of sites contained obvious anti-vaccination information, 16 (34%) had information that was anti-drug (prescription or medical use of drugs), and 14 (30%) had general anti-medical information related to the medical profession. Interestingly, no site had specific HP Focus Area information on the topic of arthritis, osteoporosis, and chronic back conditions. Complete responses from reviewers and kappa ratios of chiropractic information are listed in table 4.

Sites that mentioned 'subluxation' were more likely to have anti-vaccine information compared to sites that did not [OR = 5.7(95% CI,0.6-50.6)], were more likely to have anti-drug information [OR = 5.7(95%CI,0.6-50.6)], and to have anti-medical information [OR = 4.5(95% CI,0.5-40.3)]. However, these did not approach statistical significance due to small cell numbers. Sites that mentioned 'innate' were more likely to contain anti-vaccine information [OR = 7.5(95%CI,1.4-39.0)], were more likely to have anti-drug information [OR = 7.5(95% CI,1.4-39.0)], and more likely to have anti-medical information on them as well [OR = 2.0(95%CI,1.4-2.9)]. Sites that mentioned spinal pain were more likely to contain anti-vaccine information as well when compared to those that did not, [OR = 4.9(95%CI, 0.9-26.0)], more likely contained anti-drug information [OR = 12.1(95% CI,1.4-105.0)], and more likely to contain anti-medicine information, [OR = 9.4(95%CI,1.0-81.0)], though not all were statistically significant at the 95% confidence level.

Discussion

Reviewer agreement levels were generally good to excellent. In cases where variation occurred it was often due to the depth of site review. Some information may have appeared in the opening page of a website but on others, information was on panels that required the reviewer click several tabs to reach it. When information was not visible on the website in a prominent manner it was harder to locate and probably accounts for some variation between reviewers. In addition, reviewers used their own judgment as to whether sites contained information consistent with HP initiatives. Perhaps a good example is diet and health. Some sites contained information on diet and health. However, many of those were to market a nutritional product or supplement and may not have indicated a level of dietary information related to HP initiatives. This may have accounted for variation among reviewers in general.

The Internet will get more and more use as a potential source of information on health and wellness. Smart-phone technology now allows a search from almost anywhere. The purpose of this study was to see what wellness-oriented content would appear on sites the public would likely come across on a routine search of chiropractic wellness. The findings presented here indicate a lack of sound wellness and health promotion information available on most of the sites analyzed.

Table 3 Healthy People content information found on websites

Variable	Rater1 n (%)	Rater2 n (%)	Kappa (%)
Site mentions HP initiatives			
Yes	0(0)	0(0)	100
No	47(100)	47(100)	
HP Focus Areas mentioned			
Yes	25(53)	25(53)	100
No	22(47)	22(47)	
Access to quality health care			
Yes	0(0)	0(0)	100
No	47(100)	47(100)	
Conditions *Arthritis, osteoporosis, chronic back pain*			
Yes	9(19)	0(0)	81
No	38(81)	47(100)	
Cancer prevention			
Yes	0(0)	1(2)	98
No	47(100)	46(98)	
Kidney Disease			
Yes	0(0)	0(0)	100
No	47(100)	47(100)	
Diabetes			
Yes	3(6)	0(0)	94
No	44(94)	47(100)	
Disability, secondary cond.			
Yes	0(0)	0(0)	100
No	47(100)	47(100)	
Educ. and community-based programs			
Yes	0(0)	0(0)	94
No	44(94)	47(100)	
Vision and hearing problems			
Yes	0(0)	0(0)	100
No	47(100)	47(100)	
Select Leading Health Indicators			
Physical activity			
Yes	17(36)	25(53)	83
No	30(64)	22(47)	
Overweight/obese			
Yes	9(19)	21(45)	74
No	38(81)	26(55)	
Tobacco use			
Yes	2(4)	8(17)	87
No	45(96)	39(83)	
Responsible sexual behavior			
Yes	0(0)	0(0)	100
No	47(100)	47(100)	
Mental health			
Yes	1(2)	10(21)	81
No	46(98)	37(79)	
Injury and violence			
Yes	1(2)	1(2)	100
No	46(98)	46(98)	
Immunization			
Yes	0(0)	0(0)	100
No	47(100)	47(100)	

Research into what consumers look for to determine the credibility of an Internet site may be a cause for more concern over content. One study found that people look more at the professional design of the site, whether they can get, "a quick lay-out of the site", the user-friendliness of the site, and speedy interface times rather than if the content is evidence-based or supported by the scientific literature [17]. This is unfortunate but understandable. After all, these are laypersons and not providers. This same study found that patient markers for quality included if it "sounded plausible," sounded "scientific," looked "trustworthy." These have little to do with actual viability of content.

The depth of information on the sites analyzed was poor and was rarely evidence-based. Many sites may have mentioned one should walk for example but there was no evidence of information related to PA Guidelines for Americans [18] and information related to how one could get PA into their daily lives. This study also

Table 4 Chiropractic characteristics and demographic information from websites

Variable	Rater1 n (%)	Rater2 n (%)	Kappa (%)
Site specifically mentions subluxation			
Yes	35(75)	36(77)	99
No	12(25)	11(23)	
Site specifically mentions innate			
Yes	34(72)	28(60)	87
No	13(28)	19(40)	
Mentions preventing spine pain			
Yes	37(79)	31(66)	87
No	10(21)	16(34)	
Anti-vaccine information in website			
Yes	14(30)	16(34)	96
No	33(70)	31(66)	
Anti-medical information on website			
Yes	19(40)	14(30)	89
No	28(60)	33(70)	
Anti-drug information on website			
Yes	19(40)	16(34)	94
No	28(60)	31(66)	

demonstrates that some chiropractors (those with web sites that are highly ranked by the search engines used) apparently still support the notion that chiropractic care is a viable substitute for medical care. Anti-medical, anti-drug, and anti-vaccine rhetoric was often displayed prominently on the sites evaluated. This is concerning. Worth noting is that several sites had very near identical content apparently having purchased a pre-manufactured website from one of a small number of vendors. Many practitioners may be purchasing these and paying little attention to the information that is on the sites. Nevertheless, content was poor on most sites lacking legitimate evidence-based wellness information. This is ultimately the responsibility of the provider.

Patients need information on how to become healthy and stay healthy. Many of the health conditions listed in HP documents and that this project assessed are the common causes of premature morbidity and mortality in Americans and typically, in a minority of sites was there any information that would likely help a patient restore or gain healthy ground. The sites typically marketed the chiropractor and offered promotional materials for services offered in the clinic and not wellness measures common to preventive medicine or health promotion. Even specific information on prevention of reoccurrence of back pain was scant on most sites. The anti-public health messaging could actually be seen by some as anti-prevention, therefore anti-wellness. This was discouraging as well since it could be seen on approximately 1/3 of sites reviewed.

Limitations of the study

There are some specific limitations of this study. First, this was a review of a minimum number of sites and they may not be representative of all chiropractic sites. Second, two reviewers who are researchers made the reviews and there is bias inherent to that process. However, agreement was consistent most of the time. Third, many content areas related to HP initiatives clearly would not be expected to be found on a site to promote an individual chiropractor as was the apparent intent of most of the websites reviewed. Therefore, content like safe sex practices, vision and hearing issues are not likely to be found here even if they might benefit patients who view the sites. Lastly, all of the sites netted by the search on these most popular search engines appear to be in North America and therefore, we cannot assume any of the results would generalize to Europe, Australia, or other parts of the world.

Conclusions

Patients searching the Internet for chiropractic wellness information will often find a lot of poorly done, useless information that will not help them maintain health or become well. Most of the time it simply markets the chiropractic practice and lists services that they offer in the office or allows for a patient to provide personal information in exchange for more 'wellness' information. This equates to marketing and practice building. More research should be done on how providers determine site content, whether they pay any attention to the details presented on their sites, and whether they even agree with it. Website content could be enhanced by sharing of information from reputable sources like the US Centers for Disease Control and Prevention, the National Institutes of Health and other authoritative sources. HON certification should be sought as well. Information that is illogical or contradictory to current, accepted public health and wellness practices should be removed to better serve patients and potential patients who visit these sites. This could serve to improve the cultural authority of chiropractic as providers interested in wellness in the process. Regulatory boards should begin to evaluate the advertising content on these sites as some of it seems to violate board rules on ethics and advertising.

List of abbreviations

AOL: America Online search engine; CI: confidence interval; HON: Health on the Net Foundation; HP: Health People initiative of the United States; OR: odds-ratio; PA: physical activity; US: United States.

Author details

[1]Texas Chiropractic College, Pasadena, TX, USA. [2]University of Bridgeport, Bridgeport, CT USA. [3]Parker Research Institute, Dallas, TX, USA.

Authors' contributions

SMP conceptualized the idea for the study, developed the spreadsheet for comparative analysis, was a reviewer of websites, and helped construct and review the manuscript. MWE assisted in development of methods of assessment, reviewed the websites, assisted in data analysis and interpretation, and primarily constructed the manuscript. HN performed the statistical analysis, helped create all tables. All authors reviewed and edited the manuscript and approved the final manuscript.

Competing interests

The authors are all primarily researchers and academics and acknowledge no competing interests related to the research presented.

References

1. Shepperd S, Charnock D, Gann B: **Helping patients' access high-quality health information.** *BMJ* 1999, **319**:764-766.
2. Krempec J, Hall J, Biermann JC: **Internet use by patients in orthopedic surgery.** *Iowa Orthop J* 2003, **23**:80-82.
3. Brooks BA: **Using the Internet for patient education.** *Orthop Nurs* 2001, **20**:69-77.
4. Aslam N, Bowyer D, Wainwright A, Theologis T, Benson M: **Evaluation of Internet use by pediatric orthopeadic outpatients and the quality of information available.** *J Pediatr Orthop B* 2005, **14**:129-133.
5. Butler L, Foster NE: **Back pain online: a cross-sectional survey of the quality of web-based information on low back pain.** *Spine* 2003, **28**:395-401.

6. Impicciatore P, Pandolfini C, Casella N, Bonati M: **Reliability of health information for the public on the World Wide Web: systematic survey of advice on managing childhood fever at home.** *BMJ* 1997, **314**:1875-1879.
7. Griffiths KM, Christensen H: **Quality of web-based information on treatment of depression: cross-sectional survey.** *BMJ* 2000, **25**:2932-2939.
8. Li L, Irvin E, Guzmán J, Bombardier C: **Surfing for back pain patients: the nature and quality of back pain information on the internet.** *Spine* 2001, **26**:545-557.
9. Mathur S, Shanti N, Brkaric M, Sood V, Kubeck J, Paulino C, Merola AA: **Surfing for scoliosis: the quality of information available on the Internet.** *Spine* 2005, **30**:2695-2700.
10. Vives M, Young L, Sabharwal S: **Readability of spine-related patient education materials from subspecialty organization and spine practitioner websites.** *Spine* 2009, **34**:2826-2831.
11. The Council on Chiropractic Education: **Standards for doctor of chiropractic programs and requirements for institutional status.** Scottsdale, AZ; 2007.
12. United States Department of Health and Human Services: **Healthy People 2010. Understanding and Improving Health.** [http://www.healthypeople.gov/], [Online] [cited 2010 Aug 12].
13. American Chiropractic Association: **Wellness Model.** [http://www.acatoday.org/level2_css.cfm?T2ID=117&T1ID=10&ID=10&searchQuery=wellness+and+health+promotion#109], [Online] [cited 2011 Jan 24].
14. Association of Chiropractic Colleges: **Paradigm on Wellness.** [http://www.chirocolleges.org/paradigm_scope_practice.html], [Online] [cited 2010 Jul 10].
15. Chiropractic and Osteopathic College of Australasia: **Objectives of the college.** [http://www.coca.com.au/index.php?ID=14], [Online] [cited 2010 Oct 28].
16. Byrt T: **How good is that agreement?** *Epidemiol* 1996, **7**:561.
17. Eysenbach G, Köhler C: **How do consumers search for and appraise health information on the world wide web? Qualitative study using focus groups, usability tests, and in-depth interviews.** *BMJ* 2002, **324**:573-577.
18. United States Department of Health and Human Services: **2008 Physical Activity Guidelines for Americans: Be active, healthy, and happy.** [http://www.health.gov/paguidelines], [Online] [cited 2010 Aug 10].

2

The role of chiropractic care in older adults

Paul E Dougherty[1,2*], Cheryl Hawk[3], Debra K Weiner[4,5], Brian Gleberzon[6], Kari Andrew[7] and Lisa Killinger[7]

Abstract

There are a rising number of older adults; in the US alone nearly 20% of the population will be 65 or older by 2030. Chiropractic is one of the most frequently utilized types of complementary and alternative care by older adults, used by an estimated 5% of older adults in the U.S. annually. Chiropractic care involves many different types of interventions, including preventive strategies. This commentary by experts in the field of geriatrics, discusses the evidence for the use of spinal manipulative therapy, acupuncture, nutritional counseling and fall prevention strategies as delivered by doctors of chiropractic. Given the utilization of chiropractic services by the older adult, it is imperative that providers be familiar with the evidence for and the prudent use of different management strategies for older adults.

Introduction

By 2030, nearly one in five U.S. residents is expected to be age 65 or older [1]. An estimated 14% of patients treated by doctors of chiropractic (DCs) are 65 and older [2]. The most common reason for an older adult to see a DC is musculoskeletal pain, most often lower back pain [3]. Although the most common reason for older adults seeking chiropractic care is for musculoskeletal symptoms, DCs may also provide a diverse range of services to these patients [4]. Given this fact, for the purpose of this manuscript chiropractic care will be defined as; "the provision by a doctor of chiropractic of services related to patient assessment, maintenance of health, prevention of illness, and treatment of illness or injury". The focus of this manuscript is to describe the evidence for achievement of some of these goals in the older adult population. The purpose of this manuscript is to present an overview of information to the practicing chiropractor on utilization of specific management tools. This is not meant to be a systematic review of the literature or an evidence based guideline. The authors each have personal experience in evaluating and treating older adults as well as established expertise in research and publication in these areas. The authors recognize that there is a need for further research in the area of management of the older adult by DC's and discuss in the conclusion future research considerations.

* Correspondence: pdougherty@nycc.edu
[1]Research Department, New York Chiropractic College, 2360 State Route 89, Seneca Falls, NY 13148, USA
Full list of author information is available at the end of the article

Although chiropractic encompasses many different treatment modalities, the authors have chosen to focus on five specific interventions that are commonly utilized by DCs: spinal manipulative therapy (SMT), acupuncture, physical activity/exercise, nutritional counseling and fall prevention [5,6]. These have been chosen not only because they are commonly utilized treatments, but also because they align with certain goals of Healthy People 2020: 1) to reduce the proportion of older adults with functional limitations and 2) to increase the proportion of older adults with reduced physical or cognitive function engaging in physical activities; 3) to reduce the number of falls among older adults [7,8].

Many older adults utilize chiropractic services throughout the US and Canada. A recent longitudinal study reported 14.6% utilization over a 15 year period (1993-2007) with an annual prevalence rate of between 4.1%-5.4% [2]. The majority of older adults seek chiropractic care for back and/or neck pain, and treatment approaches for these conditions vary widely. Most DCs utilize some form of SMT. More than 90% provide nutritional advice and recommend nutritional supplements. Most also recommend therapeutic exercises and advise patients to engage in physical activity [5,6]. There is also a growing trend in the utilization of acupuncture in older adults [9]. Although few studies have specifically evaluated the role of chiropractic care in older adults, it is imperative that practicing DCs familiarize themselves with the unique nuances of dealing with older adults and understand the evidence for treatment approaches. The authors provide a brief overview of the current evidence for each of the interventions listed above as well as their commonly reported indications and contraindications.

Role of spinal manipulative therapy in older adults

Spinal pain is a significant musculoskeletal problem among older patients [10]. A recent report states the prevalence of disabling and non-disabling back pain in community-dwelling adults is 6% and 23%, respectively [11]. There are data that suggest that SMT may play an important role in the management of patients with spinal and peripheral joint pain and associated dysfunction [12]. From the perspective of the public, chiropractic care is most closely associated with SMT, which is traditionally high-velocity, low-amplitude (HVLA) maneuvers applied manually to spinal and peripheral joints [13]. These maneuvers move the joints from the end of their active and passive ranges of motion into the paraphysiological joint space, but not beyond their limit of anatomic integrity to deliver a therapeutic stimulus to the joint complex [14].

It is important to recognize that SMT used by DCs in practice may incorporate multiple techniques. These techniques may include varying levels of biomechanical force, ranging from high-velocity, low-amplitude to low-velocity, low-amplitude. SMT may also include instrument-assisted manipulation, use of specialized tables, use of padded wedges and many low-force techniques [5,6]. While it is assumed that alteration of techniques may play an important role in older adults where variation in technique and application of force is thought to aid in prevention of injury associated with a SMT, there is a need for further research to determine the most appropriate approach in this population. There are two trials that have compared outcomes in older adults comparing a higher force technique versus a lower force technique; both of these trials demonstrated comparable results with both techniques [15,16].

There is a limited but suggestive body of knowledge that supports the effectiveness of SMT for many conditions that affect older patients [17]. This body of knowledge includes expert opinion, case reports, case series, observational studies and a few randomized controlled trials [17]. The majority of studies evaluated the role of SMT for musculoskeletal pain syndromes including lower back pain with and without stenosis [15,18] neck pain with and without stenosis [19,20], knee pain [21,22] and thoracic function [23,24]. In addition there has been investigation into the role of SMT in patients with dizziness [25-28].

There are a number of case reports and case series that describe the successful management of older patients with spinal or peripheral joint pain using low-velocity, low-amplitude mobilizations and high-velocity, low-amplitude manipulations as well as instrument-assisted manipulation, padded wedges and other low force techniques [29]. Observational studies and randomized controlled trials have reported improvement of spinal pain (acute, sub-acute and chronic) among seniors using not only SMT but also low force techniques such as BioEnergetic Synchronization Technique [16] and Cox Flexion-Distraction technique [15]. The 2010 UK Report of Manual therapies reported that "SMT is effective in adults for: acute, subacute, and chronic low back pain; migraine and cervicogenic headache; cervicogenic dizziness; manipulation/mobilization is effective for several extremity joint conditions; and thoracic manipulation/mobilization is effective for acute/subacute neck pain [30]." However, the authors did not do a sub-analysis of older adults.

In addition to spinal pain, there is a limited body of evidence reporting on the role of SMT to address symptoms associated with other co-morbid clinical conditions [31], including: COPD [23,24], constipation [32], depression (associated with back pain) [33], Parkinson's disease [34,35], multiple sclerosis [36], pneumonia [37], spinal stenosis [18], urinary incontinence [38], and osteoarthritic pain and dysfunction, especially of the knee [21]. This body of evidence is limited in that is it chiefly comprised of descriptive studies–case reports and case series. There are no high quality trials reporting on these conditions. There is a need to further investigate the role of SMT in the older adult for these non-spine related conditions.

Safety

There are limited data on the safety of SMT in the older adult population. Dougherty et al. have reported on the safety of SMT in the older adult population, specifically in osteoporosis, anticoagulation therapy and spinal stenosis. These data are from two randomized controlled trials and also from retrospective data from a chiropractic clinic in a long term care facility. The retrospective file review reports on institutionalized older adults who underwent SMT. These patients had significant co-morbidities such as osteoporosis, post-stroke status, Parkinson's disease, amyotrophic lateral sclerosis and other chronic conditions [34]. The data from the randomized controlled trials showed adverse event data lower than previously reported in the literature, with only 35% of the patients experiencing any type of AE and none experiencing any serious adverse events associated with SMT [39]. It is noted that the AE's reported in this trial utilized a standard definition of AE's utilized typically in drug trials. However, these were reported utilizing different terminology than the retrospective review of older adults treated in a long-term care facility, which used recently reported manual therapy specific terminology for reporting AE's [40]. This variation in criteria for reporting adverse events highlights the need to develop a universally accepted format of reporting adverse events in studies evaluating spinal manipulation that can be used in multiple research settings.

It is felt that there may even be a lower incidence of AE's associated with SMT in older adults due to the practice by most DCs of modifying their use of SMT, often substituting lower-force for higher-force procedures to minimize the net force applied to a joint [41]. In addition to the topics discussed above, there are other non-manipulative manual procedures available to DCs [29,42]. Table 1 describes the results of a consensus project on best practices in the geriatric population concerning SMT treatment considerations in the older adult [4].

Acupuncture in older adults

For the purpose of this manuscript, "acupuncture" is defined as any of a variety of interventions that are administered using acupuncture needles. In the setting of low back pain management, this includes but is not limited to traditional Chinese acupuncture, percutaneous electrical nerve stimulation (PENS; a.k.a. percutaneous neuromodulation therapy), auricular acupuncture, trigger point deactivation, and deep intramuscular electrical stimulation. It is of note that there have been no trials conducted in which chiropractors have delivered the acupuncture to older adults. There is a need to further evaluate the role of chiropractors delivering acupuncture in a clinical setting, particularly in older adults who may not be able to tolerate more traditional manual therapy techniques. There is also a need to standardize the role of training of chiropractors to perform acupuncture in older adults. The authors have chosen to only discuss those trials that have specifically focused on older adults with LBP, since that is the most common presentation of older adults to chiropractors.

While older adults have been included in some trials evaluating the efficacy of acupuncture for the treatment of low back pain (LBP), only two have focused exclusively on older adults [43,44]. These have evaluated a more contemporary acupuncture technique, lumbar PENS. The first of these studies was a randomized controlled pilot trial involving 34 community dwelling older adults with chronic low back pain (CLBP) who received either lumbar PENS or a control procedure (acupuncture needles without electrical stimulation) twice a week for 6 weeks and participants were followed for 3 months [43]. Both groups also received physical therapy. Those randomized to lumbar PENS experienced significant pain reduction and functional improvement that was maintained at 3 months, but the group that received the control procedure experienced no improvement [43].

The second study was a randomized controlled trial of 200 older adults with CLBP who received one of four interventions twice a week for 6 weeks: 1) lumbar PENS and a general conditioning and aerobic exercise (GCAE) program, 2) lumbar PENS alone, 3) limited lumbar PENS (only 2 of 12 needles were stimulated for 5 minutes as compared with full PENS during which all needles are stimulated for 30 minutes), or 4) limited lumbar PENS and GCAE. Participants were followed for 6 months and all four groups experienced significant improvement that was maintained during the follow-up period [44]. Thus while electrical stimulation appears to be essential for therapeutic response, the minimal therapeutic dose is unknown. In addition to treatment for lower back pain, other studies have evaluated the role of acupuncture for other conditions. A recent review of the use of acupuncture for chronic musculoskeletal pain reported that there is insufficient experimental evidence to recommend the use of traditional Chinese acupuncture over other modalities for older adults with persistent musculoskeletal pain. The authors then state however that there are promising preliminary data to support the use of percutaneous electrical nerve stimulation for persistent low back pain [45].

The other acupuncture procedures noted above have not been studied exclusively in older adults, although they are not uncommonly used by practitioners trained in acupuncture. With Traditional Chinese Acupuncture, needles are strategically placed in acupuncture points to move the flow of energy or Qi (pronounced "chi"). Acupuncture points may be distant from the site of pathology. Needles may be stimulated mechanically (i.e., the acupuncturist intermittently turns the needles), with heat (e.g., lamp, moxibustion), light (e.g., laser), or electricity. Percutaneous electrical nerve stimulation uses

Table 1 Treatment considerations for older adults [4]

Patient characteristic	Treatment modification
Small body size; increased frailty	Decrease biomechanical force
Severe osteoporosis and/or other bone diseases such as infection or cancer.	High-force manipulation is contraindicated
Anticoagulation or corticosteroid medication	Soft tissue or other manual procedures which compress tissues are either contraindicated or should be used with caution and decreased biomechanical force.
Fear or anxiety related to manipulation, or preference for type of procedure	Adapt manipulation and soft tissue procedures to optimize patient comfort

electricity exclusively, and needles are placed neuroanatomically along dermatomes, myotomes and scleratomes. Duration of treatment with TCA and PENS is typically 20-40 minutes. Auricular acupuncture guides the placement of acupuncture needles according the homunculus on the ear's surface. A variety of needle types are available, some of which can be left in place for several days. Trigger point deactivation ("dry needling") and deep intramuscular electrical stimulation are targeted to localized areas of myofascial pain. There is a need for further research in evaluating the therapeutic role of these specific techniques in older adults.

A summary of the indications, relative contraindications and potential adverse effects associated with these procedures is provided in Table 2.

Nutritional counseling in older adults

Current research indicates that a large percentage of older adults do not receive adequate amounts of micronutrients in their daily diet [46,47]. Studies report that prevention strategies in the form of improvement in diet and health promotion counseling can lead to improved quality of life, significant reductions in disability, and reduction in health care costs [48,49].

The main goal for nutritional counseling should be to improve food choices, particularly with respect to increasing the intake of fruits and vegetables [48]. If consumption of adequate energy and micronutrients cannot be managed with dietary modification the use of dietary supplements may be considered. However, given the lack of rigorous clinical trials evaluating the effectiveness of dietary supplements it is difficult to make strong recommendations for or against nutritional supplements for meeting the nutritional needs of older adults.

Although multivitamin-mineral (MVM) supplements are used commonly by older adults, there is limited evidence of their impact on health outcomes [50]. Vitamin D and calcium supplements appear to have the most beneficial effects [51,52]. They have been found to be a critical adjunct to any pharmacologic regimen in the treatment of osteoporosis [52] and in the prevention of hip fractures and other non-vertebral fractures [51]. In addition, a recent systematic review on Vitamin D found that "Vitamin D treatment effectively reduces the risk of falls in older adults [53]." Recommended daily intake for calcium and vitamin D are 1,200 mg and 1,000 IU respectively [51]. All other commonly consumed supplements cannot be recommended at this time either due to inadequate evidence or due to evidence of significant side effects.

Even though a supplement may be considered "benign," providers must be aware of potential drug or disease interactions [51]. Data from the National Social Life, Health and Aging Project (NSHAP), a recent population-based survey of community-dwelling older adults in the United States, evaluated the potential impact of medication use on clinical outcomes that may result from drug interactions, including interactions between prescription and nonprescription therapies. Among prescription medication users, concurrent use of over-the-counter medications was 46% and concurrent use of dietary supplements was 52%.

A recent survey on dietary supplement use in the U.S. found that about one-half of the U.S. population and 70% of adults ≥ 71 years of age use dietary supplements;

Table 2 Acupuncture and related modalities for the treatment of CLBP

Modality	Indications	Contraindications (relative)	Potential Adverse Effects
Traditional Chinese Acupuncture (TCA)	Insufficient clinical trials evidence to recommend for older adults with CLBP	• Bleeding diathesis • Pacemaker (if leads cross chest when using electrical stimulation) • Severely immune-compromised state	• Bleeding, bruising • Infection (very rare) • Transient pain flare • Transient fatigue • Vasovagal response
Percutaneous electrical nerve stimulation (PENS)	CLBP in older adults; minimum effective dose of electrical stimulation unknown	As with TCA	As with TCA
Auricular acupuncture	Insufficient clinical trials evidence to recommend for older adults with CLBP; theoretically useful for augmenting corporeal treatments.	• Bleeding diathesis • Cartilage disease (e.g., relapsing polychondritis)	As with TCA
Trigger point deactivation	Myofascial pain; local twitch response is essential therapeutic element (ref). May be combined with other acupuncture modalities, e.g., following PENS for recalcitrant localized pain.	As with TCA	As with TCA; as compared with TCA and PENS, trigger point deactivation may be painful.
Deep intramuscular electrical stimulation	Localized myofascial pathology (e.g., piriformis, erector spinae); may be performed in addition to TCA or PENS for recalcitrant localized myofascial pain.	As with TCA	As with TCA

one-third use multivitamin-multimineral dietary supplements [54]. Overall, 68% of older adults using prescription medications are concurrently using over-the-counter medications, dietary supplements, or both. It was found that 1 in 25 older adults (approximately 2.2 million) were at risk for a major potential drug-drug interaction, and that more than half of these involved non-prescription therapies (including supplement use) [55]. Physicians are frequently unaware of their patients' nonprescription medication and/or supplement use because they do not ask patients; patients do not report such use, or both. The economic and health consequences of these potential interactions are considerable [55]. It is therefore imperative to for both the consumer and the DC to understand the benefits and risks for utilization of dietary supplements, identify potential interactions with other medications, and avoid large combinations to decreased overconsumption [52]. Adverse events associated with supplement use alone, apart from interactions, may include excess levels of iron and zinc. In addition, iron overload has been associated with coronary artery disease. Zinc overload has been associated with reduced copper status, impaired immune response, and lowered plasma high-density lipoprotein cholesterol levels [46].

These findings suggest that encouraging positive attitudes about a healthful diet in combination with nutrition guidance and appropriate supplement information may result in promoting advantageous use of supplements by this at-risk population.

Physical activity and exercise in older adults

The majority of DCs report that they utilize therapeutic exercise in their practices.[5] Physical activity and exercise are often recommended by DCs to their older adult patients. A recent population survey demonstrated that exercise recommendation was underutilized by providers of multiple disciplines [56]. Position statements for osteoarthritis recommend exercise as a key component of disease management [57]. Painful limitation of function and muscle loss (i.e., sarcopenia) are two common reasons for the recommendation of exercise in this population. The loss of muscle strength has been identified as a physiologically limiting factor to living independently among older persons [58]. Recent reviews have shown the positive effects of aerobic exercise and strength training on strength, balance, and physical functioning [59]. These reviews demonstrate a modest beneficial effect of resistive training on strength outcomes and strong evidence for the improving function, particularly gait speed and chair stands.

There are a few studies that have specifically evaluated long term improvements in disability in patients who undergo resistance training [60]. There are also strong data supporting the role of resistance exercise in improving pain associated with knee osteoarthritis [61]. A recent study reports that community dwelling older adults who were adherent to an adaptive physical activity program had lower levels of pain related disability [62]. Back pain is a common problem among the older adult population and the most common condition for which older adults seek care with a DC. DCs often combine SMT and exercise therapy. Recent studies have demonstrated the benefits of combining exercise and spinal manipulation for chronic lower back pain; however none of these studies have been specifically carried out in older adults [63].

A recent comparative effectiveness review found structured exercise and SMT appear to offer equivalent benefits in the management of pain and function for patients with nonspecific chronic LBP [64]. The recommendation from this review was, "if no clinical benefit is appreciated after using one of these approaches for 8 weeks, then the treatment plan should be reevaluated and consideration should be given to modifying the treatment approach or using alternate forms of care [64]." In addition to the use of exercise for the treatment of back pain, a recently systematic review found that there is moderate evidence on the use of exercise for fall prevention [65]. Another systematic review found that interventions with balance exercises reduced falls or fall-related fractures and improved balance in the majority of the studies reviewed. Muscle strengthening exercises were also found to be effective in improving lower extremity strength and back extensor strength; however, not all RCT's reviewed reported positive effects. Bone strength was improved by weight-bearing aerobic exercise with or without muscle strengthening exercise when the duration of the intervention was at least a year [66].

Given the evidence for the use of exercise recommendation, it is important that the clinician be aware of any risks associated with exercise therapy in older adults. A recent review article found that among 121 trials identified, 53 trials provided no comments about adverse events, 25 trials reported no adverse events occurred, and 43 trials reported some types of adverse events. Most adverse events reported were musculoskeletal problems such as muscle strain or joint pain. Adverse events were reported more often in trials that recruited participants with certain health conditions, functional limitations, or sedentary lifestyle [67]. The most important considerations in providing an exercise program for older adults is to assess their general health status and to assure that the program is tailored to their needs, whether it is strength, endurance, balance or improved motion. The older adult should be educated in warning signs such as chest pain or shortness of breath.

The most important principle in developing an exercise program for the older adult is to work with him/her in order to agree on a program to which they will adhere to. Patient centered exercise prescription involves shared goals between the patient and the provider [68]. The practitioner may also want to perform simple functional tests periodically, such as timed up and go or single leg stance [69], to demonstrate to the patient that they are making progress, which may otherwise be difficult for the patient to perceive. Finally, patients should be encouraged to participate in activities they enjoy; in fact one study found that leisure time activity was more effective than structured exercise in patients with lower back pain [70].

Fall prevention in older adults

Falls can result in decreased quality of life, disability, and/or death in older adults. Approximately one-third of those aged 65 and older fall each year, and falls are the leading cause of unintentional injuries and unintentional injury deaths in this population [71]. Related direct medical costs are at least $19 billion, expected to reach $44 billion by 2020 [65]. Of those fallers whose injuries require hospitalization, 40-50% subsequently lose their independence and enter a nursing home [72].

Fall prevention in older adults is a national priority, and is the subject of two *Healthy People 2020* objectives [8]. Fall prevention interventions are based on the identification and reduction of modifiable risk factors. The most important modifiable risk factors for falls in older adults are impaired mental status; psychotropic medications; polypharmacy; environmental hazards; poor vision; lower extremity weakness and/or dysfunction; and impairments in balance, gait and activities of daily living [73].

A 2010 systematic review funded by the Agency for Healthcare Research and Quality examined interventions designed to reduce falls in older adults [65]. Physical therapy, Vitamin D supplementation and, as stated above in the section on physical activity, exercise interventions to improve gait, balance, and/or function were found to reduce fall risk [65]. Although chiropractic care was not included in the review, these interventions are within the scope of chiropractic practice.

A consensus statement on "best practices" for chiropractic care for older adults specifically recommends that DCs collect falls history information, and states that they provide treatment and exercises for musculoskeletal conditions, which can be extrapolated to be appropriate for reducing fall risk [4]. Furthermore, recent reviews written by DCs emphasize the importance of incorporating fall prevention into chiropractic practice [74,75].

Pain-related musculoskeletal disability may influence balance, gait and the ability to accomplish daily activities, and therefore may contribute to fall risk. There is considerable evidence for positive effects of SMT for spine-related pain [30]. Because chronic musculoskeletal pain, such as that of osteoarthritis, is one factor affecting gait and balance in older people, chiropractic care may have an impact on fall prevention by treating joint pain and stiffness. Also, the literature suggests a possible positive effect of SMT on certain types of vertigo. There is limited, although promising, evidence that manual therapies may be beneficial for cervicogenic vertigo [27,28,30,31,76,77].

Discussion

DCs can play an important role in the management of health conditions in the older adult. Chiropractic care has often been associated only with the management of musculoskeletal disorders by the application of SMT. However, as we have discussed in this article, DCs often utilize multiple treatment modalities that address the patient as a whole, not only his or her musculoskeletal symptoms. It is important that the clinician evaluate the patient for any associated risks to the chosen intervention. There is a need for the practicing clinician to evaluate the most effective clinical strategy for managing the challenging older adult patient. The management of older adults is complicated by many factors such as co-morbidities that may limit the type of treatment intervention employed. These co-morbidities, as highlighted in this manuscript, include concerns of osseous weakness, interaction of nutritional supplements with current prescription medication as well as concerns about fall risk. The busy practitioner must plan to spend extra time with the older adults patient to appropriately manage this population. This is a challenge given the current healthcare system. A recent survey discussed the barriers to such things as fall prevention discussions with older adults [78]. Not only are there barriers to discussions about fall prevention, but there are concerns about the amount of time that should be taken to appropriately educate the older adult concerning exercise recommendations [79]. There is a strong case to be made for the role of multidisciplinary care in the older adult with musculoskeletal pathology, however to achieve this the practicing chiropractor must develop relationships with those outside the chiropractic profession. This integrated care model has been described and has the potential to improve the overall role of chiropractic in the healthcare system [80].

There is concern about risk in the chiropractic management of the older adult and as mentioned in the body of the manuscript there is a need for systematic evaluation of the risk associated with any management strategy. In order to facilitate this evaluation of risk there is a need to develop a common terminology for the reporting of untoward events associated with any management strategy. While there have been efforts toward this, unfortunately the proposed terminology proposed by Carnes et al. [40] are not practical in some research settings such as the Veteran's Health Administration.

Once risks have been ruled out, the DC, while being sensitive to patient preferences, can choose from a wide variety of treatment approaches within the chiropractic scope of practice. It is noteworthy that there remains a controversy concerning the role of the chiropractor in delivering acupuncture. In the US the regulations concerning the use of acupuncture vary by state and therefore it is not able to be utilized in all clinical settings. There is also a need for research further defining the role of acupuncture in the management of older adults.

As the number of older adults presenting to chiropractic practices increases it is imperative that the DC not only discuss the patient's current complaints, but also preventive strategies including fall prevention, nutritional counseling and physical activity. As the population continues to age there will be a greater need for the chiropractic profession to meet the needs of the older adult.

Conclusions

While there is already substantial published research to assist the evidence-based DC in his/her care plan for the older adult, there is a need for well designed clinical trials and large observational studies to identify the most beneficial treatments, particularly for complementary and alternative interventions such as manual therapy including, but not limited to, spinal manipulative therapy and acupuncture.

Author details
[1]Research Department, New York Chiropractic College, 2360 State Route 89, Seneca Falls, NY 13148, USA. [2]School of Medicine and Dentistry, University of Rochester, Rochester, NY 14620, USA. [3]Logan College of Chiropractic, Chesterfield, MO 63017, USA. [4]Anesthesiology & Psychiatry, VA Pittsburgh, Pittsburgh 15261, USA. [5]U. of Pittsburgh, 3550 Terrace Street Pittsburgh, PA 1526, USA. [6]Canadian Memorial Chiropractic College, 6100 Leslie Street, Toronto, ON M2H 3J1, Canada. [7]Palmer College of Chiropractic, 1000 Brady St, Davenport, IA 52803, USA.

Authors' contributions
PD conceived of the study, designed the study, drafted the manuscript, and reviewed literature. CH participated in manuscript writing and literature review. DW participated in manuscript writing and literature review. BG participated in manuscript writing and literature review. KA participated in manuscript writing and literature review. LK participated in manuscript writing and literature review. All authors read and approved the final manuscript.

Competing interests
The authors declare that they have no competing interests.

References
1. U.S. Census Bureau: **An older and more diverse population by mid-century.** *Book an Older and More Diverse Population by Mid-Century, City* 2008.
2. Weigel P, Hockenberry JM, Bentler SE, Obrizan M, Kaskie B, Jones MP, Ohsfeldt RL, Rosenthal GE, Wallace RB, Wolinsky FD: **A longitudinal study of chiropractic use among older adults in the United States.** *Chiropr Osteopat* 2010, **18**:34.
3. Coulter ID, Hurwitz EL, Adams AH, Genovese BJ, Hays R, Shekelle PG: **Patients using chiropractors in North America: who are they, and why are they in chiropractic care?** *Spine* 2002, **27**:291-296, discussion 297-298.
4. Hawk C, Schneider M, Dougherty P, Gleberzon BJ, Killinger LZ: **Best practices recommendations for chiropractic care for older adults: results of a consensus process.** *J Manipulative Physiol Ther* 2010, **33**:464-473.
5. Christensen M, Kollasch M, Hyland JK: *Practice Analysis of Chiropractic* Greeley: NBCE; 2010.
6. Christensen M, Kollasch M, Ward R, Webb K, Day A, ZumBrunnen J: *Job Analysis of Chiropractic* Greeley: NBCE; 2005.
7. U.S. Department of Health and Human Services: **Healthy people 2010: understanding and improving health.** *Book Healthy People 2010: Understanding and Improving Health.* 2 edition. Washington: U.S. Government Printing Office; 2000.
8. U.S. Department of Health and Human Services: **Healthy people 2020.** *Book Healthy People 2020* Washington: U.S. Government Printing Office; 2011.
9. Votova K, Wister AV: **Self-care dimensions of complementary and alternative medicine use among older adults.** *Gerontology* 2007, **53**:21-27.
10. Weiner DK, Sakamoto S, Perera S, Breuer P: **Chronic low back pain in older adults: prevalence, reliability, and validity of physical examination findings.** *J Am Geriatr Soc* 2006, **54**:11-20.
11. Docking RE, Fleming J, Brayne C, Zhao J, Macfarlane GJ, Jones GT: **Epidemiology of back pain in older adults: prevalence and risk factors for back pain onset.** *Rheumatology (Oxford)* 2011, **50**:1645-1653.
12. Bokarius AV, Bokarius V: **Evidence-based review of manual therapy efficacy in treatment of chronic musculoskeletal pain.** *Pain Pract* 2010, **10**:451-458.
13. Hurwitz EL, Coulter ID, Adams AH, Genovese BJ, Shekelle PG: **Use of chiropractic services from 1985 through 1991 in the United States and Canada.** *Am J Public Health* 1998, **88**:771-776.
14. Pickar JG: **Neurophysiological effects of spinal manipulation.** *Spine J* 2002, **2**:357-371.
15. Hondras MA, Long CR, Cao Y, Rowell RM, Meeker WC: **A randomized controlled trial comparing 2 types of spinal manipulation and minimal conservative medical care for adults 55 years and older with subacute or chronic low back pain.** *J Manipulative Physiol Ther* 2009, **32**:330-343.
16. Hawk C, Rupert R, Colonvega M, Boyd J, Hall S: **Comparison of Bio-Energetic Synchronization Technique and customary chiropractic care for older adults with chronic musculoskeletal pain.** *J Manipulative Physiol Ther* 2006, **29**:540-549.
17. Gleberzon BJ: **A narrative review of the published chiropractic literature regarding older patients from 2001-2010.** *J Can Chiropr Assoc* 2011, **55**:76-95.
18. Stuber K, Sajko S, Kristmanson K: **Chiropractic treatment of lumbar spinal stenosis: a review of the literature.** *J Chiropr Med* 2009, **8**:77-85.
19. Kukurin GW: **The amelioration of symptoms in cervical spinal stenosis with spinal cord deformation through specific chiropractic manipulation: a case report with long-term follow-up.** *J Manipulative Physiol Ther* 2004, **27**:e7.
20. Murphy DR, Hurwitz EL, Gregory AA: **Manipulation in the presence of cervical spinal cord compression: a case series.** *J Manipulative Physiol Ther* 2006, **29**:236-244.
21. Law A: **Diversified chiropractic management in the treatment of osteoarthritis of the knee.** *J Can Chiropr Assoc* 2001, **45**:232-240.
22. Brantingham JW, Globe G, Pollard H, Hicks M, Korporaal C, Hoskins W: **Manipulative therapy for lower extremity conditions: expansion of literature review.** *J Manipulative Physiol Ther* 2009, **32**:53-71.
23. Dougherty PE, Engel RM, Vemulpad S, Burke J: **Spinal manipulative therapy for elderly patients with chronic obstructive pulmonary disease: a case series.** *J Manipulative Physiol Ther* 2011, **34**:413-417.
24. Engel R, Vemulpad S: **The role of spinal manipulation, soft-tissue therapy, and exercise in chronic obstructive pulmonary disease: a review of the**

literature and proposal of an anatomical explanation. *J Altern Complement Med* 2011, **17**:797-801.
25. Chaibi A, Tuchin PJ: **Chiropractic spinal manipulative treatment of cervicogenic dizziness using Gonstead method: a case study.** *J Chiropr Med* 2011, **10**:194-198.
26. Strunk R, Hawk C: **Effects of chiropractic care on dizziness, neck pain, and balance: a single-group, preexperimental, feasibility study.** *J Chiropr Med* 2009, **8**:156-164.
27. Hawk C, Cambron JA: **Chiropractic care for older adults: effects on balance, dizziness and chronic pain.** *J Manipulative Physiol Ther* 2009, **32**:438-447.
28. Hawk C, Cambron JA, Pfefer MT: **Pilot study of the effect of a limited and extended course of chiropractic care on balance, chronic pain, and dizziness in older adults.** *J Manipulative Physiol Ther* 2009, **32**:438-447.
29. Mykietiuk C, Wambolt M, Pillipow T, Mallay C, Gleberzon BJ: **Technique Systems used by post-1980 graduates of the Canadian Memorial Chiropractic College practicing in five Canadian provinces: a preliminary survey.** *J Can Chiropr Assoc* 2009, **53**:32-39.
30. Bronfort G, Haas M, Evans R, Leiniger B, Triano J: **Effectiveness of manual therapies: the UK evidence report.** *Chiropr Osteopat* 2010, **18**:3.
31. Hawk C, Khorsan R, Lisi AJ, Ferrance RJ, Evans MW: **Chiropractic care for nonmusculoskeletal conditions: a systematic review with implications for whole systems research.** *J Altern Complement Med* 2007, **13**:491-512.
32. Rédly M: **The effects of chiropractic care on a patient with chronic constipation.** *J Can Chiropr Assoc* 2001, **45**:185-192.
33. Rowell R, Lawrence DJ, Hawk C: **Relief of depressive symptoms in an elderly patient with low back pain [case report].** *Clin Chiropr* 2006, **9**:34-38.
34. Dougherty P, Killinger L: **Role of chiropractic in a long-term care setting.** *Long-Term Care Interface* 2005, **6**:33-38.
35. Elster EL: **Upper cervical chiropractic management of a patient with Parkinson's disease: a case report.** *J Manipulative Physiol Ther* 2000, **23**:573-577.
36. Dougherty P, Lawrence D: **Chiropractic care of musculoskeletal pain in multiple sclerosis patients.** *Clin Chiropr* 2005, **8**:57-65.
37. Noll DR, Degenhardt BF, Fossum C, Hensel K: **Clinical and research protocol for osteopathic manipulative treatment of elderly patients with pneumonia.** *J Am Osteopath Assoc* 2008, **108**:508-516.
38. Zhang J, Haselden P, Tepe R: **A case series of reduced urinary incontinence in elderly patients following chiropractic manipulation.** *J Chiropr Med* 2006, **5**:88-91.
39. Dougherty P, Karuza J, Savino D: **Adverse event reporting in a federally funded randomized clinical trial.** *American Public Health Association Annual Meeting; November 7-11, 2009* Philadelphia: American Public Health Association; 2009.
40. Carnes D, Mullinger B, Underwood M: **Defining adverse events in manual therapies: a modified Delphi consensus study.** *Man Ther* 2010, **15**:2-6.
41. Triano J, Schultz AB: **Loads transmitted during lumbosacral spinal manipulative therapy.** *Spine (Phila Pa 1976)* 1997, **22**:1955-1964.
42. Killinger LZ: **Chiropractic and geriatrics: a review of the training, role, and scope of chiropractic in caring for aging patients.** *Clin Geriatr Med* 2004, **20**:223-235.
43. Weiner DK, Rudy TE, Glick RM, Boston JR, Lieber SJ, Morrow LA, Taylor S: **Efficacy of percutaneous electrical nerve stimulation for the treatment of chronic low back pain in older adults.** *J Am Geriatr Soc* 2003, **51**:599-608.
44. Weiner DK, Perera S, Rudy TE, Glick RM, Shenoy S, Delitto A: **Efficacy of percutaneous electrical nerve stimulation and therapeutic exercise for older adults with chronic low back pain: a randomized controlled trial.** *Pain* 2008, **140**:344-357.
45. Weiner DK, Ernst E: **Complementary and alternative approaches to the treatment of persistent musculoskeletal pain.** *Clin J Pain* 2004, **20**:244-255.
46. Sebastian RS, Cleveland LE, Goldman JD, Moshfegh AJ: **Older adults who use vitamin/mineral supplements differ from nonusers in nutrient intake adequacy and dietary attitudes.** *J Am Diet Assoc* 2007, **107**:1322-1332.
47. Ahmed T, Haboubi N: **Assessment and management of nutrition in older people and its importance to health.** *Clin Interv Aging* 2010, **5**:207-216.
48. Chernoff R: **Nutrition and health promotion in older adults.** *J Gerontol A Biol Sci Med Sci* 2001, **56(Spec No 2)**:47-53.
49. Bartali B, Semba RD, Frongillo EA, Varadhan R, Ricks MO, Blaum CS, Ferrucci L, Guralnik JM, Fried LP: **Low micronutrient levels as a predictor of incident disability in older women.** *Arch Intern Med* 2006, **166**:2335-2340.
50. Mackowiak ED, Bernstein Y, Paul SH: **The adult vitamin and mineral supplement maze.** *Consult Pharm* 2010, **25**:234-240.
51. Park S, Johnson M, Fischer JG: **Vitamin and mineral supplements: barriers and challenges for older adults.** *J Nutr Elder* 2008, **27**:297-317.
52. Buhr G, Bales CW: **Nutritional supplements for older adults: review and recommendations-part I.** *J Nutr Elder* 2009, **28**:5-29.
53. Kalyani RR, Stein B, Valiyil R, Manno R, Maynard JW, Crews DC: **Vitamin D treatment for the prevention of falls in older adults: systematic review and meta-analysis.** *J Am Geriatr Soc* 2010, **58**:1299-1310.
54. Bailey RL, Gahche JJ, Lentino CV, Dwyer JT, Engel JS, Thomas PR, Betz JM, Sempos CT, Picciano MF: **Dietary supplement use in the United States, 2003-2006.** *J Nutr* 2011, **141**:261-266.
55. Qato DM, Alexander GC, Conti RM, Johnson M, Schumm P, Lindau ST: **Use of prescription and over-the-counter medications and dietary supplements among older adults in the United States.** *JAMA* 2008, **300**:2867-2878.
56. Carey TS, Freburger JK, Holmes GM, Castel L, Darter J, Agans R, Kalsbeek W, Jackman A: **A long way to go: practice patterns and evidence in chronic low back pain care.** *Spine (Phila Pa 1976)* 2009, **34**:718-724.
57. Keysor JJ, Brembs A: **Exercise: necessary but not sufficient for improving function and preventing disability?** *Curr Opin Rheumatol* 2011, **23**:211-218.
58. Reid KF, Naumova EN, Carabello RJ, Phillips EM, Fielding RA: **Lower extremity muscle mass predicts functional performance in mobility-limited elders.** *J Nutr Health Aging* 2008, **12**:493-498.
59. Mangione KK, Miller AH, Naughton IV: **Cochrane review: Improving physical function and performance with progressive resistance strength training in older adults.** *Phys Ther* 2010, **90**:1711-1715.
60. Liu CJ, Latham N: **Can progressive resistance strength training reduce physical disability in older adults? A meta-analysis study.** *Disabil Rehabil* 2011, **33**:87-97.
61. Latham N, Liu CJ: **Strength training in older adults: the benefits for osteoarthritis.** *Clin Geriatr Med* 2010, **26**:445-459.
62. Hicks GE, Benvenuti F, Fiaschi V, Lombardi B, Segenni L, Stuart M, Pretzer-Aboff I, Gianfranco G, Macchi C: **Adherence to a community-based exercise program is a strong predictor of improved back pain status in older adults: an observational study.** *Clin J Pain* 2012, **28(3)**:195-203.
63. Bronfort G, Maiers MJ, Evans RL, Schulz CA, Bracha Y, Svendsen KH, Grimm RH Jr, Owens EF Jr, Garvey TA, Transfeldt EE: **Supervised exercise, spinal manipulation, and home exercise for chronic low back pain: a randomized clinical trial.** *Spine J* 2011, **11**:585-598.
64. Standaert CJ, Friedly J, Erwin MW, Lee MJ, Rechtine G, Henrikson NB, Norvell DC: **Comparative effectiveness of exercise, acupuncture, and spinal manipulation for low back pain.** *Spine (Phila Pa 1976)* 2011, **36**: S120-S130.
65. Michael YL, Whitlock EP, Lin JS, Fu R, O'Connor EA, Gold R: **Primary care-relevant interventions to prevent falling in older adults: a systematic evidence review for the U.S. Preventive services task force.** *Ann Intern Med* 2010, **153**:815-825.
66. de Kam D, Smulders E, Weerdesteyn V, Smits-Engelsman BC: **Exercise interventions to reduce fall-related fractures and their risk factors in individuals with low bone density: a systematic review of randomized controlled trials.** *Osteoporos Int* 2009, **20**:2111-2125.
67. Liu CJ, Latham N: **Adverse events reported in progressive resistance strength training trials in older adults: 2 sides of a coin.** *Arch Phys Med Rehabil* 2010, **91**:1471-1473.
68. Tse MM, Pun SP, Benzie IF: **Pain relief strategies used by older people with chronic pain: an exploratory survey for planning patient-centred intervention.** *J Clin Nurs* 2005, **14**:315-320.
69. Sibley KM, Straus SE, Inness EL, Salbach NM, Jaglal SB: **Balance assessment practices and use of standardized balance measures among Ontario physical therapists.** *Phys Ther* 2011, **91**:1583-1591.
70. Hurwitz EL, Morgenstern H, Chiao C: **Effects of recreational physical activity and back exercises on low back pain and psychological distress: findings from the UCLA Low Back Pain Study.** *Am J Public Health* 2005, **95**:1817-1824.
71. Tinetti ME: **Clinical practice. Preventing falls in elderly persons.** *N Engl J Med* 2003, **348**:42-49.
72. Lajoie Y, Gallagher SP: **Predicting falls within the elderly community: comparison of postural sway, reaction time, the Berg balance scale and**

the Activities-specific Balance Confidence (ABC) scale for comparing fallers and non-fallers. *Arch Gerontol Geriatr* 2004, **38**:11-26.

73. Moreland J, Richardson J, Chan DH, O'Neill J, Bellissimo A, Grum RM, Shanks L: **Evidence-based guidelines for the secondary prevention of falls in older adults.** *Gerontology* 2003, **49**:93-116.
74. Gleberzon B: **Geriatric chiropractic care as a health promotion and disease prevention initiative: focus on fall prevention.** *Top Integrative Health Care* 2010, **1**:2[http://www.tihcij.com/Articles/Geriatric-Chiropractic-Care-as-a-Health-Promotion-and-Disease-Prevention-Initiative-Focus-on-Fall-Prevention.aspx?id=0000234].
75. Larson L, Bergmann TF: **Taking on the fall: the etiology and prevention of falls in the elderly.** *Clin Chiropr* 2008, **11**:148-154.
76. Reid SA, Rivett DA: **Manual therapy treatment of cervicogenic dizziness: a systematic review.** *Man Ther* 2005, **10**:4-13.
77. Hawk C, Pfefer M, Strunk R, Ramcharan M, Uhl N: **Feasibility study of short-term effects of chiropractic manipulation on older adults with impaired balance.** *J Chiropr Med* 2007, **6**:121-131.
78. Chou WC, Tinetti ME, King MB, Irwin K, Fortinsky RH: **Perceptions of physicians on the barriers and facilitators to integrating fall risk evaluation and management into practice.** *J Gen Intern Med* 2006, **21**:117-122.
79. Schneider H, Cristian A: **Role of rehabilitation medicine in the management of pain in older adults.** *Clin Geriatr Med* 2008, **24**:313-334, vii.
80. Murphy DR, Schneider MJ, Seaman DR, Perle SM, Nelson CF: **How can chiropractic become a respected mainstream profession? The example of podiatry.** *Chiropr Osteopat* 2008, **16**:10.

3

A health care system in transformation: making the case for chiropractic

Richard Brown

Abstract

There are a number of factors that have conspired to create a crisis in healthcare. In part, the successes of medical science and technologies have been to blame, for they have led to survival where lives would previously have been cut short. An informed public, aware of these technological advances, is demanding access to the best that healthcare has to offer. At the same time the burden of chronic disease in an increasing elderly population has created a marked growth in the need for long term care. Current estimates for expenditure predict a rapid escalation of healthcare costs as a proportion of the GDP of developed nations, yet at the same time a global economic crisis has necessitated dramatic cuts in health budgets. This unsustainable position has led to calls for an urgent transformation in healthcare systems.

This commentary explores the present day healthcare crisis and looks at the opportunities for chiropractors as pressure intensifies on politicians and leaders in healthcare to seek innovative solutions to a failing model. Amidst these opportunities, it questions whether the chiropractic profession is ready to accept the challenges that integration into mainstream healthcare will bring and identifies both pathways and potential obstacles to acceptance.

Keywords: Chiropractic, Healthcare transformation, Healthcare reform

Background

A need for transformation in healthcare systems throughout the globe has long been recognised [1-3]. Social reform, improvements in living conditions and the positive impact of public health initiatives have all conspired to enhance quantity and quality of life [4]. As the baby boomers of the post World War Two era move into their twilight years enjoying a range of activities that would have left their ancestors aghast [5], western societies have experienced a steady increase in the size of the ageing population as communities dance, jog, cycle and gyrate their way into their eighties and nineties [6].

But while we celebrate the achievements of medical science in prolonging and sustaining life, health care systems have been buckling under the pressure [7]. Advances in health technologies have brought about highly sophisticated systems of investigation, surgery and medical care [8,9]. In nations where health is delivered free at the point of service and where an informed public demands access to the most advanced available care, costs of health provision have rapidly escalated [10]. At the same time, fiscal deficits and global economic crises have resulted in budgets being dramatically reduced as governments struggle to balance the pressures on the public purse [11,12] whilst at the same time demanding added value. In nations which have seen the cost of healthcare as a proportion of the nation's GDP rise steeply, in some cases by over seventy per cent [13], it is clear that within such an environment traditional models of service delivery are no longer fit for purpose.

Discussion

Global health crises

The impact of conflict between forced financial austerity and life-saving, though costly, technological advances in healthcare has been felt across the globe. The starkest example of the need for health systems transformation exists in the United States, where nearly 50 million residents live without insurance coverage [14]. Despite clear evidence supporting the need for change and the efforts of the current administration to put healthcare reform at

Correspondence: rbrown.bca@gmail.com
The Lansdown Clinic, 1, High Street, Stroud, Gloucestershire GL5 1AU, United Kingdom

the top of its agenda [15], political and establishment opposition has meant that progress has faltered to the point of stagnation [16]. Vested interests, notably of a powerful medical lobby and a dominant insurance industry have ensured that the public remain suspicious of any proposals for change. Calls for a synergy between government and large industry to reduce the burden [17] have still to produce meaningful results.

In the UK, the pressure under which the National Health Service has found itself has been compounded by national debt and a prolonged economic slump [18]. The coalition government which came to power in 2010 led to a wide ranging review of healthcare provision and a White Paper, *Equity and Excellence: Liberating the NHS* [19], set out the necessary steps for transforming the delivery of health care in the UK by setting out the need for a patient centred approach, the optimisation of outcomes, and the empowerment of clinicians to innovate in order to deliver the optimal, cost-effective services locally to their individual patient populations.

As a consequence, a new Health and Social Care Act [20] has been rapidly driven through the UK Parliament. The Act represents the biggest single reorganisation of the NHS since it was established in 1948. Despite a general acknowledgment that the current system was unsustainable, the measures contained in the Act have created much disquiet amongst mainstream health professionals [21] who under the reforms are set to be charged with independently controlling much of the £106bn healthcare budget [22].

By abolishing traditional budget-holding Primary Care Trusts and Strategic Health Authorities, the Act sets up one single Health Board (Public Health England) [23] to allocate resources and provide commissioning guidance. Under the new framework, family doctors are set to form local Clinical Commissioning Groups, with the power to prioritise budgetary spending to key identified areas of greatest health need and allocate resources on behalf of their patients as they see fit. The introduction of the Any Qualified Provider (AQP) scheme [24] allows those operating independently of the NHS framework to compete for contracts to deliver health services. Critics argue that the Act is complex, incoherent and not fit for purpose and have voiced fears that the inclusion of private individuals and organisations within service delivery will strike at the heart of an NHS that is cherished as a national public institution [25].

In Canada, while the public has expressed support for its nation's health service [26], similar pressures to those seen in the UK have resulted in a growing clamour for transformation [27,28]. Here too, the growth of the aging population amidst a sharp increase in the cost and complexity of medicine and the burden of long term care for chronic conditions have left the system in crisis as administrations are faced with having to spread the healthcare budget ever more thinly [29].

Africa is faced with similar calls for health transformation, although here the drivers for change are frequently more associated with child mortality, HIV/AIDs and high levels of poverty [30]. Even a country such as South Africa, seen as wealthy within the context of its neighbours, faces significant health disparities [31]. Fragmented health services and inaccessibility outside of the main centres mean that a significant proportion of the population receive little in the way of modern healthcare [32].

Despite the protests of those who see the transformation of healthcare systems as being fraught with negative issues, not changing cannot be an option. Not only would maintaining the status quo provoke an economic catastrophe, human resource implications of continued growth and demand for services make the current system unsustainable. It is therefore imperative that innovative ways of satisfying need must be found and, if the prophecies of impending collapse are to be believed, transformation must occur swiftly.

Opportunities for the chiropractic profession

For the chiropractic profession, the crisis provides opportunities hitherto unseen in its 117-year history. With an identified gap (some might say chasm) in the marketplace for cost-effective spine care, it is critical that these opportunities are understood.

The evolution of the profession to one that in many jurisdictions is subject to statutory regulation has meant that it should no longer be characterised as complementary or alternative medicine, but as a mainstream provider of neuromusculoskeletal services. Transformation gifts the profession opportunities to deliver solutions to critical issues of inadequate provision in the field of spinal health.

These opportunities present themselves in a range of fields. In the arena of public health, the provision of spinal health promotion can become the preserve of the chiropractic profession. Educating communities in posture, manual handling and basic self-help measures has the potential to position chiropractic as the experts in spinal health. In occupational medicine, where neuromusculoskeletal disorders are endemic, working with industry to reduce sickness absence and implement prompt return to work strategies has the potential for enormous savings to be made. In general medicine, working in multidisciplinary teams as spine care experts will assist in the provision of prompt evidence-based care and a reduced likelihood of chronic back pain through delayed access. Along with a focus on promoting health and wellness, mobility and independence within the older health sector can be supported by chiropractor-led teams.

As members of an established profession, chiropractors must rapidly wake up to the realisation that there is a void in the field of non-surgical spinal healthcare which chiropractic can fill. There must not, however, be any delay in ensuring that we are suitably prepared and able to respond in a way that makes chiropractic an attractive option for those charged with resolving the crisis in service provision. So far as health system transformation is concerned, the train is leaving the station and, as a profession, we must quickly decide whether we want to be on it. Not only that, we must also consider which class of ticket we wish to purchase and where in the train we would like to sit.

It would, of course, be inconceivable to think that chiropractic as a profession would not want to involve itself in the process of healthcare transformation. Certainly, there will be those who may seek to characterise such involvement as a malevolent shift toward a medicalisation of the profession and a loss of autonomy. These are frequently the same voices that caution against any dialogue with colleagues in other healthcare disciplines and who prefer the romanticism of a bygone era where accountability and clinical governance had not entered the chiropractic lexicon.

To grasp the opportunities at hand, chiropractors of all philosophical persuasions must recognise the critical importance of integration and multidisciplinary teamwork. There can be no place for isolationism in modern chiropractic. We can embrace what is happening in healthcare, see opportunities and become part of delivering a patient-centred model, or we can contract, shrivel up and accept that we were only ever destined to be jesters in the court of the musculoskeletal marketplace.

Strategies for inclusion

Having discussed the opportunities for chiropractic within the transformation of healthcare systems it is necessary to explore what needs to be done to ensure that the profession is a key stakeholder.

Leaders in the profession have a responsibility and an obligation to ensure that chiropractic is well represented whenever there is talk of transformation in healthcare systems. Such representation must take place at all levels and there is a need to ensure that politicians recognise the benefits to society, the medical establishment realises that chiropractic can fill a void that no one else seems inclined to occupy, and chiropractors themselves share the vision that by uniting under a banner of universal access to patient-centred, evidence-based care, they can become the default experts in their field.

Chiropractic has the means to play a key role in healthcare transformation, but the profession does have to examine itself and overcome obstacles that have historically left it vulnerable to challenge and condemnation.

Perhaps first and foremost, there is a clear need to promote a consistent message. It is a matter of great regret that chiropractic's identity is often blurred and the good work done by a hard working majority can very quickly be undone by a damaging minority of evangelists who preach a message of high volume, practitioner-centred practice building. In modern healthcare systems, there can be no place for treadmill chiropractic and organisations who seek to turn back pain into a profiteering industry cannot be allowed to flourish. While projects to define chiropractic's identity have been previously undertaken, it may be timely to revisit this controversial area and decide whether in today's environment this identity reflects the needs of a modern profession.

A strong case can be made for chiropractic, but words must be supported by actions. We must robustly condemn unethical practice, and no longer tolerate conduct which falls below acceptable standards of patient-centred care. If we are to play our part in the transformation of healthcare systems, our responsibility lies in raising the bar and ensuring that chiropractic is a profession deserving of serious consideration as a provider of mainstream healthcare.

Thanks to the researchers in our profession and to those who promote research, we can be confident in providing to those who are scrutinising our profession evidence upon which our claims of effectiveness are based. Evidence is of course the known truth at any one point in time, but evolutionary change in the profession must take place in order to survive and that change must in part be based on scientific research evidence.

Those committed to the development of the chiropractic profession have recognised the value of investment in research and there is an increasing number who have committed their careers to chiropractic research and who dedicate their working lives to ensuring that the profession is both academically recognised and respected. Through university-based affiliations, particularly in Europe and North America, the credibility of the entire profession is being steadily enhanced.

Modern, credible chiropractic researchers have entered a world which deals in finding out the truth and not being afraid of admitting that what chiropractors have done for many years may not be as good as they had previously thought. The publishing of negative as well as positive outcomes marks a maturing of the profession and better reflects the reality of healthcare.

For decades, the chiropractic profession has been blighted by myopic and defensive responses to research that challenged traditional opinions and approaches to care. That as a profession we can now be seen to be reflecting on what works and what does not and then evolving accordingly marks a maturing from an era of teenage angst. Not before time, it elevates the profession above those individuals who have traditionally misrepresented data and placed a positive spin on research in order to support an outdated and one-dimensional model of assessment and care.

Modern chiropractic: a package of evidence-based care

For chiropractic to gain credibility, we must also accept that we cannot simply be one-trick ponies. Claims by some chiropractors that we should not be diagnosticians but merely the correctors of vertebral subluxation perpetuate the myth that consulting a chiropractor will invariably involve lengthy programmes of spinal manipulation. If we are to play a part in transformational health care we must promote the fact that chiropractors are primary healthcare practitioners who utilise a package of care grounded in evidence and in the interests of their patients.

We must move away from the popular perception that as soon as you step foot inside a chiropractor's clinic you will be fast tracked into an extensive programme of spinal adjustments with or without objective evidence of improvement [33]. Fortunately, modern chiropractors are demonstrating by evidence-informed approaches and a broad range of clinical techniques that there is far more to chiropractic than spinal manipulation. The incorporation of other manual methods, exercise prescription and the promotion of active care through education all point to a patient centred care approach. The development of spinal care pathways [34,35] is increasingly seen as the future of effective management and chiropractors are ideally placed to participate in what has been historically referred to as 'the Back Pain Revolution' [36].

Collaboration in multidisciplinary teams

In our transformational world, we must also see the potential for collaborative care. Effective healthcare systems, whether in Canada, the United Kingdom, Australia or elsewhere, rely on the sharing of best practice. This necessitates a mindset for collaboration and teamwork that places patients at the heart of care delivery and provides no place for interprofessional rivalry or petty squabbling. This does not mean there cannot be constructive debate, nor is there an obligation for health professionals always to agree. What is expected, however, is an environment of mutual respect where all parties can contribute freely and the best interests of the patient are placed at the forefront.

There are already examples of chiropractors involving themselves and setting up collaborative spine care teams. In hospital-based programmes, private clinics, and community initiatives, chiropractors are working within multidisciplinary groups. For the first time, chiropractors worked as part of a multi-faceted team within the host medical services Polyclinic at the London 2012 Olympic Games. This is the result of forward-thinking chiropractors who have professionally promoted the profession and who have defended the rights of chiropractors to be part of the greatest sporting event on the planet. In doing so, they have broken down barriers, corrected misapprehensions and have overcome pockets of resistance.

Quality assurance in chiropractic healthcare

The acquisition of trust in any profession is underpinned by the quality of its education. The framework for quality assurance worldwide is provided by the Council on Chiropractic Education International (CCEI) [37]. Despite the existence of quality assurance agencies and regulatory authorities, there remains significant variation in chiropractic education across the globe, with some programmes emphasising a strongly evidence-based biomedical model of education whilst others prefer to promote a more traditional philosophically-centred approach.

While this disparity creates a rich diversity of practice within the profession, it nevertheless presents a confused message to those viewing the profession from the outside [38]. This variation may present an obstacle to the widespread acceptance of chiropractic into mainstream healthcare. While the evidence-based framework of one chiropractic degree programme may be wholly familiar to other health professions, the continued emphasis on theoretical subluxation-based models of care within other programmes leads to accusations that the evidence base for chiropractic care struggles to stand up to scrutiny [39]. A schism persists and there are growing calls to define where the future of the profession may lie [40].

We must therefore consider whether in our quest to achieve cultural authority in chiropractic our primary aim should be to ensure that there is a consistency in the delivery of education. At present, we have a somewhat anomalous situation where the portability of graduates between continents is hampered by wide variations in undergraduate education. In Europe, at the same time that Switzerland has a six year chiropractic programme leading to graduates being formally recognised as medical professionals [41], other programmes are being delivered that are far shorter and do not require full time attendance [42]. Of course we must acknowledge that modern education is outcomes- rather than hours-focused [43], but nevertheless, the gap between one programme and another and the entry requirements demanded of each suggests that not all chiropractors are the same. Styles of learning delivery can be problem-based and tutorial driven or a more traditional didactic approach [44], but if we are to compete and seize the opportunities that transformation may bring, decision-makers must be assured that minimum standards of education are being consistently delivered.

A commitment to lifelong learning

In assuring both the public and other key stakeholders, we must also confirm a commitment to lifelong learning by making it a universal mandatory requirement [45]. Patients deserve and demand assurance that their health care providers remain up to date with developments in their field of expertise [46]. 'Strongly encouraging' continuing professional development in chiropractic is not enough and to stake our place as care-givers in the changing world of neuromusculoskeletal medicine we must show leadership by ensuring that chiropractors are mandated to maintain their skills and knowledge.

Primarily driven by moves to ensure that medical doctors remain up to date, the UK government is committed to developing systems of revalidation across all of the regulated health professions. What form revalidation may take for chiropractors is yet to be seen, but the objective is to ensure consistency and affirm good practice. Early consultations were marred by accusations of misleading and inaccurate extrapolations of risk data, but in promoting a patient-centred approach, the chiropractic profession should welcome a proportionate system of revalidation.

A standardised education, coupled with an obligation to undertake continuing professional development once in practice, must be considered two essential pillars in chiropractic's quest for cultural authority. As a profession, we will be judged on the commitment to, and realisation of, high standards, continuous improvement and professional excellence.

Chiropractors as non-surgical healthcare specialists

In transforming healthcare systems, it becomes governments to develop existing collaborative models and form new ones [47]. In doing so, they must commit to prioritising areas where the human and economic burden of disease is greatest, including obesity [48], diabetes [49], elderly long term care and spine care [50]. With respect to the latter, the failure of existing models of care to address the problem is of such magnitude that improving the provision of back and neck pain services must be a critical factor in any transformational health system design.

Across western societies, disproportionate costs are incurred by the small percentage of spine patients who develop chronic conditions [51]. It is estimated that it runs into billions of dollars, the true cost is difficult to define, as the financial burden of disease extends beyond the costs of providing health care [52]. The cost to industry, and to society through long term sickness benefits, and the costs associated with providing long term formal or informal care significantly magnify the true figures [53]. Ensuring prompt access must therefore be one of the key aims of any transformational strategy to prevent acute spinal conditions becoming unnecessarily chronic [54].

Chiropractic's duty to act

For chiropractic to demonstrate that it is ready to seize the opportunities that transformational healthcare systems may bring it needs to show that it has the capacity, the consistency and the capability to satisfy the needs of a nation and the requirements of collaborative partners.

Firstly, in terms of capacity, the chiropractic profession must ensure that it has sufficient numbers across a wide geographical distribution and population demographic to ensure prompt delivery of services. Human resourcing has been part of the problem in the existing model of care [55,56], so as a profession, chiropractic must ensure that it can deliver adequate numbers to satisfy demand. This may of itself require innovative models, such as that advocated by the World Health Organisation [57] and adopted by the chiropractic profession in Brazil [58].

Secondly, the chiropractic profession must deliver its services consistently by using internationally agreed models of care. Evidence-based practice, which employs best scientific information, clinical expertise and patient values and circumstances, must be embraced by chiropractors. There can be no place in such a model for extravagant programmes of care that encourage patient dependency and routinely overstate gravity. The profession must show its integrity in clearly defining those conditions for which it is most effective, and attention should be directed towards sub grouping [59,60]. By clearly setting out the patient groups within which chiropractic can be most effective, protocols for onward referral must be identified, so that referring physicians may be assured that when treatment is not working, patients may be either referred to another discipline or back to primary care. Classification systems have already been developed to enable effective targeting of subgroups and the outcomes have been encouraging [61].

Thirdly, we must show that we are capable of justifying our place in a new health system. Capability must be demonstrated by ensuring that as a profession we are equipped to effectively meet the expectations of patients, health service managers, politicians and other key stakeholders. This will require the profession to demonstrate that not only is it capable of delivering evidence based care in a timely manner; it must do so in such a way that maximises value for money [62].

Capacity, consistency and capability must all be underpinned by trust. Relationships between chiropractic and mainstream medicine have regularly been blighted by mutual suspicion and mistrust. For chiropractic to play a part in health system transformation, historical prejudices should now be set aside and a commitment must be made to work collaboratively in a spirit of openness and transparency.

There is already evidence of collaborative models that demonstrate that chiropractic is well placed to work within an integrated setting [63-65]. Hospital outpatient integration and other models of integrative healthcare should be championed. In the UK, a collaborative pilot study using chiropractors, osteopaths and physiotherapists resulted in a 28% reduction in referrals to the orthopaedic outpatient department and a satisfaction rate exceeding 90% amongst GPs and patients [66].

The size of the profession means that we should share these examples of best practice on a global level. The World Federation of Chiropractic [67] may be well placed to facilitate this process and ensure that collaborative models exist internally as well as externally. Similarly, the production of consensus statements and clinical practice guidelines demonstrate a commitment to quality patient care and a profession supportive of research-driven, evidence-based practice [68-70].

But it is one thing to put a system in place and another to make it work. The key to success will be the adoption of a chiropractic model of non-surgical spine care by the gatekeepers - the general medical practitioners. In the presence of credible alternatives, what is it that will convince MDs to take a leap of faith and refer a patient for chiropractic care?

Much as we would like to convince ourselves otherwise, the bottom line *is* the bottom line. It could be argued that we do not have to be any better than the competition; we just have to be cheaper. However, with pressures being applied at both ends and an existing model that has been woefully inadequate, there is clearly a need for chiropractic to be both better and cheaper if it is to be seen as an attractive option. And it does not end there. We need to be better, and cheaper, and have shorter waiting times, and be accountable at a much higher level than some of our counterparts. We have to prove ourselves worthy of any referral that comes our way and that means being at the top of our game as we contend with the last-chance saloon cases that may initially comprise much of our practice as we are tested by those wary of a profession seeking to stake its claim in an already-congested marketplace.

Our challenge lies with being equipped to deliver sustainable, high levels of service [71]. While established mainstream healthcare services have embraced the concept of clinical governance, chiropractors, as an autonomous group, have not universally embraced formal systems of clinical audit, outcome measurement, care pathways and protocols that help ensure sustainability. This is by no means an insurmountable hurdle yet it will require a shift in culture to one more in line with the system into which we aspire to be accepted [72].

Conclusion

The transformation of healthcare systems provides many opportunities for chiropractic. There is now a good evidence base for the utility of the services that chiropractors provide and, coupled with the suboptimal management of non-surgical spinal disorders, chiropractors should be seriously considered as potential partners in the management of neuromusculoskeletal health.

Transformation in healthcare demands courage and leadership. It will mean plotting new courses and navigating difficult and treacherous waters. It will be brave leadership that decides that chiropractic constitutes part of the answer to the back pain crisis and it therefore befalls us to ensure that the decision is made easier by promoting a realistic, achievable model of care [73].

Just as chiropractic's leaders have a duty to promote, develop and seize the opportunities that are available, so should we encourage and develop the concept of individual leadership in chiropractic. Chiropractic in western society may shortly be presented with unique opportunities which may not come again in our professional lifetimes. Recognising the opportunity is important. Seizing the opportunity is important. But it is sustaining the opportunity and delivering on expectations that will define who and what we become as chiropractors within the healthcare community.

Competing interests

The author is the current President of the British Chiropractic Association.

References

1. Health Care Transformation Task Force: Recommendations: 2008. Accessed at http://www.health.state.mn.us/divs/hpsc/hep/transform/ttfreportfinal.pdf.
2. Leape L, Berwick B, Clancy C, Conway J, Gluck P, Guest J, Lawrence D, Morath J, O'Leary D, O'Neill P, Pinakiewicz D, Isaac T: **Transforming healthcare: a safety imperative.** *Qual Saf Health Care* 2009, **18**:424–428.
3. Denis JL, Forest PG: **Real reform begins within: an organisational approach to healthcare reform.** *J Health Polit Policy Law* 2012, **37**(4):633–645. Epub.
4. Carr AJ, Gibson B, Robinson PG: **Is quality of life determined by expectations or experience?** *BMJ* 2001, **322**:1240.
5. Hartman-Stein PE, Potkanowicz ES: **Behavioural determinants of healthy aging: good news for the baby boomer generation.** *Online J Issues Nurs* 2003, **8**(2):6.
6. Aoyagi Y, Shepherd RJ: **Steps per day: the road to senior health?** *Sports Med* 2009, **39**(6):423–438.
7. Whitcomb ME: **Commentary: Meeting future medical care needs: a perfect storm on the horizon.** *Acad Med* 2011, **86**(12):1490–1491.
8. Herndon JH, Hwang R, Bozic KH: **Healthcare technology and technology assessment.** *Eur Spine J* 2007, **16**(8):1293–1302.

9. Rossi A: **Speciality drugs, healthcare costs rise in tandem.** *Biotechnol Healthc* 2009, **6**(3):52.
10. Collier R: **Economy down, health costs up.** *CMAJ* 2010, **182**(1):E44.
11. Neville S: **Rising healthcare costs put countries at risk.** *Financ Times* 2012, Accessed at http://www.ft.com/cms/s/0/235923ca-4c0c-11e1-98dd-00144feabdc0.html.
12. Bodenheimer T: **High and rising health care costs. Part 1: seeking an explanation.** *Ann Intern Med* 2005, **142**(10):847–854.
13. Di Matteo L: **The sustainability of public health expenditures: evidence from the Canadian federation.** *Eur J Health Econ* 2010, **11**(6):569–584.
14. De Navas-Walt C, Proctor BD, Smith JC, US Census Bureau, Current Population Reports p60-243: *Income, poverty and health insurance coverage in the United States 2010.* Washington DC: US Government Printing Office; 2011.
15. Holtz-Lakin D, Ramlet MJ: **Health care reform is like to widen federal deficits, not reduce them.** *Heal Aff* 2010, **29**(6):1136–1141.
16. Blank RH: **Transformation of the US healthcare system: Why is change so difficult?** *Curr Sociol* 2012, **60**(4):415–426.
17. Barratt C, Lee PV: **Health care transformation and CEO responsibility.** *Heal Aff* 2009, **28**(2):177–179.
18. Stuckler D, Basu S, Suhrcke M, Mckee M: **The health implications of financial crisis.** *Ulster Med J* 2009, **78**(3):142–145.
19. Department of Health: *Enabling Excellence: Autonomy and accountability for healthcare workers, social care workers and social workers.* 2011. February. Cm 8008, ISBN 0101800827, 9780101800822. The Stationery Office.
20. UK Parliament: *Health and social care Act.*; 2012. c7.
21. McLellan A, Middleton J, Godlee F: **Lansley's NHS "reforms".** *BMJ* 2012, **344**:e709.
22. NHS Commissioning Board: *Towards establishment: creating responsive and accountable clinical commissioning groups.*; 2012. Accessed at www.commissioningboard.nhs.uk/files/2012/01/NHSCBA-02-2012-6-Guidance-Towards-establishment-Final.pdf.
23. UK Department of Health: *The transition to public health England: action plan for the NTA.* 2011. Crown copyright.
24. Department of Health: *Any qualified provider.* Accessed at www.healthandcare.dh.gov.uk/any-qualified-provider-2/.
25. Campbell D: **NHS reform bill 'complex, incoherent and not fit for purpose', say doctors.** *Guardian* 2012, 2012 March 1 (Accessed at http://www.guardian.co.uk/politics/2012/mar/01/nhs-reform-bill-incoherent-doctors).
26. Nanos N: *Canadians overwhelmingly support universal health care; think Obama is on right track in United States,* Institute for research on public policy. 2009. Accessed at www.medicare.ca/wp-content/uploads/2009/11/nanos-poll.pdf.
27. Hutchison B, Levesque JF, Strumpf E, Coyle N: **Primary health care in Canada: systems in motion.** *Milbank Q* 2011, **89**(2):256–288.
28. Hutchison B: **A long time coming: primary healthcare in Canada.** *Healthc Pap* 2008, **8**(2):10–24.
29. Skinner BJ, Rovere M: *Canada's medicare bubble: is government health spending sustainable without user based funding? Studies in Healthcare Policy.* Fraser Institute; 2011. Accessed at http://www.fraserinstitute.org/uploadedFiles/fraser-ca/Content/research-news/research/publications/canadas-medicare-bubble.pdf.
30. Bradshaw D, Bourne D, Nannan N: **What are the leading causes of death among South African children?** *MRC Policy Brief* 2003. Accessed at http://www.unicef.org/southafrica/SAF_publications_mrc.pdf.
31. Braveman P: **Health disparities and health equity: concepts and measurement.** *Annu Rev Public Health* 2006, **27**:167–194.
32. Health Department, Republic of South Africa: *White paper for the transformation of the health system in South Africa.* Accessed at http://www.doh.gov.za/show.php?id=3189.
33. Pincus T, Vogel S, Breen A, Foster N, Underwood M: **Persistent back pain – why do physical therapy clinicians continue treatment? A mixed methods study of chiropractors, osteopaths and physiotherapists.** *Eur J Pain* 2006, **10**(1):67–76.
34. Paskowski I, Schneider M, Stevens J, Ventura JM, Justice BD: **A hospital based standardised spine care pathway: report of a multidisciplinary, evidence based process.** *J Manipul Physiol Ther* 2011, **34**(2):98–106.
35. Fourney DR, Dettori JR, Hall H, Harti R, McGirt MJ, Daubs MD: **A systematic review of clinical pathways for lower back pain and introduction of the Saskatchewan spine pathway.** *Spine* 2011, **36**(Suppl):S164–S171.
36. Waddell G: *The back pain revolution.* 2nd edition. USA: Churchill Livingstone; 2004.
37. Councils on Chiropractic Education International: www.cceintl.org.
38. Mirtz TA, Perle SM: **The prevalence of the term subluxation in north American English language doctor of chiropractic programs.** *Chiropr Man Therap* 2011, **19**:14.
39. Reggars JW: **Chiropractic at the crossroads or are we just going round in circles.** *Chiropr Man Ther* 2011, **19**:11.
40. Simpson JK: **The five eras of chiropractic and the future of chiropractic as seen through the eyes of a participant observer.** *Chiropr Man Ther* 2012, **20**(1):1.
41. Humphreys BK, Peterson CK, Muehlemann D, Haueter P: **Are Swiss chiropractors different than other chiropractors? Results of the job analysis survey 2009.** *J Manipul Physiol Ther* 2010, **33**(7):519–535.
42. Jones-Harris AR: **Are chiropractors in the UK primary healthcare or primary contact practitioners? A mixed methods study.** *Chiropr Osteopat* 2010, **18**:28.
43. Scicluna HA, Grimm MC, O'Sullivan AJ, Pilotto LS, Jones PD, McNeill HP: **Clinical capabilities of graduates of an outcomes-based integrated medical programme.** *BMC Med Educ* 2012, **12**(1):23.
44. Costa ML, van Rensburg L, Rushton N: **Does teaching style matter? A randomised trial of group discussion versus lectures in orthopaedic undergraduate teaching.** *Med Educ* 2007, **41**(2):214–217.
45. Dauphinee WD, Tamblyn R, Cruess SR, Cruess RL: **Commentary: one strategy for building public trust in changing times.** *Acad Med* 2010, **85**(6):941–944.
46. Fleet LJ, Kirby F, Cutler S, Dunikowski L, Nasmith L, Shaughnessy R: **Continuing professional development and social accountability: a review of the literature.** *J Interprof Care* 2008, **22**(Suppl1):15–29.
47. Sundberg T, Halpin J, Warenmark A, Falkenberg T: **Towards a model for integrative medicine in Swedish primary care.** *BMC Health Serv Res* 2007, **7**:107.
48. Tarride JE, Haq M, Taylor VH, Sharma AM, Nakhai-Pour HR, O'Reilly D, Xie F, Dolovich L, Goeree R: **Health status, hospitalisations, day procedures and physician costs associated with body mass index levels in Ontario. Canada.** *Clinicoecon Outcomes Res* 2012, **4**:21–30.
49. Hex N, Bartlett C, Wright D, Taylor M, Varley D: **Estimating the current and future costs of Type 1 and Type 2 diabetes in the UK, including direct health costs and indirect societal and productivity costs.** *Diabet Med* 2012, **29**(7):855–862.
50. Gore M, Sadosky A, Stacey BR, Tai KS, Leslie D: **The burden of chronic low back pain: clinical co-morbidities, treatment patters and healthcare costs in usual care settings.** *Spine* 2012, **37**(11):E668–E677.
51. Mehra M, Hill K, Nicholl D, Schadack J: **The burden of chronic low back pain with and without a neuropathiccomponent: a healthcare resource use and cost analysis.** *J Med Econ* 2012, **15**(2):245–252.
52. Wiesar S, Horisberger B, Schmidhauser S, Eisenring C, Brugger U, Ruckstuhl A, Dietrich J, Mannion AF, Elfering A, Tamcan O, Muller U: **Cost of low back pain in Switzerland in 2005.** *Eur J Health Econ* 2011, **12**(5):455–467.
53. Dagenais S, Caro J, Haldeman S: **A systematic review of low back pain cost of illness studies in the United States and internationally.** *Spine J* 2008, **8**(1):8–20.
54. Becker A, Held H, Redaelli M, Strauch K, Chenot JF, Leonhardt C, Keller S, Baum E, Pfigsten M, Hildebrandt J, Basler HD: **Low back pain in primary care: costs of care and prediction of future hedalth care utilisation.** *Spine* 2010, **35**(18):1714–1720.
55. Grover A: **Critical care workforce: a policy perspective.** *Crit Care Med* 2006, **34**(3 Suppl):S7–S11.
56. Sheldon GF, Ricketts TC, Charles A, King J, Fraher EP, Meyer A: **The global health workforce shortage: role of surgeons and other providers.** *Adv Surg* 2008, **42**:63–85.
57. World Health Organisation: *WHO guidelines on basic training and safety in chiropractic.* Geneva: WHO Press; 2005. ISBN 9241593717.
58. Chapman-Smith D: **An identity battle in Latin America.** *The Chiropractic Report* 2007, **21**(2):1–6.
59. Foster NE, Mullis R, Young J, Doyle C, Lewis M, Whitehurst D, Hay EM, IMPaCT Back Study Team: **IMPaCT Back study protocol. Implementation of subgrouping for targeted treatment systems for low back pain patients in primary care: a prospective population-based sequential comparison.** *BMC Musculoskelet Disord* 2010, **11**:186.

60. Kent P, Keating JL, Leboeuf-Yde C: **Research methods for subgrouping low back pain.** *BMC Med Res Methodol* 2010, **10:**62.
61. Hebert JJ, Koppenhaver S, Walker BF: **Subgrouping patients with low back pain. A treatment based approach to classification.** *Sports Health: A Mulitdisciplinary Approach* 2011. Accessed at www.sph.sagepub.com/content/3/6/534.full.pdf.
62. Michaleff ZA, Lin CW, Maher CG, van Tulder MW: **Spinal manipulation epidemiology: systematic review of cost effectiveness studies.** *J Electromyogr Kinesiol* 2012, **22**(5):655–662.
63. Dunn AS, Green BN, Gilford S: **An analysis of the integration of chiropractic services within the United States military and veterans' health care systems.** *J Manipulative Physiol Ther* 2009, **32**(9):749–757.
64. Branson RA: **Hospital-based chiropractic integration within a large private hospital system in Minnesota: a 10 year example.** *J Manipul Physiol Ther* 2009, **32**(9):740–748.
65. Cohen MM, Penman S, Pirolla M, Da Costa C: **The integration of complementary therapies in Australian general practice: results of a national survey.** *J ALtern Complement Med* 2005, **11**(6):995–1004.
66. Gurden M, Morelli M, Sharp G, Baker K, Betts M, Bolton J: **Evaluation of a general practitioner referral service for manual treatment of back and neck pain.** *Prim Health Care Res Dev* 2012, **30:**1–7.
67. Bryans R, Descarreaux M, Duranleau M, Marcoux H, Potter B, Ruegg R, Shaw L, Watkin R, White E: **Evidence-based guidelines for the chiropractic treatment of adults with headache.** *J Manipul Physiol Ther* 2011, **34**(5):274–289.
68. World Federation of Chiropractic: www.wfc.org.
69. Farabaugh RJ, Dehen MD, Hawk C: **Management of chronic spine-related conditions: consensus recommendations of a multidisciplinary panel.** *J Manipul Physiol Ther* 2010, **33**(7):484–492.
70. Bishop PB, Quon JA, Fisher CG, Dvorak MF: **The chiropractic hospital-based interventions research outcomes (CHIRO) study: a randomised controlled trial on the effectiveness of clinical practice guidelines in the medical and chiropractic management of patients with acute mechanical low back pain.** *Spine J* 2010, **10**(12):1055–1084.
71. Mootz RD, Hansen DT, Souza TA, Triano JJ, Wiese BC: **Application of incremental change strategies in chiropractic and multidisciplinary clinical settings for quality improvement.** *Qual Manag Health Care* 2000, **8**(3):42–64.
72. Triano JJ, Goertz C, Weeks J, Murphy DR, Kranz KC, Kopansky-Giles D, Morgan W, Nelson CF: **Chiropractic in North America: toward a strategic plan for professional renewal – outcomes from the 2006 Strategic Planning Conference.** *J Manipul Phyiol Ther* 2010, **33**(5):395–405.
73. Hansen DT, Adams AH, Meeker WC, Phillips RB: **Proposal for establishing structure and process in the development of implicit chiropractic standards of care and practice guidelines.** *J Manipul Physiol Ther* 1992, **15**(7):430–438.

4

Prognostic factors for short-term improvement in acute and persistent musculoskeletal pain consulters in primary care

Jennifer E Bolton[1*] and Hugh C Hurst[2]

Abstract

Background: Given the costs associated with the management of musculoskeletal pain in primary care, predicting the course of these conditions remains a research priority. Much of the research into prognostic indicators however considers musculoskeletal conditions in terms of single pain sites whereas in reality, many patients present with pain in more than one site. The aim of this study was to identify prognostic factors for early improvement in primary care consulters with acute and persistent musculoskeletal conditions across a range of pain sites.

Methods: Consecutive patients with a new episode of musculoskeletal pain completed self-report questionnaires at baseline, and then again at the 4/5th treatment visit, and if they were still consulting, at the 10th visit. The outcome was defined as patient self-report improvement sufficient to make a meaningful difference. Independent predictors of outcome were identified using multivariate regression analyses.

Results: Acute (<7 weeks) patients, on average, had more severe conditions in terms of pain, disability, anxiety and work fear-avoidance behaviour than patients with persistent (≥7 weeks) pain, but were more likely to be better by the 4/5th visit. Several variables at baseline were associated with improvement at the 4/5th visit, but the predictive models were weak and unable to discriminate between patients who were improved and those who were not. In contrast, it was possible to elicit a predictive model for improvement later on at the 10th visit, but only in patients with persistent pain. Being employed, reporting a decline in work fear-avoidance behaviour at the 4/5th visit, and being better by the 4/5th visit, were all independently associated with improvement. This model accounted for 34.3% ($p < 0.001$) of the variation in observed improvement, and had good discriminative ability (the area under receiver operating characteristic (ROC) curve was 0.80 (95%CI 0.73 to 0.86)) and approximate balance in correctly identifying improved and non-improved cases (79.0% and 68% respectively).

Conclusions: We were unable to identify baseline characteristics that predicted early outcome in musculoskeletal pain patients. However, early self-reported improvement and decline in work fear-avoidance behaviour as predictors of later improvement highlighted the importance of speedy recovery in persistent musculoskeletal pain consulters. Our findings reinforce the elusive nature of baseline predictors, and the need for more emphasis on early changes as prognostic predictors in musculoskeletal conditions.

Keywords: Musculoskeletal, back pain, neck pain, primary care, prognosis, improvement, prospective cohort

* Correspondence: jbolton@aecc.ac.uk
[1]Anglo-European College of Chiropractic, Parkwood Road, Bournemouth BH5 2DF, UK
Full list of author information is available at the end of the article

Background

Musculoskeletal disorders, including back, leg, neck, shoulder and arm pain, are costly and prevalent conditions most of which are managed in primary care [1]. The impact of these conditions has ramifications not only for the individual, but at a population level for healthcare utilisation and society at large. In spite of this, our biomedical understanding of the majority of these conditions is poor, and treatment effects are modest at best [2]. Moreover, although the consensus once was that acute episodes recovered within six weeks, it is now known that the clinical course of acute back and neck pain is not that simple, and more often than not beset with frequent recurrences and flare-ups [3-5].

It is apparent that musculoskeletal disorders are highly individualised and multidimensional, and that patients differ both in their response to treatment and in their recovery patterns. This presents enormous challenges to researchers using methodologies in the quantitative paradigm. For example, the modest average treatment effects may mask individual differences with some patients responding a great deal, and others hardly at all. This led, almost a decade ago, to calls for the identification of subgroups of patients either with more favourable prognoses or more likely to respond to particular treatments [2,6].

Unfortunately what was described then as the 'holy grail' of back pain research [7] has yet to produce clear answers in terms of either prognostic or treatment modifier factors. Consistent factors identified between exploratory studies remain elusive, and those factors that have been identified tend to explain relatively little of the variance in the outcome suggesting as yet unidentified predictors. Consequently, research into subgroups has faltered at the derivation stage and has yet to move on significantly to validation and impact studies [6,8].

Nevertheless, given the potential of clinical prediction research in improving patient care in musculoskeletal disorders, the pursuit of prognostic factors continues apace, predominantly in low back and neck and/or shoulder pain. Most recently, investigators in this field have distinguished between acute and chronic patients, arguing that predictors may differ given the different prognostic characteristics of these two groups [4,9,10]. Moreover, others have suggested that prognostic indicators may be common across different pain sites, and rather than distinguish between pain regions, predictors should be identified for musculoskeletal conditions in general [1].

The aim of this study therefore was to identify prognostic factors for short-term improvement in a large cohort of patients with acute and persistent musculoskeletal conditions across different pain sites, typical of those managed in primary care by GPs, physiotherapists, osteopaths and chiropractors.

Methods

Data from new or new episode patients consulting for a range of musculoskeletal conditions at a chiropractic practice in Bristol, UK from November 2001 to December 2009 were collected prospectively. The only exclusion criteria were patients below the age of 17, and those not able to read and understand the questionnaires either because of limited fluency in the English language or being considered too elderly and frail to do so. Patients were asked to complete questionnaires in the reception area prior to their first consultation (baseline), then again in the reception area after their 4th or 5th treatment session and, if they were still consulting, after their 10th visit. The data from these questionnaires were primarily used to inform the clinician and guide his/her decision-making during the course of treatment. However, patients were informed that the information would also be used anonymously for research purposes and that completion of the questionnaires was indicative of their consent. Ethics approval was given by the local ethics committee. Over the period of data collection, there were a number of chiropractors employed in the practice, and patients were treated pragmatically according to individual needs, including advice, spinal manipulation and mobilisation, dry needling and exercise in keeping with current guidelines [11].

Questionnaires

The baseline questionnaire collected patient information relating to demographics, work status, lifestyle behaviours and attitudes, and clinical characteristics of the presenting complaint. Areas that the patient felt 'most pain' were categorised as: 'low back'; 'leg(s)'; 'neck'; 'shoulder(s)/arm (s)'; 'head' and 'other'. Patients were allowed to mark more than one area. The questionnaire also included the Bournemouth Questionnaire (BQ), a validated outcome measure for use in routine practice settings in back [12] and neck [13] pain patients. The BQ is a multidimensional instrument that can be used as either individual scores on each of seven 11-point numerical rating subscales covering (i) pain, (ii) disability (activities of daily living (ADL)), (iii) disability (social activities), (iv) anxiety, (v) depression, (vi) work, both inside and outside the home, fear-avoidance and (vii) locus of control, or as the total score (maximum 70). Additionally, patients completed a pain diagram. An overlay grid was used to measure the total area of pain anteriorly and posteriorly (each with a maximum score of 52 units). Inappropriate marking of the pain diagram, for example sporadic, non-physiological patterns, pain markings outside the body, and use of additional words or symbols to describe the pain, was recorded by the clinician. At the 4/5th and 10th visits, patients completed the BQ as well as the Patient Global Impression of Change (PGIC) scale [14].

Prognostic (predictor) variables

A priori discussion between clinicians and researchers identified sociodemographic, biopsychosocial and clinical variables likely to be associated with prognosis in musculoskeletal conditions. Potential predictors were defined either as baseline variables, or as change (between visit) variables. Age, total area of body pain marked on the anterior and posterior pain drawings, and BQ scores and change scores were analysed as continuous variables. All other potential predictors recorded at baseline were dichotomised for ease of interpretation and clinical utility. Area of pain was dichotomised using the mean score for the sample (<8/≥8 units); injury/trauma as a perceived cause of the pain (yes/no/don't know) was collapsed by 'don't know' responses recoded to 'no', expectation of change in condition over the next few weeks (recover or improve/stay about the same/get worse) by recoding to recovery (yes/no), and employment status (employed/working in the home/retired/seeking work) by recoding to paid employment (yes/no). All other variables, which did not require recoding, included pain all over (yes/no), a similar complaint in the past (yes/no), medication use (a lot of the time/occasionally or never), satisfaction with current work status (yes/no), expectation of working normally in six months' time (yes/no), smoker (yes/no), alcohol consumption (regularly/never or hardly ever), level of physical activity compared to people of a similar age (more or about the same/less) and general health and well-being (excellent or good/fair or poor).

Outcome

Outcomes were monitored using BQ total and subscale raw change (i.e. baseline minus treatment visit) scores. The outcome (improvement) for the prediction analysis was defined as those patients scoring either 6 (better, and a definite improvement that has made a real and worthwhile difference) or 7 (a great deal better, and a considerable improvement that has made all the difference) on the PGIC. All other patients (1 = no change or worse, 2 = almost the same, hardly any change, 3 = a little better but no noticeable change, 4 = somewhat better but no noticeable change, 5 = moderately better and a slight and noticeable difference) were categorised as reporting no (meaningful) improvement.

Data analysis

Baseline characteristics were compared between acute (current episode <7 weeks) and persistent (current episode ≥7 weeks) pain patients using the χ^2 test and unpaired t test for categorical and continuous variables respectively. Within-patient differences in continuous variables were analysed using the paired t test.

For the prediction analysis, univariate logistic regression was carried out to determine those variables that were significantly associated with improvement at the 4/5th visit and at the 10th visit. The significance level was set at $p \le 0.10$ to avoid excluding potential predictor variables. Significant variables ($p \le 0.05$) independently associated with the outcome were subsequently entered into a forward stepwise multivariate logistic regression model. Variables were checked for redundancy by noting the correlation coefficients ($r \ge 0.8$) between variables in the presence of the other variables in the model. The independence of the variables was also assessed by noting the condition index (<20) of each variable calculated by re-running the final model using linear regression. The ability of the final model to discriminate between improvers and non-improvers was calculated from the area under the receiver operating characteristic curve (AUC) using patient self-report improvement as the external criterion. An AUC of 0.5 indicates no discrimination, 0.7 to 0.8 acceptable discrimination, and 0.9 excellent discrimination [15]. The adjusted %R^2 was used as the index of the percentage of the variance in the outcome explained by the model. All analyses were conducted using SPSS v17.

Results

The baseline questionnaire was completed by 2,422 patients with musculoskeletal complaints amenable to chiropractic treatment. Patients reported pain in the following region(s), which were not mutually exclusive: 1,691 (70.0%) back pain, 973 (40.3%) neck pain, 686 (28.4%) shoulder and/or arm pain, 472 (19.6%) leg pain and 210 (8.7%) headache. Of 1,706 back pain patients, 420 (24.6%) reported accompanying leg pain, and 504 (29.6%) also had neck and/or shoulder/arm pain. Of 1,216 patients presenting with neck and/or shoulder/arm pain, 522 (42.9%) had only neck pain and 231 (19.0%) had only shoulder/arm pain. Almost half (555, 45.8%) of patients with neck and/or upper extremity pain also reported pain in the back and/or leg.

The mean age of the sample was 40.8 (SD ± 14.21) years and the gender split was approximately equal (males: 1,184, 48.9%). The majority of the sample was in paid employment (1,899, 79.4%) with 221 (9.2%) retired, 146 (6.1%) working in the home, 63 (2.6%) seeking work and 62 (2.6%) students. The mean times between baseline and the 4/5th visit, and between baseline and the 10th visit, were 16.8 (± 10.49) and 51.6 (± 15.36) days respectively.

Acute vs. persistent pain

The characteristics of acute (n = 1,335, 56%) and persistent (n = 1,059, 44%) musculoskeletal pain patients are shown in table 1. Although significant, the difference in

Table 1 Baseline characteristics

Characteristic	Acute (<7 weeks) (n = 1,335)	Missing data	Persistent (≥7 weeks) (n = 1,059)	Missing	*p-value
Gender (male)	674 (50.5)	0	498 (47.0)	0	0.092
Age (years)	40.2 (± 13.09)	0	41.4 (± 15.43)	0	0.032
Pain diagram					
Shaded area (mm):	7.0 (± 5.51)	0	8.3 (± 7.30)	0	<0.001
Posterior	1.5 (± 3.58)	0	2.6 (± 4.79)	0	<0.001
Anterior					
Pain diagram: ≥8 mm	484 (36.3)	0	486 (45.9)	0	<0.001
Pain diagram: Inappropriate marking	145 (10.9)	2 (0.15)	193 (18.2)	2 (0.19)	<0.001
Back pain	984 (73.8)	1 (0.08)	685 (64.9)	4 (0.38)	<0.001
Leg pain	228 (17.2)	6 (0.45)	242 (23.0)	5 (0.47)	<0.001
Neck pain	465 (34.9)	2 (0.15)	501 (47.4)	3 (0.28)	<0.001
Headache	71 (5.3)	2 (0.15)	137 (13.0)	3 (0.28)	<0.001
Shoulder/arm pain	318 (23.9)	3 (0.22)	362 (34.2)	1 (0.09)	<0.001
Widespread pain	23 (1.7)	19 (1.4)	89 (8.6)	28 (2.6)	<0.001
Caused by injury/trauma	354 (26.7)	10 (0.75)	250 (23.9)	11 (1.0)	0.112
Past similar complaint	891 (67.4)	13 (0.97)	640 (62.4)	34 (3.2)	0.012
Taking medication	299 (22.7)	17 (1.3)	279 (26.6)	10 (0.94)	0.028
Expectation of recovery	1,048 (79.1)	10 (0.75)	505 (48.1)	10 (0.94)	<0.001
Paid employment	1,108 (83.8)	13 (0.97)	773 (74.2)	17 (1.6)	<0.001
Satisfied with work	1,191 (93.4)	60 (4.5)	846 (86.6)	82 (7.7)	<0.001
Smoker (ever)	700 (52.5)	2 (0.15)	550 (52.0)	2 (0.19)	0.816
Alcohol (regularly)	1,032 (77.5)	3 (0.22)	718 (68.2)	6 (0.57)	<0.001
Physically active	1,136 (85.3)	4 (0.30)	794 (75.4)	6 (0.57)	<0.001
In good general health	1,204 (90.4)	3 (0.22)	866 (81.8)	7 (0.66)	<0.001

Values are numbers (%) for categorical and mean (± SD) for continuous variables. N = number of observations.

* Chi^2 test for categorical and unpaired t test for continuous variables.

age between the two groups was small, and there was no difference in gender distribution. Compared with acute patients, the persistent pain group had a lower proportion in paid employment and a lower proportion satisfied with their work status. As expected, a significantly lower proportion of patients with persistent pain expected to make a good recovery, considered themselves as physically active as people of a similar age and rated themselves in overall good health. Additionally, the mean area of the body shaded in pain was higher in patients with persistent pain, and a higher proportion described their pain as widespread. When reporting the area of their pain, more acute patients reported pain in the back. In contrast a higher proportion of persistent pain patients reported neck pain, upper extremity pain, leg pain and headache. Medication use was significantly higher in the persistent pain group. Interestingly, a statistically significantly higher proportion of acute patients described having similar complaints in the past. Baseline scores on the BQ for acute and persistent pain patients are shown in table 2. Patients in the acute group had statistically higher mean levels of pain and disability in ADL and in social activities, anxiety and work fear-avoidance beliefs.

All patients completed a follow-up questionnaire at the $4^{th}/5^{th}$ visit. There was a significant ($p < 0.001$) decline in all seven BQ sub-scales from baseline to follow up in both groups of patients (table 2). The magnitude of this change however, was significantly greater in the acute group for all seven subscales of the BQ. In terms of improvement (i.e. scoring 6 or 7 on the PGIC scale), as expected a significantly ($p < 0.001$) higher proportion (941, 70.6%) of patients in the acute group considered themselves as better at the $4/5^{th}$ visit compared to that (468, 44.3%) in the persistent pain group.

Prognostic variables

Thirty potential predictor variables for improvement at the $4/5^{th}$ and at the 10th visits were investigated.

Improvement at $4/5^{th}$ visit

Acute patients

In acute patients, being male, taking medication for the pain complaint, being in paid employment, being a smoker and expecting to make a good recovery were all

Table 2 Bournemouth Questionnaire (BQ) scores at baseline and change scores at 4/5th visit

BQ scores:	Baseline					Change scores at 4/5th visit				
	Acute (n = 1,335)	Missing data	Persistent (n = 1,059)	Missing data	*p-value	Acute (n = 1,335)	Missing data	Persistent (n = 1,059)	Missing data	*p-value
Pain	6.0 (2.12)	14	5.5 (2.21)	3	<0.001	3.4 (2.44)	16	2.1 (2.32)	4	<0.001
Disability in activities of daily living	5.6 (2.69)	13	4.5 (2.75)	1	<0.001	3.5 (2.88)	14	1.8 (2.64)	3	<0.001
Disability in social activities	5.3 (3.07)	18	4.0 (3.03)	6	<0.001	3.4 (3.17)	20	1.7 (2.68)	9	<0.001
Anxiety	5.0 (2.78)	8	4.7 (2.90)	5	0.025	2.7 (2.97)	11	1.8 (2.97)	6	<0.001
Depression	3.2 (2.90)	10	3.3 (2.96)	4	0.504	1.7 (2.81)	13	1.3 (2.89)	8	<0.001
Fear-avoidance beliefs	4.7 (3.06)	34	4.4 (3.02)	16	0.007	2.3 (3.23)	38	1.5 (3.03)	21	<0.001
Locus of control	5.0 (2.59)	20	4.9 (2.78)	12	0.689	2.8 (2.97)	28	1.8 (2.86)	16	<0.001
Total score	34.8 (13.69)	60	31.2 (14.45)	29	<0.001	19.7 (14.67)	77	12.0 (13.29)	43	<0.001

Values are means (± SD). * unpaired t test.

positively associated with improvement (table 3). Similarly, scoring high at baseline on the BQ sub-scales, apart from depression, increased the odds of improvement at the 4/5th visit. In contrast, having a high area marked on the pain drawing and having upper extremity pain reduced the odds of improvement.

In the subsequent multivariate analysis (table 4) being male, expecting to make a good recovery, being in paid employment and high levels on the BQ disability scales (ADL and social activities) were all independently associated with improvement. Marking a high area on the pain drawing was independently associated with reduced odds of improvement. However, the model only explained a small amount (7.4%) of variance in the outcome and showed little ability (AUC 0.64) to discriminate between improved and non-improved patients.

Persistent pain patients

Fewer variables were associated with improvement at the 4/5th visit (table 3). Patients with neck pain were significantly more likely to be improved, as were patients expecting to make a good recovery and those patients who considered themselves to be in good general health. Patients who reported drinking alcohol had reduced odds of improvement.

In the multivariate analysis (table 4), having neck pain, expecting to make a good recovery and being in good general health were independently associated with improvement at the 4/5th visit. Drinking alcohol was independently associated with reduced odds of improvement. However, the final model again explained very little (3.9%) of the variance in observed improvement, and poor discriminative ability (AUC 0.60).

Improvement at 10th visit

At the 10th visit, the number of patients still consulting was significantly reduced. Of the 1,335 acute patients, improvement data at the 10th visit were available on 168 (11.4%) patients, of whom only 25 (14.9%) reported they were not improved. As a result, there was insufficient data for multivariate regression analysis in this group.

Persistent pain patients

For patients with persistent pain, of the original group of 1,059, data were available on 185 (17.5%), of whom 76 (41.1%) were not improved at the 10th visit. Table 5 shows the univariate association between baseline variables, BQ change variables and PGIC data at the 4/5th visit, and improvement at the 10th visit. Reporting a similar condition in the past at baseline was negatively associated with improvement. Being in paid employment, being a smoker and higher baseline BQ scores in disability in ADL and social activities, and in work fear-avoidance behaviour, were all associated with increased odds of improvement at the 10th visit. Considering the change variables, the BQ total and sub-scale change scores, and being better at the 4/5th visit, were all associated with improvement at the 10th visit.

To avoid over-fitting the model given the relatively small number of patients (109 outcome events (improvement)), only those predictor variables significant at the 5% level were entered in the multivariate model. The change in total BQ was excluded to avoid colinearity between this and the BQ sub-scale scores. From the 12 variables entered, three variables were independently associated with improvement at the 10th visit (table 5). These were improvement at the 4/5th visit, being in paid employment, and decline in work fear-avoidance behaviour at the 4/5th visit. The model correctly predicted 74.4% of patients (compared to the observed 58.3%) improving at the 10th visit. The predictive model accounted for 34.3% of the variation in observed improvement, had good discriminative ability (AUC 0.80) and an approximate balance of correctly identifying improved and non-improved cases (79.0% and 68% respectively).

Table 3 Univariate logistic regression analysis of potential predictors at baseline for improvement at 4/5th visit

	Acute (n = 1,335)		**Persistent (n = 1,059)**	
Predictor variable	**Unadjusted OR (95% CI)**	**p-value**	**Unadjusted OR (95% CI)**	**p-value**
Gender (male)	**1.31 (1.03 to 1.66)**	**0.025**	0.92 (0.72 to 1.18)	0.514
*Age (higher)	0.99 (0.99 to 1.00)	0.192	1.00 (0.99 to 1.01)	0.955
*Posterior area body pain (higher)	0.99 (0.97 to 1.01)	0.231	0.99 (0.97 to 1.01)	0.213
*Anterior area body pain (higher)	1.02 (0.98 to 1.06)	0.275	0.99 (0.96 to 1.01)	0.360
Marked area of posterior body pain (high)	**0.77 (0.59 to 0.95)**	**0.018**	0.92 (0.72 to 1.17)	0.494
Inappropriate markings	0.99 (0.68 to 1.44)	0.938	0.81 (0.59 to 1.11)	0.195
Back pain	1.16 (0.89 to 1.51)	0.275	0.81 (0.63 to 1.05)	0.113
Leg pain	0.84 (0.62 to 1.14)	0.268	0.96 (0.72 to 1.28)	0.784
Neck pain	0.90 (0.70 to 1.14)	0.374	**1.34 (1.05 to 1.70)**	**0.020**
Headache	0.80 (0.49 to 1.34)	0.409	1.19 (0.83 to 1.71)	0.342
Shoulder and/or arm pain	**0.69 (0.53 to 0.90)**	**0.007**	1.01 (0.78 to 1.30)	0.968
Widespread pain	0.79 (0.33 to 1.87)	0.584	0.87 (0.56 to 1.35)	0.533
Trauma	1.03 (0.79 to 1.35)	0.804	1.07 (0.80 to 1.42)	0.648
Similar complaint in past	0.94 (0.73 to 1.21)	0.632	0.94 (0.73 to 1.22)	0.657
Taking medication	**1.43 (1.06 to 1.92)**	**0.019**	1.03 (0.78 to 1.36)	0.835
Expect to recover	**1.68 (1.27 to 2.23)**	**0.001**	**1.57 (1.23 to 2.01)**	**0.001**
Paid employment	**1.41 (1.04 to 1.93)**	**0.028**	1.00 (0.76 to 1.33)	0.981
Satisfied with work status	0.80 (0.48 to 1.33)	0.391	1.19 (0.82 to 1.73)	0.368
Smoke	**1.28 (1.01 to 1.62)**	**0.042**	1.02 (0.80 to 1.30)	0.882
Alcohol	0.95 (0.72 to 1.26)	0.728	**0.74 (0.57 to 0.96)**	**0.023**
Physically active	1.18 (0.85 to 1.63)	0.326	1.01 (0.76 to 1.34)	0.948
In good health	1.19 (0.81 to 1.76)	0.384	**1.66 (1.19 to 2.30)**	**0.003**
*BQ Pain	**1.11 (1.05 to 1.17)**	**0.001**	1.03 (0.97 to 1.09)	0.340
*BQ Disability	**1.16 (1.11 to 1.21)**	**0.001**	1.03 (0.99 to 1.08)	0.194
*BQ Social disability	**1.14 (1.10 to 1.19)**	**0.001**	1.02 (0.98 to 1.06)	0.407
*BQ Anxiety	**1.07 (1.03 to 1.12)**	**0.001**	1.03 (0.99 to 1.07)	0.197
*BQ Depression	0.99 (0.95 to 1.03)	0.510	1.01 (0.97 to 1.06)	0.494
*BQ WFAB	**1.06 (1.02 to 1.10)**	**0.003**	1.00 (0.96 to 1.04)	0.962
*BQ LOC	**1.06 (1.02 to 1.11)**	**0.010**	0.98 (0.94 to 1.02)	0.324
*BQ Total	**1.02 (1.01 to 1.03)**	**0.001**	1.00 (1.00 to 1.01)	0.334

*Continuous variables

Table 4 Multivariate logistic regression analysis of prognostic predictors at baseline for improvement at 4/5th visit

	Coefficient	**OR**	**95% CI**	**p-value**	**Sensitivity; Specificity; Percentage correctly predicted; Area under ROC (95% CI); Adjusted R^2**
Acute N = 1,335					
Gender (male)	0.26	1.30	1.01 to 1.68	0.044	97.2%; 9.6%; 70.8%; 0.64 (0.61 to 0.68); 7.4%
High area marked on pain drawing	0.27	0.76	0.59 to 0.99	0.040	
Expect to recover	0.34	1.40	1.04 to 1.89	0.025	
In paid employment	0.34	1.40	1.00 to 1.95	0.050	
BQ (ADL disability)	0.085	1.09	1.02 to 1.16	0.012	
BQ (Social disability)	0.072	1.08	1.01 to 1.14	0.016	
Persistent N = 1,059					
Neck pain	0.29	1.34	1.04 to 1.73	0.022	37.0%; 74.1%; 57.7%; 0.60 (0.56 to 0.63); 3.9%
Expect to recover	0.42	1.53	1.19 to 1.96	0.001	
In good health	0.51	1.67	1.19 to 2.35	0.003	
Alcohol	0.29	0.75	0.57 to 0.98	0.034	

Table 5 Univariate and multivariate logistic regression analysis of prognostic predictors (baseline and change) for improvement at 10th visit (persistent pain patients only)

Persistent N = 185	Univariate		Multivariate		
Predictor variable:	**Unadjusted OR (95% CI)**	**p-value**	**Adjusted OR (95% CI)**	**p-value**	**Model**
Baseline:					
Gender (male)	1.17 (0.65 to 2.10)	0.602			
*Age (higher)	1.00 (0.98 to 1.01)	0.615			
*Posterior area body pain (higher)	0.98 (0.94 to 1.02)	0.320			
*Anterior area body pain (higher)	0.99 (0.93 to 1.05)	0.732			
Marked area of posterior body pain (high)	1.22 (0.68 to 2.19)	0.510			
Inappropriate markings	0.59 (0.29 to 1.23)	0.158			
Back pain	0.94 (0.49 to 1.78)	0.846			
Leg pain	1.14 (0.57 to 2.29)	0.706			
Neck pain	0.74 (0.41 to 1.34)	0.319			
Headache	0.97 (0.41 to 2.32)	0.950			
Shoulder and/or arm pain	1.28 (0.67 to 2.40)	0.435			
Widespread pain	0.77 (0.27 to 2.22)	0.628			
Trauma	1.44 (0.69 to 2.96)	0.330			
Similar complaint in past	**0.56 (0.28 to 1.09)**	**0.085**			
Taking medication	0.59 (0.31 to 1.13)	0.113			
Expect to recover	1.59 (0.87 to 2.88)	0.130			
Paid employment	**2.06 (1.07 to 3.98)**	**0.031**	**2.26 (1.03 to 4.99)**	**0.043**	
Satisfied with work status	0.80 (0.33 to 1.92)	0.613			
Smoke	**1.85 (1.01 to 3.36)**	**0.045**			
Alcohol	0.67 (0.37 to 1.24)	0.207			
Physically active	1.32 (0.66 to 2.63)	0.429			
In good health	1.77 (0.86 to 3.63)	0.121			
*BQ Pain	1.07 (0.93 to 1.24)	0.338			
*BQ Disability	**1.19 (1.05 to 1.34)**	**0.006**			
*BQ Social disability	**1.10 (0.99 to 1.22)**	**0.086**			
*BQ Anxiety	1.02 (0.93 to 1.13)	0.668			
*BQ Depression	0.99 (0.89 to 1.09)	0.784			
*BQ WFAB	**1.14 (1.02 to 1.27)**	**0.017**			
*BQ LOC	1.00 (0.89 to 1.12)	0.973			
*BQ Total	1.02 (0.99 to 1.04)	0.156			
At 4/5th visit:					
*Change BQ Pain	**1.33 (1.13 to 1.56)**	**0.001**			
*Change BQ Disability	**1.37 (1.19 to 1.58)**	**0.001**			
*Change BQ Social disability	**1.19 (1.05 to 1.35)**	**0.005**			
*Change BQ Anxiety	**1.16 (1.05 to 1.29)**	**0.004**			
*Change BQ Depression	**1.16 (1.04 to 1.29)**	**0.008**			
*Change BQ WFAB	**1.30 (1.16 to 1.47)**	**0.001**	**1.26 (1.11 to 1.44)**	**0.001**	
*Change BQ LOC	**1.27 (1.11 to 1.44)**	**0.001**			
*Change BQ Total	**1.07 (1.04 to 1.10)**	**0.001**			
Improved 4/5th visit	**6.24 (3.15 to 12.36)**	**0.001**	**5.42 (2.59 to 11.35)**	**0.001**	Sensitivity; Specificity; Percentage correctly predicted; Area under ROC (95% CI); Adjusted R2 79.0%; 68.0%; 74.4%; 0.80 (0.73 to 0.86); 34.3%

*Continuous variables

Discussion

This study identified prognostic variables in patients consulting for acute and persistent musculoskeletal pain conditions. We chose to use patient self-report improvement as the outcome, and used a rigorous cut-off for improvement that was meaningful to the patient. It has been shown that patients' perception of improvement is multi-factorial and more complex than either alleviation of symptoms or improvement in function alone [16,17]. We made the distinction between acute and persistent pain in line with the NICE guideline on the management of pain greater than 6 weeks [11]. Our results showed clear differences, on average, between these two groups in terms of more area in pain, widespread pain and lower expectations of recovery in those with persistent pain. In contrast, acute patients were more likely to be in employment, satisfied with their work status, and consider themselves to be physically active and in general good health. Musculoskeletal conditions in acute patients were more severe at baseline, with higher levels of pain, disability, anxiety and work fear-avoidance behaviour than those with persistent pain. In spite of greater severity however, acute patients got better faster, and by the 4/5th visit (approximately 2 weeks on average) a greater proportion reported that they were better.

A significant proportion of patients in this study reported pain in more than one site, illustrating the difficulty of investigating musculoskeletal disorders on the basis of regional pain. In spite of this, most musculoskeletal research in primary care confines itself to single pain sites, for example low back pain, even though inevitably a proportion of participants will have musculoskeletal pain elsewhere. In spite of this, in a systematic review of prognostic factors in musculoskeletal pain, only 4 out of 45 included studies investigated patients with general musculoskeletal pain [1].

Expecting to make a good recovery was strongly associated with early improvement by the 4/5th visit in both acute and persistent pain patients, but apart from this no other predictors were the same in these two groups. This contrasts with the study by Grotle et al. [10] that suggested considerable overlap in prognostic indicators for outcome between acute (<3 months) and chronic (>3 months) low back pain patients. Similar overlap in prognostic factors was found in patients with acute (<2 weeks) [4] and chronic (> 3 months) [9] low back pain. In the present study, being male, being in paid employment, being a smoker, high BQ baseline levels and taking medication were all associated with early recovery in acute patients, while marking a higher area on the pain drawing and having upper extremity pain were negatively associated. In patients with persistent pain, having neck pain and reporting being in good health were positively associated, whereas alcohol consumption was negatively associated. However, in both acute and persistent pain patients the predictive models explained very little of the variance in improvement by 4/5th visit, suggesting that other factors, not measured in this study, are important. For example, longer pain duration has been identified as one of the few consistent predictive factors in back and neck pain [1]. However, as we used this variable to subgroup our population, it was not entered as a potential predictor. Similarly, we did not measure improvement before the 4th visit, which in another prognostic study in chiropractic patients, being better at the 2nd visit was identified as a strong predictor of improvement at the 4th [18]. It may also be the case that it is not possible to predict early recovery from baseline variables, particularly in acute patients with generally rapid recovery.

We were unable to investigate prognostic factors for improvement at the 10th visit in acute patients because most of these patients had ceased to consult. Although this might be presumed to be because they were no longer in pain, this may not be the case [3]. In contrast, sufficient numbers of persistent pain patients still consulting allowed us to proceed with analysis. Being in paid employment, being a smoker, and high levels of baseline disability and work fear-avoidance behaviour were all positively associated with improvement by the 10th visit, while having a similar condition in the past was negatively associated. Declines in all the BQ subscales between baseline and the 4/5th visit, and reporting improvement on the PGIC scale at the 4/5th visit, were also positively associated with improvement at the 10th visit. In the final predictive model, being better at the 4/5th visit was by far the strongest predictor, together with being in paid employment and reporting a decline in work fear-avoidance behaviour at the 4/5th visit. This result echoes that shown by others [18,19] that early changes may be more important as predictors in musculoskeletal conditions than variables measured at baseline. In other words, that unless a patient improves quickly, the prognosis, at least in the short-term, is poor. It also calls into question the use of screening tools at baseline to identify patients at risk of poor prognosis, and the need for inclusion of early changes in addition to baseline factors in future prognostic research. The other factors that were independently associated with improvement were a decline in work fear-avoidance behaviour and being in paid employment. In a recent study, fear of pain was found to be a significant predictor of outcome in back pain patients [10], although a systematic review of fear-avoidance behaviour and prognosis in back pain [20] reported no convincing evidence of a link. In support of our findings on employment status as a prognostic factor, Grotle and co-workers [10] showed that being non-employed was associated with long term disability in both acute and chronic low back pain patients. In overall terms, when comparing our findings with the existing literature, it is clear that there remains a lack of consistency in prognostic factors identified between studies, and that identifying useful factors, particularly at baseline, remains a challenge.

This study has several limitations, not least because it was a pragmatic study conducted in real time everyday clinical practice. First, it is restricted to relatively early outcomes (up to seven weeks on average) and in the relatively small proportion of patients that were still consulting. We therefore do not know if the predictive model presented here holds true either in the longer term or in those patients who had stopped consulting. Second, there was no control group, and therefore we are only able to present prognostic factors for the clinical course of these conditions, and not for treatment effects. Third, all variables were self-reported by patients in the chiropractic practice, which may have been subject to reporting bias. Fourth, all patients attended one chiropractic practice, and as such may not be representative either of musculoskeletal patients in general seeking chiropractic care, or of those seeking care from other primary care practitioners. Finally, while it may be considered a strength of the study to include patients with musculoskeletal complaints in general, there still remains the question of why should prognostic factors be common across musculoskeletal pain sites. Many of these conditions share similar characteristics, such as co-morbidities, non-specific aetiologies, recurrent and episodic courses, and prognostic factors such as duration of pain and previous episodes. Nevertheless, clumping these conditions together may be a step too far, or alternatively beg the question as to why not more musculoskeletal research is conducted on this basis.

Conclusions

Patients with acute musculoskeletal pain consulting a chiropractor were more severe, on average, than those with persistent pain, but more likely to get better quicker. Although a number of variables were associated with a favourable outcome in acute and persistent pain patients by the $4/5^{th}$ visit, the predictive models were weak and we were unsuccessful in identifying baseline variables as predictors of early recovery. In contrast, the model constructed to predict self-reported improvement later on in persistent musculoskeletal pain patients showed good discriminative ability. In this model, reporting improvement at the $4/5^{th}$ visit, a decline in work fear-avoidance behaviour at the $4/5^{th}$ visit and being in paid employment at baseline were all independently associated with improvement at the 10th visit. These results highlight the importance of early recovery in persistent musculoskeletal pain consulters, and the need to include change variables in addition to baseline variables in future prognostic research.

Acknowledgements

The authors wish to thank the chiropractors and staff at Clifton Chiropractic Clinic for their assistance with data collection for this study. No funding was either sought or received.

Author details

[1]Anglo-European College of Chiropractic, Parkwood Road, Bournemouth BH5 2DF, UK. [2]Clifton Chiropractic Clinic, 123 Pembroke Road, Clifton BS8 3EU, UK.

Authors' contributions

JB and HH conceived and designed the study; HH collected the data; JB and HH analysed and interpreted the data. JB was responsible for the first draft of the manuscript; JB and HH were responsible for revisions and approval of the final manuscript.

Competing interests

The authors declare that they have no competing interests.

References

1. Mallen CD, Peat G, Thomas E, Dunn KM, Croft PR: **Prognostic factors for musculoskeletal pain in primary care: a systematic review.** *Br J Gen Prac* 2007, **57**:655-661.
2. Foster NE, Hill JC, Hay EM: **Subgrouping patients with low back pain in primary care: are we getting any better at it?** *Man Ther* 2011, **16**:3-8.
3. Croft P, Macfarlane GJ, Papageorgiou AC, Thomas E, Silman AJ: **Outcome of low back pain in general practice: a prospective study.** *BMJ* 1998, **316**:1356-1359.
4. Henshcke N, Maher CG, Refshauge KM, Herbert RD, Cumming RG, Bleasel J, York J, Das A, McAuley JH: **Characteristics of patients with acute low back pain presenting to primary care in Australia.** *Clin J Pain* 2009, **25**:5-11.
5. Hush JM, Lin CC, Michaleff ZA, Verhagen A, Refshauge KM: **Prognosis of acute idiopathic neck pain is poor: a systematic review.** *Arch Phys Med Rehabil* 2011, **92**:824-829.
6. Kent P, Keating JL, Leboeuf-Yde C: **Research methods for subgrouping low back pain.** *BMC Med Res Meth* 2010, **10**:62.
7. Bouter LM, Penniick V, Bombardier C: **Cochrane Back Review Group.** *Spine* 2003, **28**:1215-1218.
8. Moons KGM, Royston P, Vergouwe Y, Grobbee DE, Altman DG: **Prognosis and prognostic research: what, why and how?** *BMJ* 2009, **338**:1317-1320.
9. Costa LC, Maher CG, McAuley JH, Hancock MJ, Herbert RD, Refshauge KM, Henschke N: **Prognosis for patients with chronic low back pain: inception cohort study.** *BMJ* 2009, **339**:b3829.
10. Grotle M, Foster NE, Dunn KM, Croft P: **Are prognostic indicators for poor outcome different for acute and chronic low back pain consulters in primary care?** *Pain* 2010, **151**:790-797.
11. National Institute for Health and Clinical Excellence: **Guideline CG 88:Early management of persistent non-specific low back pain.** 2009 [http://guidance.nice.org.uk/CG88].
12. Bolton JE, Breen AC: **The Bournemouth Questionnaire: a short-form comprehensive outcome measure:I. Psychometric properties in back pain patients.** *J Manipulative Physiol Ther* 1999, **22**:503-510.
13. Bolton JE, Humphreys BK: **The Bournemouth Questionnaire: a short-form comprehensive outcome measure:II. Psychometric properties in neck pain patients.** *J Manipulative Physiol Ther* 2001, **25**:141-148.
14. Hurst HC, Bolton JE: **Assessing the clinical significance of change scores recorded on subjective outcome measures.** *J Manipulative Physiol Ther* 2004, **27**:26-35.
15. Hosmer DW, Lemeshow S: **Applied Logistic Regression.** New York, NY: John Wiley;, 2 2000.
16. Beaton DE, Tarasuk V, Katz JN, Wright JG, Bombardier C: **'Are you better?' A qualitative study of the meaning of recovery.** *Arth Care Res* 2001, **45**:270-279.

17. Hush JM, Refshauge K, Sullivan G, de Souza L, Maher CG, McAuley JH: **Recovery: what does it mean to patients with low back pain?** *Arth Rheum* 2009, **61**:124-131.
18. Malmqvist S, Leboeuf-Yde C, Ahola T, Andersson O, Ekstrom K, Pekkarinen H, Turpeinen M, Wederkopp N: **The Nordic back pain subpopulation program: predicting outcome among chiropractic patients in Finland.** *BMC Chiro Osteo* 2008, **16**:13.
19. Axen I, Rosenbaum A, Robech R, Larsen K, Leboeuf-Yde C: **The Nordic back pain subpopulation program: can patient reactions to first chiropractic treatment predict early favourable treatment outcome in non-persistent low back pain?** *J Manipulative Physiol Ther* 2005, **28**:153-158.
20. Pincus T, Vogel S, Burton AK, Santos R, Field A: **Fear avoidance and prognosis in back pain: a systematic review and synthesis of current evidence.** *Arth Rheum* 2006, **54**:39999-4010.

Subtle clinical signs of a meningioma in an adult: a case report

Andrée-Anne Marchand[1] and Julie O'Shaughnessy[2*]

Abstract

Background: Meningiomas are the most common brain tumor in the adult population. This case report describes the epidemiology, the clinical presentation as well as the current treatment options for this condition.

Case presentation: A 49 year-old man attended a chiropractic clinic with non-specific chronic low back pain. Upon the history taking and the systems review, he reported a loss of both smell and taste for which investigations conducted by two different otolaryngologists did not yield a specific diagnosis. The patient was referred to a neurologist who ordered a computer tomography scan that eventually revealed a compression brain tumor.
Brain tumors can produce a large variety of clinical presentations, such as upper motor neuron lesion symptoms, altered consciousness or vital functions which are easy to identify. However, subtle signs, such as those presented in this case, can be neglected.

Conclusion: Clinicians should be aware of uncommon clinical presentations including cranial nerve or neurological dysfunction and refer their patient to a specialist when detected.

Keywords: Meningioma, Brain tumor, Chiropractic, Cranial nerve, Neurological dysfunction

Résumé (French language)

Introduction: Les méningiomes sont les tumeurs cérébrales les plus fréquemment rencontrées dans la population adulte. Cette étude de cas décrit l'épidémiologie, la présentation clinique ainsi que les options de traitement pour cette condition.

Présentation du cas: Un homme de 49 ans, s'est présenté à une clinique chiropratique ayant comme motif principal une lombalgie chronique non spécifique. L'anamnèse et la revue des systèmes ont révélé une perte de l'odorat et du goût, pour laquelle des examens menés par deux otolaryngologistes différents n'ont mené à aucun diagnostic précis. Le patient fut ensuite référé à un neurologue qui a ordonné une tomographie axiale révélant une tumeur compressive localisée au cerveau.
Les tumeurs cérébrales peuvent être responsables d'une grande variété de manifestations cliniques incluant des symptômes facilement reconnaissables, tels qu'une lésion des motoneurones supérieurs et une altération de la conscience ou des fonctions vitales. Toutefois, des signes plus subtils, tels que ceux présentés dans ce cas, peuvent être négligés.

Conclusion: Les cliniciens devraient être familiers avec les présentations cliniques inhabituelles liées aux méningiomes, y compris les désordres neurologiques. La référence des patients à un spécialiste est souhaitable aussitôt la problématique découverte.

* Correspondence: julie.o'shaughnessy@uqtr.ca
[2]Département de chiropratique, Université du Québec à Trois-Rivières (UQTR), Trois-Rivières, Québec, Canada
Full list of author information is available at the end of the article

Background

Meningiomas arise from arachnoidal cells of the leptomeninges and are the most common primary tumors of the central nervous system in adults [1]. Over the past decades, improved and more frequent use of brain imaging has resulted in an increase in the diagnostic incidence and prevalence of meningiomas [1]. According to the United States Central Brain Tumor Registry, meningiomas had the highest incidence and accounted for 35.5% of all primary brain tumors between 2005 and 2009 [2]. Age-adjusted incidence is more than twice as common in females and increases dramatically after age 65 [2]. Ninety–eight percent of meningiomas are reported to be non–malignant and are usually confirmed by either histological or radiographical studies [2]. The following case report highlights the importance of primary contact practitioners awareness to the presence of abnormal symptoms related to meningiomas. It also presents the crucial clinical findings that warrant referral for further investigation.

Case presentation

History

A 49 year-old male attended a chiropractic clinic with a history of nonspecific chronic low back pain. Upon further questioning, the patient mentioned a progressive decrease in sense of smell and taste which was reported as complete since the last two and a half years. Following medical consultation for this matter since a year ago, two otolaryngologists had been consulted and both conducted nasal and oesophageal endoscopies that were considered normal. Lifestyle review revealed an average consumption of four alcoholic beverages daily and sometimes up to forty-eight to seventy-two beverages weekly. The result of the CAGE questionnaire [3] which yielded two positive answers (need to cut down on drinking (C) and need a drink first thing in the morning (E: eyes opener)) out of four (annoyed by people criticizing your drinking (A) and ever felt guilty about drinking (G)) was in accordance with the patient acknowledgement of his alcohol problem. Past medical history revealed bilateral knee meniscectomy, right carpal tunnel surgical decompression, L4-L5 discectomy and excision of a benign cervical lipoma. The patient reported his health status as otherwise healthy and denied the presence of any constitutional symptoms.

Physical examination

Upper and lower limb neurological examination was bilaterally present, symmetric and rated as unremarkable for deep tendon reflexes, sensation and motor strength. Pathological reflexes were absent bilaterally. A cranial nerve exam revealed anosmia. In accordance with diagnostic imaging practice guidelines [4] cervical spine radiographs were ordered in light of the presence of central nervous system sign and symptoms. The radiological examination revealed postural anomalies, cervical degenerative disc disease and congenital non-union of the posterior arch of the atlas. Given the patient's age, his non-smoking status, absence of trauma, unremitting nature of the symptoms and lack of previous invasive investigation the chiropractor suspected a neurological compression from internal cause. The decision was made to refer the patient to a neurologist for further investigation of the decreased sense of smell and taste.

Intervention and outcome

A computer tomography (CT) scan ordered by the neurologist upon initial assessment revealed a 6 cm planum sphenoidale mass located in the frontal lobe, suggesting a benign meningioma (Figures 1 and 2). The tumor was well circumscribed and no osseous abnormalities were detected. The patient underwent a frontolateral craniotomy with complete resection of the tumor mass. Post-surgical complication of a cerebrospinal fluid (CSF) leakage through the nasal cavity occurred 3 days later. A spinal tap was initially used to drain the CSF, but subsequent air accumulation within the intracranial cavity as visualized on CT led to a second surgical intervention. The dural breach was repaired through reconstruction of the anterior base of the ethmoid. No other surgical complication was reported and the pathological analysis confirmed a diagnosis of meningioma.

At one year follow-up, the patient did not report any neurological symptoms, except anosmia. No further surgical complications were reported. He had no limitations to his daily living activities and he returned back to work full time. Of interest, the patient's problem with alcohol resolved without treatment after the surgery.

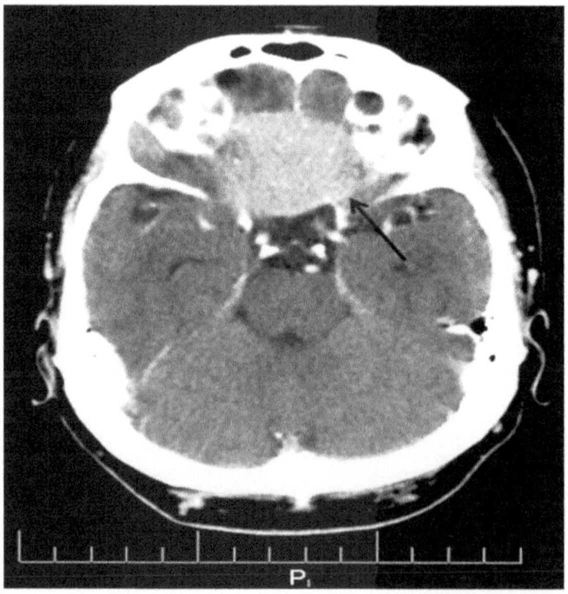

Figure 1 Axial view, CT of the head, soft tissue window reveals a 6x6 cm well marginated meningioma extending into the planum sphenoidale.

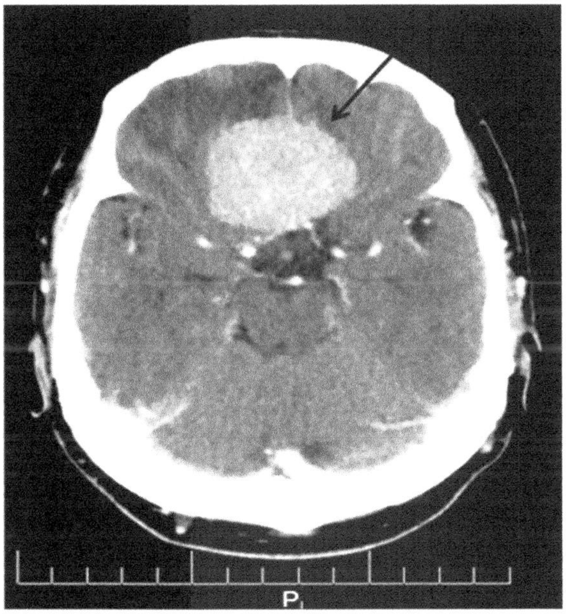

Figure 2 Axial view, CT of the head, soft tissue window reveals compression of the frontal lobe by the meningioma.

Discussion

Meningiomas of the midline anterior skull base such as the olfactory groove meningioma presented in this case report are a rare clinical entity and represent about 10% of all intracranial meningiomas [5]. Olfactory groove meningioma (OGM) originates from the anterior cranial base, commonly at the cribriform plate of the ethmoid bone, planum sphenoidale or the frontospenoidal suture [6]. Arising from the weakest part of the skull base makes it prone to infiltration of the underlying bone. It also sometimes extend into the paranasal sinuses and nasal cavity, displacing the olfactory tracts laterally and the optic chiasm posteriorly [7]. The tumors are generally encapsulated and attached to the dura. OGMs receive their vascular supply primarily from the anterior and posterior ethmoidal arteries. Vascular contribution from the dura, anterior branches of the middle meningeal artery and the meningeal branches of the ophthalmic artery are also often seen [8].

Although there are several meningioma subtypes, (meningotheiomatous, fibrous, psammomatous) their identification has little prognostic value. Only clear cell meningiomas are thought to have clinical significance due to their aggressive behaviour [8]. Histologic features are used to classify meningiomas into one of the three World Health Organization (WHO) grades and are useful in predicting recurrence and survival rate. About 90% of tumors are grade I (benign) with a risk of recurrence after post-surgical resection of 7% to 20%. Incidence of grade II meningiomas (atypical) is 5% to 7%, with a recurrence rate of 40% whereas less than 3% are classified as grade III (malignant or anaplastic). Between 50% to 80% of malignant cases will recur [9].

Several risk factors for the development of meningiomas have been hypothesized, and until now, the literature does not reveal any clear association. Environmental risk factors such as exposure to ionizing radiation are currently acknowledged as the leading cause underlying meningioma formation [8]. As such, low dose exposure as it is the case in dental x-rays, is a common source of radiation in the general population. Increased risks of developing meningioma have been identified with having had a bitewing examination at any age (Odd ratio: 2.0) and panoramic films under the age of 10 years old (Odd ratio: 4.9) [10]. A population-based prospective cohort study which included 27,791 post-menopausal women has determined that low levels of physical activity, history of oophorectomy (unilateral or bilateral), high height and body mass index (BMI) in the years preceding diagnosis and history of uterine fibroids were associated with an increased risks of meningioma [11]. In a large case–control study examining the relationship between family, personal medical history and meningioma, the results suggested a positive association between meningioma and first-degree family members diagnosed at a young age, female related hormone and ionization radiation [12].

Clinical presentation

Although they usually remain clinically quiescent during the early phase of growth, meningiomas localized to the frontal lobe result in a variety of alterations in cognitive and functioning behaviours [5]. The most common symptoms reported are headaches, visual disturbances and anosmia, often leading to incorrect diagnosis such as sinusitis, migraine and neuralgia [13]. In a retrospective study of 56 cases of olfactory groove meningioma, preoperative signs and symptoms screening revealed mental changes, headache, visual disturbance, dizziness, seizure, papilledema and hemiparesis [7]. Of interest in our present case, the patient reported spontaneous resolution of his alcoholism following the surgical intervention. To the best of our knowledge no previous report of a possible association between meningioma and alcoholism exits in the literature. Although other factors could explain the sudden patient's sobriety, it seems unlikely that heavy drinking habits could have stopped without any withdrawal effects. Given that tumours located in the frontal region are responsible for mental alterations such as attention deficits, disinterest and emotional detachment we hypothesize that alcoholism may have been the initial symptom experienced by the patient as a result of the meningioma growth.

Physical examination

Within the primary care setting, the suspicion of olfactory groove meningioma may be based solely on information gathered in the history. Although anosmia is thought to be an early symptom, surprisingly few patients complain of olfactory dysfunction, making its detection extremely difficult during routine clinical examination. Proposed explanations for the lack of suspicion include natural gradual decline in olfactory function and lateralised anosmia in which case olfactory function is maintained by the contralateral side [14]. When particular attention is brought to the olfactory function, the "sniffin' sticks" test can be performed to identify any odour threshold, discrimination, and identification deficits [14]. It has been suggested that in order to promptly diagnose at an early stage, CT scan "should be used in all patients presenting with loss of sense of smell that cannot be explained by head injury, other disease or previous surgical procedures of the olfactory region" [13]. Physical examination should include nasal endoscopy, as up to 15% of patients with OGMs are reported to have an intranasal component [15].

Imaging

Diagnosis and decision on the best surgical approach are usually made with the use of magnetic resonance imaging, due to its ability to show the tumor's dural origin, along with perifocal edema and location or encasement of major vessels [16]. In addition, meningiomas display a strong homogeneous enhancement when gadolinium contrast is used. Images displayed by CT show meningiomas as well-defined extra-axial masses associated with brain displacement and allow for identification of characteristics such as intratumoral calcification or hyperostosis [8,16].

Treatment

Treatment options for OGMs follow those in other skull base tumors. It is generally accepted that a small tumor, stable in size over time and asymptomatic, should be monitored through serial imaging. However, for meningiomas occurring in patients younger than 65 years of age, surgery is usually recommended. Curative treatment of meningiomas can usually be achieved by surgery alone when the tumor, its dural attachment and infiltrated bone can be completely resected. Even large size tumors can be totally removed due to the arachnoid membrane creating a separation from nearly all surrounding critical neurovascular structures [8]. Despite numerous surgical approaches that have been described in the literature and the refinement of technologies, removal of meningiomas of the anterior cranial base remains a challenge due to complex anatomical relations and surrounding of important neurovascular structures. One common theme discussed in the literature is that regardless of the technique used and tumor size, preservation of olfactory or visual function ipsilateral to the location of the tumor has a very poor outcome.

Radiation therapy comes into play in the management of meningioma when gross total resection cannot be safely achieved, such as in optic nerve sheath meningiomas, when tumors recur after surgery and in radiographically diagnosed tumors when biopsy is not possible. Radiotherapy is also provided as adjuvant therapy following resection of atypical and malignant meningiomas [8,9]. The role of chemotherapy is limited to treatment of tumors that recur after surgery and only when radiotherapy options are exhausted due to its reported minimal impact against this type of neoplasm [9].

Prognosis

When OGM resection results were initially reported, mortality ranged from 17.3% to 22.7% [8]. Recent literature revealed decreased mortality associated to meningioma with a 3-year post diagnosis survival estimate of 93.4% in patients treated with resection compared to 88.3% in patients not surgically treated. Younger patient age, female gender, unilateral tumors and surgical resection appear to be potential predictors of improved prognosis in patients with meningiomas [17]. The recurrence rate at 10 years has been reported to vary from 9% to 20% for totally resected meningiomas, and from 18.4% to 50% for meningiomas following subtotal resection. The mean time to recurrence of meningiomas has been determined to be 2.5 years to 5 years [18]. Although limited evidence is available on the prognosis of untreated meningiomas, low growth rate tumors have been reported not to be an obstacle to patients function and well being even in presence of slight neurological symptoms [19].

Conclusion

Although meningioma is the most common primary tumor in the nervous system in adults, it is a rare condition. In the presence of subtle clinical signs such as those presented in this case report, clinicians should keep a high index of suspicion for brain tumor. In the presence of uncommon neurological signs and symptoms, cranial nerve dysfunction or failed conservative therapy, clinicians should not hesitate to refer the patient for further evaluation as part of a complete management program.

Informed consent

Written informed consent was obtained from the patient for publication of this Case report and any accompanying images. A copy of the written consent is available for review by the Editor-in-Chief of this journal.

Competing interest

The authors declare that they have no competing interests.

Authors' contributions

AAM and JO contributed to the literature review and writing of the manuscript. All authors read and approved the final manuscript.

Author details

[1]Canadian Memorial Chiropractic College (CMCC), Toronto, Ontario and Université du Québec à Trois-Rivieres (UQTR), Trois-Rivieres, Québec, Canada. [2]Département de chiropratique, Université du Québec à Trois-Rivières (UQTR), Trois-Rivières, Québec, Canada.

References

1. Saraf S, McCarthy BJ, Villano JL: **Update on meningiomas.** *Oncologist* 2011, **16**:1604–1613.
2. Dolecek TA, Propp JM, Stroup NE, Kruchko C: **CBTRUS statistical report: primary brain and central nervous system tumors diagnosed in the United States in 2005–2009.** *Neuro Oncol* 2012, **14**(Suppl 5):v1–v49.
3. Ewing JA: **Detecting alcoholism. The CAGE questionnaire.** *JAMA* 1984, **252**:1905–1907.
4. Bussieres AE, Taylor JA, Peterson C: **Diagnostic imaging practice guidelines for musculoskeletal complaints in adults-an evidence-based approach-part 3: spinal disorders.** *J Manipulative Physiol Ther* 2008, **31**:33–88.
5. Gazzeri R, Galarza M, Gazzeri G: **Giant olfactory groove meningioma: ophthalmological and cognitive outcome after bifrontal microsurgical approach.** *Acta Neurochir (Wien)* 2008, **150**:1117–1125.
6. Pepper JP, Hecht SL, Gebarski SS, Lin EM, Sullivan SE, Marentette LJ: **Olfactory groove meningioma: discussion of clinical presentation and surgical outcomes following excision via the subcranial approach.** *Laryngoscope* 2011, **121**:2282–2289.
7. Bassiouni H, Asgari S, Stolke D: **Olfactory groove meningiomas: functional outcome in a series treated microsurgically.** *Acta Neurochir (Wien)* 2007, **149**:109–121.
8. Adappa ND, Lee JY, Chiu AG, Palmer JN: **Olfactory groove meningioma.** *Otolaryngol Clin North Am* 2011, **44**:965–980. ix.
9. Norden AD, Drappatz J, Wen PY: **Advances in meningioma therapy.** *Curr Neurol Neurosci Rep* 2009, **9**:231–240.
10. Claus EB, Calvocoressi L, Bondy ML, Schildkraut JM, Wiemels JL, Wrensch M: **Dental x-rays and risk of meningioma.** *Cancer* 2012, **118**:4530–4537.
11. Johnson DR, Olson JE, Vierkant RA, Hammack JE, Wang AH, Folsom AR, Virnig BA, Cerhan JR: **Risk factors for meningioma in postmenopausal women: results from the Iowa Women's Health Study.** *Neuro Oncol* 2011, **13**:1011–1019.
12. Claus EB, Calvocoressi L, Bondy ML, Schildkraut JM, Wiemels JL, Wrensch M: **Family and personal medical history and risk of meningioma.** *J Neurosurg* 2011, **115**:1072–1077.
13. Tsikoudas A, Martin-Hirsch DP: **Olfactory groove meningiomas.** *Clin Otolaryngol Allied Sci* 1999, **24**:507–509.
14. Welge-Luessen A, Temmel A, Quint C, Moll B, Wolf S, Hummel T: **Olfactory function in patients with olfactory groove meningioma.** *J Neurol Neurosurg Psychiatry* 2001, **70**:218–221.
15. Derome PJ, Guiot G: **Bone problems in meningiomas invading the base of the skull.** *Clin Neurosurg* 1978, **25**:435–451.
16. Rachinger W, Grau S, Tonn JC: **Different microsurgical approaches to meningiomas of the anterior cranial base.** *Acta Neurochir (Wien)* 2010, **152**:931–939.
17. Cahill KS, Claus EB: **Treatment and survival of patients with nonmalignant intracranial meningioma: results from the surveillance, epidemiology, and end results program of the National Cancer Institute. Clinical article.** *J Neurosurg* 2011, **115**:259–267.
18. Snyder WE, Shah MV, Weisberger EC, Campbell RL: **Presentation and patterns of late recurrence of olfactory groove meningiomas.** *Skull Base Surg* 2000, **10**:131–139.
19. Bindal R, Goodman JM, Kawasaki A, Purvin V, Kuzma B: **The natural history of untreated skull base meningiomas.** *Surg Neurol* 2003, **59**:87–92. discussion 92.

6

Dietary supplement recommendations by Saskatchewan chiropractors: results of an online survey

Kent Stuber[1*], Paul Bruno[2], Kevyn Kristmanson[3] and Zara Ali[1]

Abstract

Background: Chiropractors receive training in nutrition during their education, previous surveys have found that chiropractors frequently provide recommendations to patients relating to nutrition and dietary supplement intake. However, it has not been ascertained which specific supplements chiropractors recommend or the types of health conditions for which supplement recommendations are made.

Objective: The purpose of this study was to determine which dietary supplements are most commonly recommended by chiropractors in the province of Saskatchewan,Canada and the health conditions for which supplement recommendations are made.

Design: An online survey of licensed chiropractors practicing in the province of Saskatchewan, Canada was distributed three times following online and in-person notifications of the survey.

Statistical analyses performed: Descriptive statistics were reported, predominantly in the form of means and proportions.

Results: A response rate of 45% was obtained. All of the respondents (100%) indicated providing nutritional advice or counselling to patients, while nearly all (99%) indicated providing dietary supplement recommendations to patients. Respondents estimated that they provide nutritional advice or counselling to 31% of their patients on average, and recommend dietary supplements to an average of 25% of their patients. The most commonly recommended supplements were glucosamine sulfate, multivitamins, vitamin C, vitamin D, calcium, omega-3 fatty acids, and probiotics. The most common reasons to recommend dietary supplements were for "general health and wellness" (82% of respondents), "bone health" (74%), "rheumatologic, arthritic, degenerative, or inflammatory conditions' (72%), and "acute and/or chronic musculoskeletal conditions" (65%).

Conclusion: The majority of respondents indicated providing nutritional counselling and recommendations for dietary supplements to their patients. Respondents generally recommend a small number of dietary supplements and provide these recommendations and counselling to fewer than half of their patients on average, while tending to focus on conditions most closely related to the scope of practice of chiropractors. The findings of this study may have been limited by selection bias owing to the low response rate and as those who respond to surveys are often more likely to respond positively.

Keywords: Chiropractic, Nutrition, Survey, Dietary supplement

* Correspondence: kstuber@cmcc.ca
[1]6100 Leslie Street, Toronto, ON M2H 3J1, Canada
Full list of author information is available at the end of the article

Background

Use of dietary supplements is quite common throughout North America, with surveys indicating a past year usage prevalence of up to 73% in the general public [1]. The most commonly utilized supplements are multivitamins/multi-minerals, followed by single vitamin or mineral supplements; other supplements (e.g. herbal/botanical) are less commonly utilized [1]. In this manuscript we will define *dietary supplements* as encompassing both *herbal supplements* (i.e. those obtained from a botanical source) and *nutritional supplements* (e.g. vitamin and/or mineral formulations, amino acids, and hormones not derived from a botanical source) [2].

Chiropractors are among the numerous health care professionals who provide nutritional and dietary advice to patients. In the typical North American chiropractic educational program students complete two courses in nutrition, one providing the foundations of biochemistry and nutrition, followed by a clinical nutrition course [3,4]. Some chiropractors will continue to additional specialization in nutrition, obtaining post-graduate certificates, graduate degrees, or diplomate status in clinical nutrition [3,4].

A 2009 survey of chiropractors across the United States indicated that approximately 94% make nutritional or dietary recommendations to patients [5]. This is higher than previous surveys of American chiropractors which have typically shown 80% of chiropractors incorporate nutritional counselling in their practices [4,6]. A 2001 survey [6] indicated that the most commonly recommended nutritional products by chiropractors were vitamins (by 78% of chiropractors), followed by minerals (65%), herbal preparations (54%), and nutrient combinations for specific conditions (54%). Previous surveys of registered dietitians indicate that 74% to 97% recommend dietary supplements, while only 13% recommend herbal-based supplements [7,8]. This is compared with 40% of pharmacists [2], 79% of physicians [9], 82% of nurses [9], 72% of cardiologists, 66% of dermatologists, and 91% of orthopedists who have indicated recommending dietary supplements to patients [10].

We conducted an online survey, the primary purpose of which was to determine which dietary supplements are most commonly recommended by chiropractors in the province of Saskatchewan, Canada. The current survey is unique compared with previous surveys of chiropractors on this topic in that it asked the frequency with which chiropractors recommend numerous specific dietary supplements and the health conditions for which they recommend supplements, in addition to inquiring about professional behaviours and post-graduate training related to nutrition.

Methods

This study consisted of an online survey conducted in September 2012. The inclusion criteria consisted of all chiropractors who were actively practicing in the province of Saskatchewan and members of the Chiropractors' Association of Saskatchewan (CAS). The CAS distributed the e-mail messages for the authors so that confidentiality of their members' contact information was not violated. All qualified participants were contacted up to a total of five times, including four e-mail messages and one in-person invitation. Participants were initially contacted by a pre-notification e-mail message. Five days later, two of the authors (PB and KK) attended the CAS Annual General Meeting and announced that the initial e-mail invitation would be distributed two days after the meeting (seven days after the pre-notification message). Subsequently, two reminder e-mail invitations were distributed at further two week intervals (14 and 28 days after the initial e-mail invitation message).

The survey e-mail invitation and reminder messages contained the objective and purpose of the study (as part of a study information sheet), which then linked interested participants to an informed consent form via one of the authors' (KS) Survey Monkey™ account. Participants who agreed to be involved in the study and agreed to the terms of the informed consent were asked to click on an "I Agree" button, which then directed them to the rest of the survey. The survey consisted of several questions including those related to: demographic and nutrition educational background, professional behaviours related to nutrition, how often they recommend different dietary supplements, and the types of conditions for which they recommend supplements (see Additional file 1). Respondents answered the survey in complete anonymity. There was no compensation for participation in this survey. Survey results were summarized with descriptive statistics, expressed as either means or proportions of respondents, depending on the question's structure. Ethics approval was received from the Canadian Memorial Chiropractic College Research Ethics Board.

Prior to commencement of the survey study, a convenience sample of three clinicians at the HK Lee Clinic on the Canadian Memorial Chiropractic College campus were asked to review and complete the questionnaire to ensure appropriate question quality, style, and content and to allow for revisions to be made. Minor changes were made to survey questions based on the feedback, producing the final survey that was accessed by respondents. The data provided by the clinicians is not included in the data reported herein.

Results

Of the 182 active CAS members who were contacted, 81 participated in the survey (45% response rate).

Demographic information for the survey respondents and for all chiropractors registered with the CAS at the time the survey was conducted are presented in Table 1. With regards to these demographic data, the survey respondents appear to be representative of the target population of chiropractors.

The respondents indicated varying levels of continuing education course involvement related to nutrition and dietary supplements: 17% had not completed any such courses, 54% had taken between one and five courses, 12% had taken between six and ten courses, and 16% had taken 11 or more courses. The vast majority (94%) did not have or were not in the process of completing a post-graduate certificate, fellowship, diplomate, or Master's degree in nutrition, while 5% had a post-graduate certificate in nutrition, and 2.5% had a post-graduate fellowship or diplomate in nutrition (one of the respondents had both a post-graduate certificate and fellowship or diplomate).

All of the respondents (100%) indicated providing nutritional advice or counselling to patients, while nearly all (99%) also indicated providing dietary supplement recommendations to patients. On average, the respondents estimated that they provide nutritional advice or counselling to 31% of their patients, and recommend dietary supplements to 25% of their patients. In addition, respondents estimated that they refer an average of 6% of their patients to medical doctors and 11% of their patients to naturopathic doctors for dietary or nutrition-related concerns. The average estimated percentage of patients referred to registered dieticians, nutritionists, and homeopathic doctors was 3% (each).

Table 2 depicts the number of respondents who indicated recommending different dietary supplements to their patients, as well as the number of respondents who sell those supplements in their clinics. The supplements that were recommended most often (i.e. recommended "almost always or all of the time" or "often" by ≥25% of respondents) were glucosamine sulfate, multi-vitamins, vitamin C, vitamin D, calcium, omega-3 fatty acids, and probiotics.

When asked for the types of conditions or reasons for which they recommend dietary supplements, the most common response was for "general health and wellness" (82% of respondents), followed by "bone health" (74%), "rheumatologic, arthritic, degenerative, or inflammatory conditions' (72%), "acute and/or chronic musculoskeletal conditions" (65%), "weight loss or management" (36%), "digestive conditions" (35%), "neurologic conditions" (35%), "reproductive conditions such as menopause or premenstrual symptoms management" (27%), and "skin conditions" (25%). The remaining reasons for recommending dietary supplements were indicated by fewer than 25% of the respondents and included "anti-aging" (22%), "hormone imbalances" (20%), "cardiovascular conditions" (17%), "nutritional cleansing or colon health" (16%), "weight gain" (15%), "endocrine conditions" (14%), and "psychological conditions" (10%).

Discussion

All of the respondents to this survey indicated that they provide nutritional advice or counselling to patients, and 99% provide dietary supplement recommendations. Similarly, a 2009 survey of 2371 chiropractors across the United States indicated that 94% provided nutritional and dietary recommendations [5]. In a survey of 125 New York chiropractors, Holtzman and Burke found that 80% of respondents utilized nutritional counseling

Table 1 Demographic information for survey respondents (n=81) and for all chiropractors registered with the Chiropractors' Association of Saskatchewan (CAS) at the time the survey was conducted (n=182)

		Survey respondents	All CAS members
Gender	*Female*	34%	30%
	Male	66%	70%
College of graduation	*Canadian Memorial Chiropractic College*	75%	69%
	Other college	25%	31%
Years in practice	*0-5 years*	17%	20%
	6-10 years	11%	12%
	11-15 years	16%	17%
	16-20 years	22%	18%
	21-25 years	10%	10%
	26-30 years	7%	8%
	31-35 years	5%	7%
	≥ 36 years	11%	8%

Table 2 Number of survey respondents (n=81) who recommend (almost always or all of the time, often, sometimes, rarely, never) and sell the following dietary supplements

Dietary supplement	Number of respondents who provided a response	Number of respondents who recommended the supplement			Sold in the respondents' clinic
		"Almost always or all the time" or "Often"	*"Sometimes"*	*"Rarely" or "Never"*	
Glucosamine sulfate/ other forms of glucosamine	81	30*	35	16	23
Chondroitin sulfate	64	7	16	41	6
Methylsulfonylmethane (MSM)	67	15	18	34	13
White willow bark	61	3	13	45	6
Boswellia	61	6	10	45	6
Bromelain	65	6	21	38	9
Quercetin	61	3	14	44	8
Multi-vitamins	72	27*	28	17	21
Any B vitamins	66	13	29	24	10
Niacin specifically	55	3	11	41	6
Folic acid specifically	57	5	13	39	6
Vitamin B12 specifically	57	7	12	38	6
Vitamin C	61	26*	16	19	15
Vitamin D	73	40*	17	16	18
Vitamin E	62	7	19	36	7
Calcium	71	32*	19	20	18
Chromium	59	5	13	41	7
Iron	61	6	17	38	5
Magnesium	63	18	21	24	7
Potassium	59	3	14	42	5
Selenium	58	3	9	46	4
Zinc	59	5	12	42	5
Co-enzyme Q10	64	8	13	43	11
Omega-3 fatty acids	75	41*	15	19	20
Omega-6 fatty acids	65	13	11	41	13
Garlic pills	57	3	8	46	3
Saw palmetto	62	5	13	44	11
Black cohosh	56	2	6	48	6
St. John's Wort	53	0	5	48	1
Ginkgo biloba	54	0	7	47	3
Echinacea	53	3	11	39	4
Ginseng	53	2	3	48	2
Creatine	52	0	4	48	4
Protein powders	56	6	8	42	6
Homeopathic formulations	56	5	5	46	5
Probiotics	67	20*	18	29	14

* indicates the supplements that were recommended "almost always or all the time" or "often" by ≥25% of respondents.

in their practices, and dietary supplement prescription was the most common form of such counselling [4]. Respondents were asked to estimate the percentage of their patients to whom nutritional advice or counselling was provided (31% on average) as well as the percentage of patients who received dietary supplement recommendations (25% on average). These rates are lower than those reported by 74 American chiropractors in a 2001 survey, who provided nutritional counselling to an average of 37% of their patients, and recommended dietary supplements to an average of 50% of their patients [6].

Although dietary supplement recommendation to patients appears to be common amongst Saskatchewan chiropractors, only a small number of dietary supplements are frequently recommended (glucosamine sulfate, multivitamins, vitamin C, vitamin D, calcium, omega-3 fatty acids, and probiotics). These results are not substantially different from the findings of Hetherwick et al. that the most commonly recommended nutrient-based dietary supplements by California dietitians were calcium, multivitamins with or without minerals, vitamin E, vitamin C, and iron [7]. Their most commonly recommended herbal supplement was Echinacea, a finding supported by Cashman et al. in their survey of Massachusetts dietitians [7,11]. Conversely, nearly half of the current survey respondents indicated that they "rarely" or "never" recommend Echinacea. Interestingly, a recent review indicates that Echinacea may be effective in reducing the duration and severity of a cold [12].

When considering the types of health conditions for which respondents recommend dietary supplements, there was a level of concurrence with the specific supplements being recommended. The most common reason for recommending supplements to patients was for "general health and wellness" (by 82% of respondents), which is reflected by multi-vitamins, vitamin C, and probiotics being among the most recommended supplements. Vitamin C has been found effective in preventing the common cold [12], however there is conflicting and insufficient evidence to date regarding the use of multivitamins [13-15] and probiotics [16,17] for the prevention and treatment of different health conditions. The next most common reason to recommend supplements was for "bone health" (74%), which is reflected by vitamin D and calcium being frequently recommended and well supported in the literature and by clinical practice guidelines [18-20]. Omega-3 fatty acids and glucosamine sulfate were also commonly recommended by respondents, and this may be a reflection of their frequently recommending supplements for "rheumatologic, arthritic, degenerative, or inflammatory conditions" (72%) and "acute and/or chronic musculoskeletal conditions" (65%). However, there is conflicting evidence surrounding the use of both omega-3 fatty acids [21-24] and glucosamine sulfate [25-27] for such conditions. Holtzman and Burke found that the most common conditions for which New York chiropractors provided nutritional counselling were osteoarthritis (by 76% of respondents) and osteoporosis (71%), followed by obesity, diabetes, coronary artery disease, fibromyalgia, and allergies (each at least 50%) [4].

In comparing the current results to other health professions, a recent survey of American dietitians found that the most common reason for recommending supplements by this group was bone health (70%), followed by filling nutrition gaps (69%), overall health and wellness (49%), lowering cholesterol (46%), cardiac health (46%), dietary pattern reasons (for vegetarians or vegans for example, 43%), and digestive health (39%) [8]. Dickinson et al. surveyed 900 physicians (including 300 general practitioners) and 277 nurses, and the three most common reasons these groups recommend dietary supplements to patients were for overall health and wellness (41% of physicians and 62% of nurses), followed by bone health (41% and 58%, respectively) and joint health (37% and 37%) [9]. In a survey of 300 cardiologists, 300 dermatologists, and 300 orthopedists, the most common reasons that each group provided for recommending dietary supplements was reflected in their professional specialty [10]. For example, the cardiologists' most common reason for recommending dietary supplements was to lower cholesterol (58%), followed by heart health (55%) and maintaining healthy cholesterol (36%) [10]. Dermatologists most frequently recommended dietary supplements for skin, hair, and nails (81%), followed by overall health and wellness (30%) and bone health (25%). Orthopedists most frequently recommended dietary supplements for bone health (75%), followed by joint health (73%) and musculoskeletal pain (53%) [10]. The findings from the current survey reflect the trends observed in these surveys in that "general health and wellness" was the most commonly cited reason for Saskatchewan chiropractors to recommend supplements to patients, followed by "bone health", "rheumatologic, arthritic, degenerative, or inflammatory conditions", and "acute and/or chronic musculoskeletal conditions." It is reasonable to expect chiropractors' recommendations to parallel those of orthopedists as both groups predominantly treat patients with musculoskeletal and degenerative conditions, and this does appear to be the case. However, chiropractors seem to have a substantially greater tendency to recommend supplements for "general health and wellness" than do orthopedists (82% versus 25%) [10].

Postgraduate education in nutrition

Smith and Spillman found that their chiropractor respondents had completed 84 postgraduate nutrition hours on average [6], while the majority of respondents to the current survey had taken between one and five postgraduate courses on nutrition and 28% had completed at least six postgraduate nutrition courses. A small minority of respondents (6%) had completed formal postgraduate qualification (certificate, fellowship, diplomate, graduate degree) in nutrition. Holtzman and Burke [4] found that 65% of their chiropractor respondents did not feel that they had received adequate education in nutrition, and 47% of the respondents in Smith and Spillman [6] felt similarly. Although the current survey's respondents were not asked to rate the perceived adequacy of the nutritional education in their chiropractic training, these previous survey findings may in part explain why so many respondents have augmented their education with postgraduate training in nutrition.

Referral rates to and from other health professionals

A 2009 survey of chiropractors in the United States indicated that chiropractors refer patients to nutritionists and receive patient referrals from nutritionists at a frequency between "Never" and "Rarely" (<1/month), while patient referrals to and from family practitioners occurred at a frequency between "Rarely" and "Sometimes" (1-3/month) [28]. The findings from the current survey are in line with these, as respondents indicated referring a higher percentage of their patients to medical doctors (6% of their patients on average) and naturopathic doctors (11%) for dietary or nutrition-related concerns than to dietitians or nutritionists (3% each).

Study strengths and weaknesses

The response rate of this survey was 45%, which is low, but still within the anticipated range for surveys of chiropractors [29]. Previous surveys of chiropractors regarding nutritional and dietary supplement recommendations have obtained response rates varying between 13% and 34%. The current study actually had the highest response rate of chiropractors thus far on this topic, making it difficult to necessarily validate the results of the current survey against those conducted previously [4-6]. Numerous steps were taken to encourage a higher response rate, such as pre-notification, and multiple contacts, both in person and through e-mail messages [29]. Respondents to this survey were practicing chiropractors from only one jurisdiction in Canada, which limits the ability to generalize results to other North American jurisdictions. Additionally, not all of respondents answered all of the survey questions, creating a level of uncertainty for those particular results.

Furthermore, while this survey did inquire about different reasons for respondents to recommend dietary supplements, it did not ask respondents to directly relate these reasons to specific supplements. Additionally, the list of supplements occasionally did not necessarily correspond to those different reasons. For example, none of the listed supplements would be considered to be specifically targeted towards "weight loss or management", which was mentioned as a reason for recommending supplements by 36% of respondents. In addition, all of the survey respondents indicated providing nutritional advice or counselling to patients, and nearly all respondents provide dietary supplement recommendations to patients. These data lead to a concern of some degree of selection bias where only those who do recommend supplements or provide nutritional advice or counselling chose to complete the survey. As mentioned previously Table 1 indicates that the survey respondents do not appear to be essentially different from the entire population of Saskatchewan chiropractors from a demographic standpoint, thus it is unclear if there is any bias in the results due to non-response.

Conclusions

The majority of respondents to this survey indicated providing nutritional counselling and recommendations for dietary supplements to patients. They provide these recommendations and counselling to fewer than half of their patients on average and tend to focus on conditions most related to the chiropractic scope of practice, including general health and wellness, along with musculoskeletal and degenerative conditions. Respondents mainly recommend a small number of dietary supplements such as multivitamins, vitamin C, vitamin D, calcium, probiotics, glucosamine sulfate, and omega-3 fatty acids. Most of the responding chiropractors have completed postgraduate courses on nutrition, and generally do not refer a high proportion of patients for nutritional counselling to other health professionals. Future research should be directed towards larger jurisdictions which may be more representative of North American chiropractors and should include qualitative research which elucidates the reasons for different professional behaviours relating to nutrition.

Additional file

Additional file 1: Online Nutritional Survey.

Competing interests

The authors declare that they have no competing interests.

Authors' contributions

KS conceived and designed the study, participated in data collection and analysis, and drafted the manuscript. PB contributed to study design, data collection, data analysis, and revisions of the manuscript. KK contributed to study design, data collection, and revisions of the manuscript. ZA contributed to study design and revisions of the manuscript. All of the authors have given their approval of the final version to be published.

Acknowledgements
The authors wish to acknowledge the Board members and administrative staff of the Chiropractors' Association of Saskatchewan (CAS) for their assistance with survey invitation distribution to members of the CAS.

Author details
[1]6100 Leslie Street, Toronto, ON M2H 3J1, Canada. [2]3737 Wascana Parkway, Regina, Saskatchewan S4S 0A2, Canada. [3]102 - 12 Cheadle St. West Swift Current, Saskatchewan S9H 0A9, Canada.

References

1. Timbo BB, Ross MP, McCarthy PV, Lin C-TJ: **Dietary supplements in a national survey: prevalence of use and reports of adverse events.** *J Am Diet Assoc* 2006, **106:**1966–1974.
2. Howard N, Tsourounis C, Kapusnik-uner J: **Dietary supplement survey of pharmacists: personal and professional practices.** *J Altern Complement Med* 2001, **7:**667–680.
3. Christensen MG, Kollasch MW, Hyland JK: **Chapter 1 - the chiropractic profession.** In *Practice analysis of chiropractic 2010.* Edited by Christensen MG, Kollasch MW, Hyland JK. Greeley: National Board of Chiropractic Examiners; 2009:1–12.
4. Holtzman D, Burke J: **Nutritional counseling in the chiropractic practice: a survey of New York practitioners.** *Journal of Chiropractic Medicine* 2007, **6:**27–31.
5. Christensen MG, Kollasch MW, Hyland JK: **Chapter 9 - professional functions and treatment procedures.** In *Practice analysis of chiropractic 2010.* Edited by Christensen MG, Kollasch MW, Hyland JK. Greeley: National Board of Chiropractic Examiners; 2009:121–136.
6. Smith D, Spillman D: **A survey of chiropractors ' use of nutrition in private practice.** *Journal of Chiropractic Humanities* 2001, **10:**1–6.
7. Hetherwick C, Morris MN, Silliman K: **Perceived knowledge, attitudes, and practices of California registered dietitians regarding dietary supplements.** *J Am Diet Assoc* 2006, **106:**438–442.
8. Dickinson A, Bonci L, Boyon N, Franco JC: **Dietitians use and recommend dietary supplements: report of a survey.** *Nutr J* 2012, **11:**14.
9. Dickinson A, Boyon N, Shao A: **Physicians and nurses use and recommend dietary supplements: report of a survey.** *Nutr J* 2009, **8:**29.
10. Dickinson A, Shao A, Boyon N, Franco JC: **Use of dietary supplements by cardiologists, dermatologists and orthopedists: report of a survey.** *Nutr J* 2011, **10:**20.
11. Cashman LS, Burns JT, Otieno IM, Fung T: **Massachusetts registered Dietitians' knowledge, attitudes, opinions, personal Use, and recommendations to clients about herbal supplements.** *J Altern Complement Med* 2003, **9:**735–746.
12. Nahas R, Balla A: **Complementary and alternative medicine for prevention and treatment of the common cold.** *Canadian Family Physician* 2011, **57:**31–36.
13. Frank E, Bendich A, Denniston M: **Use of vitamin-mineral supplements by female physicians in the United States.** *Am J Clin Nutr* 2000, **72:**969–975.
14. Greenwald P, Anderson D, Nelson Sa, Taylor PR: **Clinical trials of vitamin and mineral supplements for cancer prevention.** *Am J Clin Nutr* 2007, **85:**314S–317S.
15. Stratton J, Godwin M: **The effect of supplemental vitamins and minerals on the development of prostate cancer: a systematic review and meta-analysis.** *Fam Pract* 2011, **28:**243–252.
16. Ritchie ML, Romanuk TN: **A meta-analysis of probiotic efficacy for gastrointestinal diseases.** *PLoS One* 2012, **7:**e34938.
17. Rowland I, Capurso L, Collins K, Cummings J, Delzenne N, Goulet O, Guarner F, Marteau P, Meier R: **Current level of consensus on probiotic science–report of an expert meeting–London, 23 November 2009.** *Gut Microbes* 2010, **1:**436–439.
18. Papaioannou A, Morin S, Cheung AM, Atkinson S, Brown JP, Feldman S, Hanley DA, Hodsman A, Jamal SA, Kaiser SM, Kvern B, Siminoski K, Leslie WD: **2010 clinical practice guidelines for the diagnosis and management of osteoporosis in Canada: summary.** *Can Med Assoc J* 2010, **182:**1864–1873.
19. Eisman J, Ebeling P, Ewald D, Flicker L, Holborow B: *Clinical guideline for the prevention and treatment of osteoporosis in postmenopausal women and older men.* South Melbourne: Royal Australian College of General Practitioners; 2010:1–76.
20. Stránský M, Rysavá L: **Nutrition as prevention and treatment of osteoporosis.** *Physiol Res* 2009, **58**(Suppl 1):S7–S11.
21. Calder PC: **Omega-3 fatty acids and inflammatory processes.** *Nutrients* 2010, **2:**355–374.
22. Wardhana, Surachmanto ES, Datau Ea: **The role of omega-3 fatty acids contained in olive oil on chronic inflammation.** *Acta Medica Indonesian* 2011, **43:**138–143.
23. March L, Barrett C, Gale F, Lassere M, McQuade J: *Clinical guideline for the diagnosis and management of early rheumatoid arthritis.* South Melbourne: Royal Australian College of General Practitioners; 2009:1–46.
24. Myhrstad MCW, Retterstøl K, Telle-Hansen VH, Ottestad I, Halvorsen B, Holven KB, Ulven SM: **Effect of marine n-3 fatty acids on circulating inflammatory markers in healthy subjects and subjects with cardiovascular risk factors.** *Inflamm Res* 2011, **60:**309–319.
25. Brand C, Buchbinder R, Wluka A, Ruth D, McKenzie S, Jones K: *Guideline for the non-surgical management of hip and knee osteoarthritis.* South Melbourne: Royal Australian College of General Practitioners; 2009:1–68.
26. Black C, Clar C, Henderson R, MacEachern C, McNamee P, Quayyum Z, Royle P, Thomas S: **The clinical effectiveness of glucosamine and chondroitin supplements in slowing or arresting progression of osteoarthritis of the knee: a systematic review and economic evaluation.** *Health Technol Assess* 2009, **13:**1–148.
27. Wandel S, Juni P, Tendal B, Nuesch E, Villiger PM, Welton NJ, Reichenbach S, Trelle S: **Effects of glucosamine, chondroitin, or placebo in patients with osteoarthritis of hip or knee: network meta-analysis.** *BMJ* 2010, **341:**c4675–c4675.
28. Christensen MG, Kollasch MW, Hyland JK: **Chapter 7 - the chiropractic practitioner.** In *Practice analysis of chiropractic 2010.* Edited by Christensen MG, Kollasch MW, Hyland JK. Greeley: National Board of Chiropractic Examiners; 2009:73–94.
29. Russell M, Verhoef M, Injeyan H, McMorland DG: **Response rates for surveys of chiropractors.** *J Manipulative Physiol Ther* 2004, **27:**43–48.

English language proficiency and the accommodations for language non-concordance amongst patients utilizing chiropractic college teaching clinics

Richard P Saporito

Abstract

Background: The number of households in the United States that are not proficient in the English language is growing and presenting a challenge to the health care system. Over nineteen percent of the US population speak a language other than English in the home. This increase in language discordance generates a greater need to find and implement accommodations in the clinical setting to insure accurate and efficient diagnosis and treatment as well as provide for patient safety. Aim: The purpose of this study is to determine the percentage of patients accessing the chiropractic college teaching clinics who are not proficient in the English language and to what extent the colleges provide accommodations for that language disparity.

Methods: The clinic directors and deans of the Association of Chiropractic Colleges were surveyed via an on-line survey engine. The survey queried the percentage of the patient population that is not English language proficient, the accommodations the college currently has in place, if the college has a language specific consent to treat document and if the college has a written policy concerning patients without English proficiency.

Results: Fifty percent of the contacted chiropractic colleges responded to the survey. In the respondent college clinics 16.5% of the patient population is not proficient in English, with over 75% speaking Spanish. All but one of the respondents provide some level of accommodation for the language non-concordance. Forty five percent of the responding colleges employ a language specific consent to treat form. The implementation of accommodations and the use of a language specific consent to treat form is more prevalent at colleges with a higher percentage of non-English speaking patients.

Conclusions: The percentage of patients with limited English proficiency accessing services at the teaching clinics of the chiropractic colleges mirrors the numbers in the general population. There is a wide disparity in the accommodations that the individual colleges make to address this language discordance. There is a need to further develop accurate and meaningful accommodations to address language disparity in the chiropractic teaching clinics.

Keywords: English language proficiency, Language concordance, Accommodations, Informed consent, Chiropractic teaching clinics

Correspondence: rsaporit@bridgeport.edu
Assistant Professor of Clinical Sciences, University of Bridgeport College of Chiropractic, 75 Linden Avenue, Bridgeport, CT 06604, USA

The ethnic diversity in the United States is expanding. Persons born outside the country comprise 12.5% of the resident population with just under one third arriving in the past 10 years [1]. In addition to those whom have entered the United States legally, there is an estimated 10.8 million additional persons who have equivocal resident status. Coincident with this change in ethnic composition is an increase in the number of households in which the primary language is not English. The 2010 U.S. Census reveals that over 55 million individuals, 19.9% of all those 5 years of age and older, speak a language other than English in the home with 45% indicating that they speak English less than "Very Well" [1].

This deficiency in English language proficiency may have a significant impact on the health care system. Quality patient care is dependent upon obtaining a thorough history, accurate feedback during the physical examination and a valid informed consent. Without a reasonable level of communication with the patient, compliance with treatment recommendations may also become problematic [2,3]. Effective communication has a positive effect on symptom response, pain control and physiological and functional improvement [4-7].

The risk of adverse effects of treatment is increased by communication difficulties. Divi, et al. found that 49.1% of adverse events involving patients with limited English language proficiency resulted in some level of physical harm, versus 29.5% in English speaking patients. Further, in those patients experiencing detectable physical harm, the level of that harm was more significant in the English non-proficient patients with 46.8% suffering, "moderate temporary harm," or worse, compared to 24.4% in those speaking English [8].

When services are provided to address language disparities, the nature of the interpreter service can affect the overall clinical outcome. Flores, et al. found that in all encounters involving language interpreters, errors of translation occurred. They found no statistical difference in the frequency of error attributable to whether the translator was a professional or ad hoc. Their analysis of the error rates revealed that 52% were errors of omission, 16% false fluency, 13% substitution, 10% editorializing and 8% additions. Sixty-three percent of the translational errors were potentially of clinical significance with the incidence 1.45 times more likely when the translation was performed by an ad hoc interpreter versus a professional translator [9]. Jackson, et al., found a similar distribution of error type although the clinical significance was much lower. They attribute this to a "best case" scenario where the interpreter was professionally trained, the topic was familiar and the doctor / patient relationship was established [10].

The level of satisfaction with care in patients without English language proficiency is significantly associated with the level of language concordance [11,12]. Ferguson and Candib, in a review of the literature, present evidence that when the physician and patient speak the same language the patient receives more information concerning his or her health and treatment and is more likely to be encouraged to participate in medical decision making [11]. Patients report an expectation of information concerning their condition and express dissatisfaction when they perceive that the lack of information from their physician has limited their participation in their care [11,13,14]. Carlesso, et al., in assessing the patient's perspective on adverse events involving manual therapy, found that contextual factors such as education concerning the nature and possibility of adverse events and trust in the provider improved the patient's attitude about the adverse event [6]. The trust patients express towards their physician is directly dependent on the degree to which they perceive socio-ethnic concordance with the physician [15,16]. Patient satisfaction has also been shown to be associated with the method used to address language issues. Lee, et al. found the greatest encounter satisfaction in Spanish speaking patients with a professional translator via a telephone service and with language concordant providers, and the least satisfaction when translation was provided by a family member or ad hoc interpreter [17]. The chiropractic profession places a high regard on the issue of satisfaction and often references studies demonstrating the high level reported by patients [18-20]. Incorporating accommodations to cultural and language dis-concordance in the teaching clinics would be consistent with this focus.

Currently no literature exists on the effect of language disparity in the chiropractic college teaching clinics. Many of the chiropractic colleges in the United States have outpatient care facilities located in ethnically diverse population centers and, as such, may serve a population with a variable level of English language proficiency. The purpose of this study is to establish baseline data on the utilization of chiropractic teaching clinics by non-English language proficient patients and the resources those clinics provide to address language non-concordance.

Methods

A survey instrument consisting of 9 questions was posted on an on-line survey engine (www.SurveyMonkey.com), allowing for anonymity of the respondents. The study design and survey instrument were approved for use by the Institutional Review Board of the University of Bridgeport. A request to complete the survey was sent to the clinic directors and / or deans of the member colleges of the Association of Chiropractic Colleges. The request asked the person filling out the survey to aggregate data from all clinics that the college directly administrates. Community based clinical training sites, hospital rotations and all other clinical training opportunities not under the direct control of the chiropractic college were excluded. While these alternative training sites may provide a greater exposure to language diversity, the college may not be able to affect accommodations for those disparities. The survey consisted of open ended, multiple choice, categorical and Likert-scale questions (Figure 1). A 5 level Likert scale was used to assess the level of satisfaction each respondent had with his or her institution's language accommodation strategies. The responses were quantified by assigning a value of −2 for Very Dissatisfied, -1 for Dissatisfied, 0 for Neither Satisfied or Dissatisfied, +1 for Satisfied and +2 for Very Satisfied. Approximately one month following an initial request for participation a second request was sent via electronic mail.

Respondents were given the following choices of accommodations for patients with limited English language proficiency and asked to indicate which are used in their clinic(s): professional translator, student or staff (ad hoc) translator, language specific forms, language specific educational materials, appropriate signage and educational presentations.

Results

Nine responses were obtained from the 18 colleges contacted for a response rate of 50%. The nine colleges participating represent a total of 37 clinical locations ranging from one to eight with a mean of five. The percentage of patients with limited proficiency in English varied widely from a low of 1% at one institution to a high of 50% at another. One college responded with a range of 10 – 15%. For statistical purposes this was averaged to 12.5%. The average percent of the limited English language population is 16.5% across all respondent institutions. There appears to be no correlation between the number of clinic sites and the concentration of language non-concordance. The college reporting the highest percentage of non-English language proficient patients only operates one clinical site while the school with the greatest number of clinical locations, eight, indicates a non-English proficient population of 5%. The Spanish language comprises the greatest cohort of non-English language proficient patients making up 75.6% of the total. Asian languages made up the majority of the remainder constituting 19.5% of the population. The remaining 4.9% were not specifically identified by the respondents (Table 1).

Of the colleges reporting, 55.6% indicate that they do not use a language specific consent to treat form. An analysis of the colleges that do not employ a language specific form reveals that they utilize 13.9% of the available accommodations listed on the survey. The four colleges that do incorporate a language specific consent to treat form on average apply 58.3% of the available accommodations (Figure 2). Further, three of the four schools that have language specific consent to treat forms also have a written policy pertaining to addressing language discordance in their teaching clinics as compared to none of the five colleges without a language specific form. Of those five colleges, three report that they have a plan to develop a written policy.

On the question of the level of satisfaction with their institution's accommodation strategies for patients that are non-English language proficient, five schools reported that they are, "Satisfied," three reported, "Neither Satisfied nor Dissatisfied," and one college responded they are, "Dissatisfied." The average level of satisfaction for those colleges who have implemented a language specific consent to treat form is, "Satisfied," (a Likert score of +1) while an average response of, "Neither Satisfied nor Dissatisfied," (a Likert scores of zero) is obtained for the five schools not employing a language specific form.

There also exists a wide disparity in the methods by which the different institutions accommodate the language needs of their patient populations. Figure 3 illustrates the responses for this survey question. The most prevalent strategy, employed by 77.8% of the colleges, is to utilize existing staff, including interns, with multilingual ability, as translators. Five of the nine respondents have language specific forms with 33.3% also incorporating translated patient educational materials. Two of the institutions provide patient education presentations for non-English proficient patients. Two of the colleges responding, 22.2%, report that they do not provide any accommodations for their non-English speaking patient population. Only one institution reported employing a professional translator.

Discussion

Language concordance is an important factor in patient compliance, treatment efficacy and risk management. A failure to adequately address a communication disparity can have significant impact on outcome and the frequency and severity of any adverse effects of treatment. Engaging the patient in an active discourse and insuring patient comprehension is an ethical imperative. The doctrine of informed consent states that the physician has an obligation, both ethical and legal, to have an appropriate conversation, or its equivalent, with the patient. According to the published policy statement by the general counsel of the American Medical Association, "It is a process of communication between a patient and physician that results in the patient's authorization or agreement to undergo a specific medical intervention." The content of that conversation should be thorough enough, "...so that he or she can make an informed decision to proceed or to refuse a particular course of medical intervention." [21].

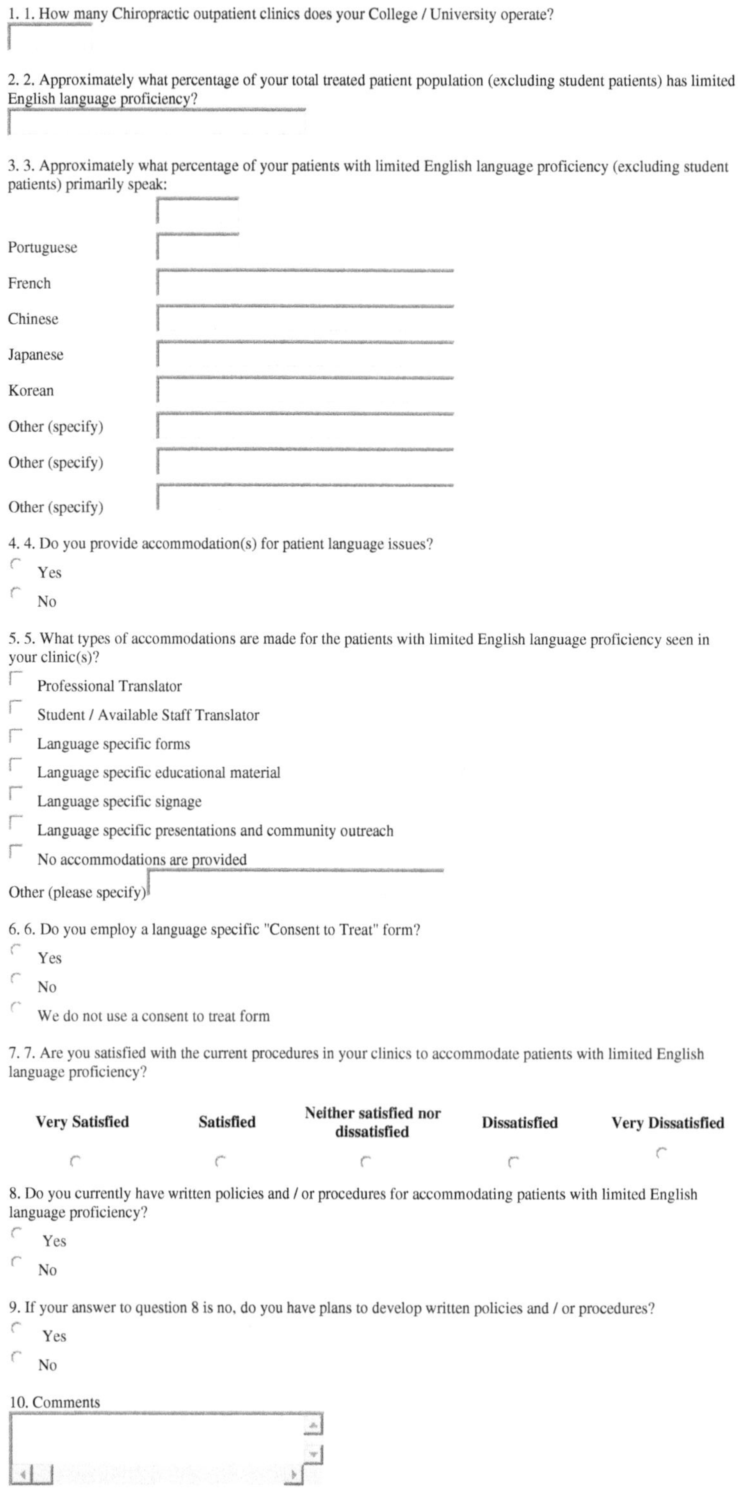

1. 1. How many Chiropractic outpatient clinics does your College / University operate?

2. 2. Approximately what percentage of your total treated patient population (excluding student patients) has limited English language proficiency?

3. 3. Approximately what percentage of your patients with limited English language proficiency (excluding student patients) primarily speak:

Portuguese

French

Chinese

Japanese

Korean

Other (specify)

Other (specify)

Other (specify)

4. 4. Do you provide accommodation(s) for patient language issues?

Yes

No

5. 5. What types of accommodations are made for the patients with limited English language proficiency seen in your clinic(s)?

Professional Translator

Student / Available Staff Translator

Language specific forms

Language specific educational material

Language specific signage

Language specific presentations and community outreach

No accommodations are provided

Other (please specify)

6. 6. Do you employ a language specific "Consent to Treat" form?

Yes

No

We do not use a consent to treat form

7. 7. Are you satisfied with the current procedures in your clinics to accommodate patients with limited English language proficiency?

Very Satisfied	Satisfied	Neither satisfied nor dissatisfied	Dissatisfied	Very Dissatisfied

8. Do you currently have written policies and / or procedures for accommodating patients with limited English language proficiency?

Yes

No

9. If your answer to question 8 is no, do you have plans to develop written policies and / or procedures?

Yes

No

10. Comments

Figure 1 The survey instrument.

Table 1 Survey results

Question		School	1	2	3	4	5	6	7	8	9
1	# of clinics		1	4	1	8	1	6	5	6	5
2	% non-English		50	1	10-15	5	5	20	25	10	20
3	Language	Spanish	80	90	0	100	85	40	100	95	90
		Portuguese	0	0	0	0	0	0	0	0	0
		French	1	0	1	0	0	0	0	0	0
		Chinese	5	0	40	0	0	15	0	0	0
		Japanese	1	0	1	0	0	10	0	0	0
		Korean	2	0	55	0	15	5	0	0	10
		Other	1	10	3	0	0	30	0	5*	0
4	+ Accommodations		N	N	Y	Y	nr	Y	Y	Y	Y
5	Method	Professional	N	N	N	N	N	N	Y	N	N
		Student/Staff	N	N	Y	Y	Y	Y	Y	Y	Y
		Forms	N	N	N	Y	N	Y	Y	Y	Y
		Ed Material	N	N	N	Y	N	N	Y	N	Y
		Signs	N	N	N	N	N	N	Y	N	N
		Presentations	N	N	N	N	N	Y	N	N	√
6	Consent Form		N	N	N	N	N	Y	Y	Y	Y
7	Satisfaction		0	−1	0	1	0	1	1	1	1
8	Policy		N	N	N	N	N	Y	N	Y	Y
9	Plan		Y	N	Y	N	Y	n/a	N	n/a	n/a
										*Vietnamese	

Y = a positive response.
N = a negative response.
n/r = no response provided.

Satisfaction is both a reflection of the patient's perception of the efficacy of the specific interventions provided as well as their assessment of the interpersonal components of the doctor-patient encounter. To a limited extent the level of satisfaction a patient has can also influence outcome measurement. In their 2005 observational study on satisfaction as a predictor of outcome in patients enrolled in the UCLA low back pain study, Hurwitz, et. al. found a short term decrease in reported pain and a longer term improvement in disability in patients generally satisfied with the care they received. The study also found a greater level of satisfaction in patients receiving care from a chiropractic physician versus from a medical provider. This increased satisfaction was attributed to the greater amount of information about their condition and treatment that was provided by the chiropractor. The difference in satisfaction between provider types disappeared when the patient received more self-care advice and an explanation of their treatment [22].

The interpretation of the results of this survey are limited by the response rate. Given the small sample size, extrapolating the results to the entire profession should be done with caution. For the data acquired, there are some identifiable trends. The patient population served by the chiropractic clinics is slightly less representative of the language diversity present in the population at large, 16.5% versus 19.9%. There is a wide percentage distribution of non-English proficient patients across the clinical sites responding, from near zero to half of all patients served. Spanish is the predominant language constituting 75% of all the non-English language proficient population.

Less than half of the colleges responding provide any significant accommodation to address language non-concordance. One institution provides a professional translator, five schools provide clinic forms in language appropriate format and only four colleges utilize a non-English consent to treat form. The four responding institutions that do provide a language appropriate consent to treat form also provide a significantly greater number of other accommodations. Seventy-five percent of these schools also have a written policy concerning accommodations for non-English proficient patients.

The data show that the colleges that place a priority on addressing language non-concordance employ a number of different strategies, from professional translators to patient education. In comparing colleges that provide many

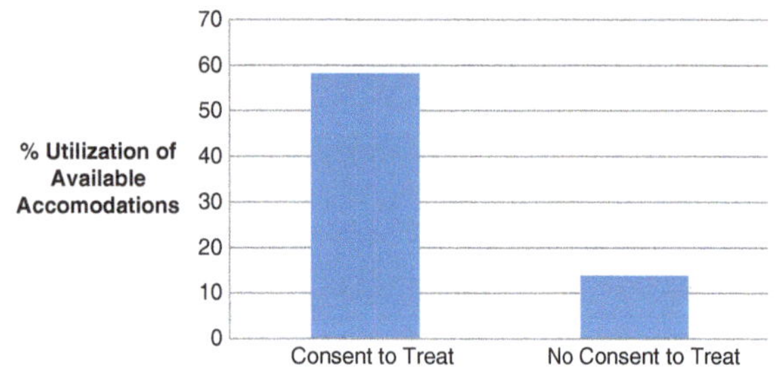

Figure 2 **Accommodation utilization as a function of the use of a language specific consent to treat form.**

accommodations to those that supply few there appears to be only a slight difference in the percentage of non-English language proficient patients served, (18.7% versus 14.7%). The results, however, may be skewed. One low accommodation college is also the institution with the highest percentage of non-English speaking patients (50%). If this response is excluded from the data, the difference in patient population served is 18.7% versus 5.9%. The observations from the survey bear out the expectation that chiropractic college teaching clinics that serve a higher percentage of patients that are not proficient in the English language employ more strategies to accommodate for that language disparity.

The most commonly employed methods of addressing language discordance is to use ad hoc interpreters; these may be other interns, staff members or family members. This is certainly a convenient and cost effective approach, but does it produce the same outcome in terms of clinical results and patient satisfaction? Seven of the nine reporting schools (77.8%) use this ad hoc strategy. There are a number of difficulties that emanate from this solution. The language ability of the ad hoc translator may not be adequate. There may exist a lack of understanding of the information being requested or provided by the physician / intern and by the patient. There can be a tendency of family members, when acting as a translator, to interject their own observations, opinions, interpretations and questions and to change the questions, comments and advice of the physician [23]. A similar tendency to alter the translation was found by Elderkin-Thompson et al. in their investigation of the use of nurses as interpreters in a primary care setting [24]. A study by Hunt and de Voogd revealed that some physicians, in response to the increased time associated with the use of ad hoc or undertrained interpreters, abbreviate their consultations to compensate for the time loss. The study further demonstrated that even though the translations provided were incomplete and inaccurate, the patients perceived the encounter as successful and felt they understood their condition and treatment [25].

Regardless of whether an institution employs a professional translator or relies on an ad hoc solution, training the physicians, interns and staff is an important consideration [9]. Hudelson, et al. found that 58.6% of the physicians in their study considered themselves, "highly competent," at working with interpreters. When asked to identify good practice behaviors, those same, self-assessed, "highly competent," providers did no better than those who self-assessed as moderate and poor in the use of interpreters [26]. Shriner and Hickey found that following completion of a training program for third year medical students in working with a translator there were significant changes in behavior. The most notable changes were: instructing the interpreter of their role, making eye contact with the patient for a majority of the encounter, using the first person and speaking directly to the patient, and avoiding side conversations with the interpreter [27]. Cha-Chi, et al. in a study of second year medical students found similar behavioral issues regarding working with an interpreter, including confidentiality and patient / translator positioning [28].

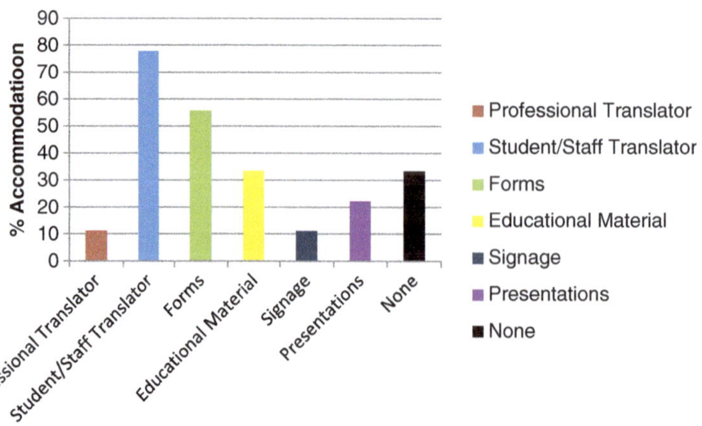

Figure 3 **Language accommodation stratagies.**

Conclusions

This study's major shortcoming is the small sample size. From the limited number of responses the findings cannot be extrapolated across all ACC member chiropractic college teaching clinics. Certain trends can be identified and highlight the need for further investigation. Further development of the survey instrument should include: inquiries into curriculum content specific to language and cultural discordance, the training of clinical supervisory staff in language and cultural issues and the content of specific written policies concerning non-English proficient patients.

The chiropractic profession continues to search for cultural authority and a larger influence in the health care system [29]. An integral part of that effort must be focused on reaching out to and providing services for the ever growing population for whom English is not the primary language spoken in the household. The chiropractic colleges should address that issue in their approaches to the non-English language proficient patient utilizing their teaching clinics, through a better understanding of best practices and a focus on cultural sensitivity.

The need to insure patient safety, effective and efficient treatment, appropriate and authentic informed consent and patient satisfaction require optimal patient - provider communication. The data confirm that while physician - patient cultural and language concordance is the optimal situation, this is often not practical. How to incorporate accurate and meaningful accommodations to address language disparity remains the challenge in all of health care, including the chiropractic profession.

Competing interests

The author declare that they have no competing interests.

Authors' contributions

All authors read and approved the final manuscript.

Acknowledgements

The author would like to thank Matthew F. Funk, DC, FIAMA for his assistance in survey distribution and his advice and support in the study design and preparation. The author also thanks Stephen M. Perle, DC, MS, FICC for his invaluable direction, encouragement and assistance in editing this manuscript.

References

1. *Promotions C for NM and, public information staff UCB. US census bureau 2010 census [internet]. [cited 2012 Aug 20].* Available from: www.census.gov/2010census/data/.
2. Manson A: **Language concordance as a determinant of patient compliance and emergency room use in patients with asthma.** *Med Care* 1988, **26**(12):1119–28.
3. Hattori N, Fulimoto K, Kondo T, Murata M, Stacy M: **Patient perspectives on Parkinson's disease therapy in Japan and the United States: results of two patient surveys.** *Patient Relat Outcome Meas* 2012, **3**:31–8.
4. Stewart MA: **Effective physician-patient communication and health outcomes: a review.** *CMAJ* 1995, **152**(9):1423–33.
5. Pérez-Stable EJ, Nápoles-Springer A, Miramontes JM: **The effects of ethnicity and language on medical outcomes of patients with hypertension or diabetes.** *Med Care* 1997, **35**(12):1212–9.
6. Carlesso LC, Cairney J, Dolovich L, Hoogenes J: **Defining adverse events in manual therapy: An exploratory qualitative analysis of the patient perspective.** *Man Ther* 2011, **16**(5):440–6.
7. Karliner LS, Jacobs EA, Chen AH, Mutha S: **Do professional interpreters improve clinical care for patients with limited English proficiency? A systematic review of the literature.** *Health Serv Res* 2007, **42**(2):727–54.
8. Divi C, Koss RG, Schmaltz SP, Loeb JM: **Language proficiency and adverse events in US hospitals: a pilot study.** *Int J Qual Health Care* 2007, **19**(2):60–7.
9. Flores G, Laws MB, Mayo SJ, Zuckerman B, Abreu M, Medina L, *et al*: **Errors in medical interpretation and their potential clinical consequences in pediatric encounters.** *Pediatrics* 2003, **111**(1):6–14.
10. Jackson JC, Nguyen D, Hu N, Harris R, Terasaki GS: **Alterations in medical interpretation during routine primary care.** *J Gen Intern Med* 2011, **26**(3):259–64.
11. Ferguson WJ, Candib LM: **Culture, language, and the doctor-patient relationship.** *Fam Med* 2002, **34**(5):353–61.
12. Carrasquillo O, Orav EJ, Brennan TA, Burstin HR: **Impact of language barriers on patient satisfaction in an emergency department.** *JGIM: J Gen Intern Med* 1999, **14**(2):82–7.
13. Verbeek J, Sengers M-J, Riemens L, Haafkens J: **Patient expectations of treatment for back pain: a systematic review of qualitative and quantitative studies.** *Spine* 2004, **29**(20):2309–18.
14. McIntosh A, Shaw CFM: **Barriers to patient information provision in primary care: patients' and general practitioners' experiences and expectations of information for low back pain.** *Health Expect* 2003, **6**(1):19–29.
15. Banerjee A, Sanyal D: **Dynamics of doctor–patient relationship: a cross-sectional study on concordance, trust, and patient enablement.** *J Family Community Med* 2012, **19**(1):12–9.
16. Fernandez A, Schillinger D, Grumbach K, Rosenthal A, Stewart AL, Wang F, *et al*: **Physician language ability and cultural competence: an exploratory study of communication with Spanish-speaking patients.** *J Gen Intern Med* 2004, **19**(2):167–74.
17. Lee LJ, Batal HA, Maselli JH, Kutner JS: **Effect of Spanish interpretation method on patient satisfaction in an urban walk-in clinic.** *J Gen Intern Med* 2002, **17**(8):641–5.
18. Eriksen K, Rochester RP, Hurwitz EL: **Symptomatic reactions, clinical outcomes and patient satisfaction associated with upper cervical chiropractic care: a prospective, multicenter, cohort study.** *BMC Musculoskelet Disord* 2011, **12**:219.
19. Beattie PF, Nelson R, Murphy DR: **Development and preliminary validation of the MedRisk instrument to measure patient satisfaction with chiropractic care.** *J Manipulative Physiol Ther* 2011, **34**(1):23–9.
20. Butler RJ, Johnson WG: **Satisfaction with low back pain care.** *Spine J* 2008, **8**(3):510–21.
21. *Office of the general counsel of the American medical association. Informed consent [cited October 28, 2007].* Available from http://www.ama-assn.org/ama/pub/category/4608.html (2007).
22. Hurwitz EL, Morgenstern H, Yu F: **Satisfaction as a predictor of clinical outcomes among chiropractic and medical patients enrolled in the UCLA low back pain study.** *Spine* 2005, **30**(19):2121–8.
23. Kuo D, Fagan MJ: **Satisfaction with methods of Spanish interpretation in an ambulatory care clinic.** *J Gen Intern Med* 1999, **14**(9):547–50.
24. Elderkin-Thompson V, Silver RC, Waitzkin H: **When nurses double as interpreters: a study of Spanish-speaking patients in a US primary care setting.** *Soc Sci Med* 2001, **52**(9):1343–58.
25. Hunt LM, de Voogd KB: **Are good intentions good enough? Informed consent without trained interpreters.** *J Gen Intern Med* 2007, **22**(5):598–605.
26. Hudelson P, Perneger T, Kolly V, Perron NJ: **Self-Assessed Competency at Working with a Medical Interpreter Is Not Associated with Knowledge of Good Practice.** *PLoS One* 2012, **7**(6):1–6.
27. Shriner CJ, Hickey DP: **Teaching and assessing family medicine clerks' use of medical interpreters.** *Fam Med* 2008, **40**(5):313–5.
28. Cha-Chi F, Lagha RR, Henderson P, Gomez AG: **Working with interpreters: how student behavior affects quality of patient interaction when using interpreters.** *Med Educ Online* 2010, **15**(1):1–7.
29. Murphy DR, Schneider MJ, Seaman DR, Perle SM, Nelson CF: **How can chiropractic become a respected mainstream profession? The example of podiatry.** *Chiropr Osteopat* 2008, **16**(1):10.

The perspectives of educators, regulators and funders of massage therapy on the state of the profession in British Columbia, Canada

Farah M Shroff[1*] and Inderjeet S Sahota[2]

Abstract

Background: Registered Massage Therapists (RMTs) are valuable members of the healthcare team who assist in health promotion, disease prevention and treatment, rehabilitation and palliation. RMT visits have increased across Canada over the past decade with the highest increase in British Columbia (BC). Currently, RMTs are private practitioners of healthcare operating within a largely publicly funded system, positioning them outside of the dominant system of healthcare and making them an important case study in private healthcare. In another paper we examined the perspectives of RMTs themselves. Here, we offer perspectives of regulators, educators and funders of Massage Therapy (MT) on advancement of the profession.

Methods: We interviewed 28 stakeholders of MT in BC – including members of the MT regulatory board, representatives from MT colleges in BC and public and private health insurers.

Results: All three groups identified research, particularly on efficacy of MT, as playing a vital role in enhancing the professional credibility of MT. However, participants noted that presently research is not a large feature of the current MT curricula and we analyze why this may be and how it can improve. Finally, conferral of baccalaureate degree status could assist RMTs in gaining recognition with the general public and other healthcare professionals.

Conclusion: RMTs have potential to ameliorate population health in a cost-effective manner. Their role in British Columbias healthcare landscape could be expanded if they produce more research and earn degree status.

Keywords: Health care professionals, Professional education, Alternative and complementary health care, Massage therapy

Background

Registered Massage Therapists (RMTs) in British Columbia (BC) are autonomous, self-regulating professionals. The majority of their practices operate as privately funded businesses providing mainly musculoskeletal healthcare services [1]. The majority of their funding comes from public and private insurance companies and their educational institutions are also for-profit businesses [2].

Massage Therapy (MT) regulation varies across Canada. Only BC, Ontario and Newfoundland currently regulate the practice of MT [3]. RMTs in BC must register with the College of Massage Therapists of British Columbia (CMTBC). There are three levels of legislation governing MT in the province: 1) the Health Professions Act of BC, 2) The Massage Therapists Regulation and 3) the By laws of the College of Massage Therapists in BC [4]. In BC, membership requires a minimum of 3000 hours, or approximately three years of training, making the approximately 2600 RMTs [5] in BC some of the best trained massage therapists in the world [6]. With cutbacks to provincial healthcare coverage, limited MT treatments are available for low income individuals [7]. Those who seek MT services due to motor vehicle or workplace accidents also receive some, albeit minimal, coverage through government administered insurance agencies with a physicians referral [7]. Presently, most RMTs clients have coverage through privately funded extended health plans. Other patients pay for MT out of pocket. Therefore,

* Correspondence: farah.shroff@ubc.ca
[1]Department of Family Practice and School of Population and Public Health, University of British Columbia, Third Floor David Strangway Bldg, 5950 University Blvd, Vancouver, BC V6T 1Z3, Canada
Full list of author information is available at the end of the article

RMTs are typically providers of private healthcare within BC. In recent years, the CMTBC has been lobbying the provincial government to reincorporate MT as a publicly insured service, citing cost-effectiveness and increased efficacy in the use of MT for the treatment of soft-tissue and other musculoskeletal disorders [8]. Many RMTs, on the other hand, feel they were inadequately compensated under government funded insurance and are not interested in returning to the previous funding scheme.

MT, physiotherapy and chiropractic have overlapping scopes of practice; however, compared to these other two professional groups, RMTs experience a number of difficulties. The general public and other healthcare providers often misunderstand RMTs. Conflation with sex-trade workers is a threat to the professional reputation of RMTs [9]. Furthermore, they face competition from unregulated bodyworkers who claim to do the same work, particularly relaxation and stress reduction massage. Touch therapies are generally misunderstood in Canada; in other countries, such as Thailand and India, massage is a time-honoured tradition understood by the majority of the population as beneficial for health [10].

Canadian RMTs typically have a relatively short career span due to the physically demanding nature of their work [2]. Moreover, RMTs depend on referrals from Medical Doctors (MDs) for clientele. Without a note from an MD, most RMTs clients would not receive insurance coverage [2,7]. Finally, RMTs are almost completely dependent on private insurers for their livelihood and while many RMTs feel they are sufficiently compensated, tensions between RMTs and private health insurers exist. These complexities render the study of MT important because they provide a popular service currently outside the realm of publicly-funded healthcare for most people. We asked the question: how can the MT profession advance given these constraints? In examining these issues we illustrate various challenges faced by RMTs as privately funded healthcare providers.

In this study we interviewed various stakeholders who were involved in the current practice of MT in BC: colleges of MT, regulators of MT and private and public healthcare insurers. In investigating avenues for greater success for this profession we learned about market-forces at play within MT; RMT education and practice are mainly privately funded so this profession relies to a great extent on financial backing from business people. In Canada, since the early 1960s many healthcare professionals are publicly funded; this includes physicians, nurses and other professionals [11]. The spiralling costs of drugs, hospital administration and doctors earnings, among other factors, threaten the financial sustainability of the Canadian public healthcare system [12]. While approximately 30% of healthcare [13] services are currently contracted to private companies, this percentage will likely increase in the future. It is, therefore, insightful to explore the contours of privatized healthcare as it currently exists in Canada.

Purpose

In assessing how this profession could move forward within a privately-funded system we sought to gain a comprehensive perspective on MT within the province. In another paper [2] we summarized the perspectives of RMTs in regards to their own profession. The purpose of this paper is to examine the perspectives of other stakeholders-- MT educational institutions, regulators and funders – soliciting their views on the advancement of this profession.

Methods

Recruitment

The research team compiled a list of all stakeholders in MT and contacted them via phone and email. All stakeholders who responded to our requests were keen to be involved. While the research team attempted to contact both elected officials as well as staff within the provincial government we received no response. We were, therefore, unable to include the voice of government in this study. Participants were not financially compensated for their participation.

Protocol

Questions were presented to study participants in written form and are appended here (Additional file 1:Appendix). Each participant signed a consent form. Ethical approval was granted by the University of British Columbia Behavioural Research Ethics Board. We employed self-completed questionnaires, focus groups and one-on-one interviews. The first author of this paper conducted all interviews and focus groups. All responses were digitally recorded and partially transcribed in order to capture participants exact words. We employed qualitative methods of questionnaire design, interviewing and analysis.

Participants

Ten members of the organization responsible for regulating the practice of MT within the province, the MT regulatory body (MTRB) were interviewed. We distributed questionnaires in advance and collected responses during the focus group. We interviewed twelve administrators representing all MT colleges within the province. All interviews were conducted at the college campuses, except one which was interviewed via email.

We interviewed members of one private and two public insurance companies. Where possible, we held interviews with insurance company representatives in charge of MT claims. We conducted focus groups with four staff members of a private insurance company. We thus interviewed six representatives from public and private insurance companies across the province.

In total, 28 people participated in this study.

Data analysis

Members of our research team partially transcribed all interviews and answers to each question were inserted into appropriate sections. For example, we had section headings of "Do you believe research can advance the profession of massage therapy?", "Are you satisfied with the current regulation of MT research curricula in schools?" and "In your opinion, what aspects of MT require further research?". From the categorized sections, we analyzed responses using qualitative techniques of coding, diagramming and thematic analysis. In addition to audio-recording, the principal investigator took notes throughout the interviews. Interviews lasted from 30 to 90 minutes.

Results & discussion

Although many ideas were presented, almost all stakeholders felt that increased research on the benefits of MT would help elevate the profession. Stakeholders views on advancing the profession are summarized below. As they identified research as a particularly important facet in moving MT forward, we discuss it in more detail.

Advancing the profession: regulators and educators

Members of the MTRB felt that acceptance from other health professionals, respect from government as well as strong validation of what RMTs do through research would advance the profession.

> "[RMTs would benefit from] strong validation of what we do through research [in addition to] greater acceptance by other health professions, greater referrals [and] no GST."

> "If we had national professional recognition wed be able to move forward."

> "[We need to] integrate evidence into practice."

> "[We would benefit from respect from] other health professionals, respect from government."

The response of MT colleges to "what steps do RMTs need to take in order to elevate the status of the profession" included the following: increasing research in the area of MT and health and educating the public on the qualifications and roles of RMTs.

> "People dont know how well educated RMTs are. RMTs have excellent training – lets talk to the public!"

> "[We need to] establish evidence-based research."

One MT college administrator felt that providing leadership to spearhead the needs of RMTs as well as establishing best business practice courses in colleges could help RMTs succeed in their careers.

> "Resistance to business practices in colleges. Chiros realised this and train to be both a good business person and practitioner. The MTA (Massage Therapists Association) could look at AMTA (American Massage Therapy Association) and invite them to speak at conferences – they know how to help members."

> "Leadership! We need better leadership to raise [the] status of our profession. Lets bring in the expertise to help us move forward. It would be good to have leaders setting direction for the program [but] we need all the stakeholders working together!"

Massage colleges and the MTRB recognized the significant role of research in getting greater acceptance for MT from other healthcare professionals and respect from the government. All stakeholders highlighted the importance of research in moving the profession forward. However, although the importance of research was frequently cited, peer-reviewed literature and research education practices are minimal. This topic is discussed in more detail next.

Role of research in moving MT forward

The importance of research in advancing the profession

The MTRB was interested in research on safety and efficacy of MT as well as cost-effectiveness. Research on safety of MT was cited by 6 of the MTRB respondents as an important component of MT that requires further research. The primary role of regulatory bodies is to protect the public. It is therefore understandable that safety is a top concern for regulators. However, there is currently no documented evidence of side effects of MT [14]. It is, therefore, considered to be safe.

"[Research is important] to help produce evidence or risk of harm in order to communicate more effectively with the government. It would be helpful in our negotiations with the Ministry of Health."

Research on efficacy was cited as important by 3 MTRB respondents and the remaining one thought cost-effectiveness would be the most valuable aspect of MT to research. Interestingly, if responses were analyzed by summing the total of the top two responses to the question, "what aspect of MT should be researched further," 9 MTRB respondents cited efficacy. This highlights the importance of researching efficacy of MT; an issue echoed in later statements by members of public and private insurers. Understandably, people want to prove that MT improves health status; therefore, research on efficacy is essential to the advancement of this profession.

"If we want the profession to grow and advance, [research] has to be very important."

"We cant expect physios and others to view us (RMTs) as their peers when we dont do research."

All participants representing MT colleges indicated that they believe research is very important to the profession of MT. One MT college administrator noted:

"If we want the profession to grow and advance, research has to be very important. If were saying our training and our practice in the health field is equal to others we have to be doing it too. For RMTs to take it to the next step theyd need a researcher to work with."

Both MT colleges and the MTRB identified research as an important component in advancing the profession. For many, research proving the efficacy and safety of MT would be beneficial in enhancing the professions image in the eyes of the provincial government. More research was also cited as important in gaining recognition from their peers, such as physiotherapists, chiropractors and importantly, medical doctors, as valuable members of the healthcare team.

Research education in MT colleges

Responses of MTRB participants with the current regulation of research education in MT colleges varied from somewhat satisfied to extremely unsatisfied. Most MTRB participants (8) were somewhat satisfied with the current regulation of MT research curricula in MT colleges whereas 1 was extremely unsatisfied and 1 was undecided.

"[Its a] work in progress. Faculty needs to buy into research with their world view."

"Extremely unsatisfied [with the current regulation of MT curricula]; further integration is needed."

MT colleges devote very little time in their curriculum, approximately 30–40 hours of the 3,000 hours, to teaching research methodologies. Some conduct a lecture-based research and statistics course which focuses on research literacy, validity and research design. Typically the research training consists of a single course taken in the advanced years of the program. However, many MT schools report that research training courses are not well received by the students. One college reported that 80% of students ask "why do we have to take this course?" Others reported that those with degrees tend to be more interested in research while other students could see the value of being able to search the literature.

MT colleges provided contradictory reflections regarding the status of their students research capabilities. Participants reported that their students had varying levels of research literacy, with some students studying the literature regularly while others rarely doing so and lacking critical thinking skills. In contrast, half the colleges stated that the majority of their graduates could design and conduct independent research. However, this sentiment was not echoed in statements given made by MT college participants. For example, one college representative stated that students do not have the experience or the time (while in college) to participate in research. Their college had only one student in a class of 33 that actually participated in their study last summer.

It is unlikely that a substantial portion of MT college graduates could indeed design and conduct independent research for a number of reasons. Firstly, courses regarding research design and statistical analyses form only a small percentage of the total courses taken during MT college training: approximately 30–40 of the total 3000 hours. This is largely due to MT colleges focus on accrediting their graduates to practice under the MTRB regulations. Secondly, as noted above, RMT students do not seem keen on conducting research; instead, their focus is on clinical practice. The reason they choose to enter MT is to work with patients and secondly MT research is often less lucrative than clinical practice [2]. Also, some administrators noted that most of their faculty do not have a research background and, therefore, are not willing or able to implement new research courses into the curricula. If faculty are not able to teach MT students about research design and/or literacy skills it is unlikely that many graduates could conduct MT research projects themselves. For half of the MT colleges to state, therefore, that their graduates could design and conduct independent research is questionable.

Barriers to incorporating research education in MT colleges

Participants noted that the greatest barriers to MT research in colleges were time, money and lack of research expertise. One MT college board member summarized these barriers:

> "One, our curriculum [is] designed to be a clinical model. My job is to prepare students to pass board exams. They have 30–40 hours out of 3000 hours to spend on research. I have a 5 year plan which includes research. Two, the majority of our faculty are not well versed on how to [conduct] research. Three, time. Four, our goal is to get accredited [by the provincial MTRB]; therefore, our main goal is accreditation."

To overcome these barriers, college representatives said that it would be helpful if someone was designated at the colleges or other MT professional associations to review the literature, organize new research by category and then convey summaries of the information to the staff and members. Another representative said that RMTs and researchers should work together: therapists could form partnerships with people who are knowledgeable in research to grow research competency and increase the facultys interest. However, all felt that the college curricula were already so full that it would be difficult to incorporate another module on advancing research capacity.

The MTRB participants believed that encouraging members to enroll in research-based courses for continuing education credits (CEC) is an important step in improving research literacy within the RMT community. Other ideas included increasing the amount of information provided on MT-related websites and making research literacy a mandate for MT colleges.

All the colleges were interested in collaborating with organizations such as the MTRB or other MT professional associations to develop, test and evaluate a best practice guideline to mentor students to carry out research. However, one wasnt sure how it would work or fit into the current curriculum. Another stated that the medical model does not appeal to them and that they would prefer a broader model that would encompass all facets of MT including the wellness and holistic aspects. One college representative said that they would prefer to work with the MT professional organizations to benefit all RMTs not just students. From their experience, they were better off using just a few well-trained RMTs for studies.

When interviewing the MTRB, the majority of respondents (9) were also interested in pursuing cooperative research projects with other MT-related organizations. They emphasized that their organization would likely play a funding-provider role as conducting research was not a mandate of the organization.

All the colleges needed funding to support their ability to integrate the research competencies throughout the curriculum. This would have to be mandated by the MTRB and supported by them, said one college. Ultimately it was felt that the board examination process drove everything. This is echoed in a statement from one MT college representative below:

> "In the end, the issues are time, money and motivation. Ultimately the board examination process drives everything. If the board examiners dont incorporate research into the process, the motivation isnt there."

Other college representatives felt that there were too many who would be resistant to such a move. As all MT colleges felt that the current curriculum is tight, creating space for the development of research literacy means removing other courses which they are unwilling or unable to do.

> "We need a curriculum review. Do we need 4000 hours or do we pull out stuff to make space for research? We cant lose manual skills [and] the university recognizes what we are doing [but] what will it take [for us] to become a degree-granting institution?"

In general, the most significant barriers to incorporating research training in MT colleges were time and the focus of the MTRB board examination. Both MT colleges and the MTRB stated they were keen on collaborating with each other and with other MT-related organizations to increase the quantity and quality of research currently being conducted in the field.

Role of research in the advancement of other professions

Increasing the number and quality of studies examining the efficacy and safety of physiotherapy, nursing and chiropractic practice have helped these professions gain recognition from both other healthcare professionals and governing bodies of healthcare. RMTs and stakeholders of MT feel these issues are of great importance in advancing the profession of MT within British Columbia [2]. Chiropractic, physiotherapy and nursing have advanced partly through research. Each of these professions emphasizes research literacy and other research skills in their curricula. A significant number of their practitioners are actively engaged in evidence-based studies producing a number of robust research articles annually. This has been discussed in detail previously [15].

Why is evidence-based MT lagging behind?

Both RMTs [2] and other stakeholders of MT recognize the importance of high quality research in advancing MTs professional recognition with other healthcare professionals, governmental healthcare organizations as well as the general public. Lack of research capacity is a substantial obstacle to moving MT forward. There is a lack of research training in MT colleges and consequently, a lack of research personnel. Ideally, academic researchers and RMTs ought to be working in teams in order to conduct research studies on the effects of MT. Part of this problem stems from the fact that research skills and literacy are not emphasized in MT colleges. The focus of these colleges is to have their graduates become accredited RMTs by the MTRB which means passing the MTRB board examinations. As this is the final goal for most MT colleges and as the examination process is focused on clinical knowledge and skills and less on research, there is little motivation to pursue research literacy and development.

Another reason has to do with the limited funding opportunities available to RMTs who wish to involve themselves in MT research. Only two organizations across Canada directly provide funding for MT research: the Holistic Health Research Foundation of Canada and the Massage Therapy Foundation. The limited funding opportunities, coupled with the fact that clinical MT practice is more lucrative and MT college graduates are often saddled with large debts means the incentive to pursue MT research is low.

Degree status for MT education could help advance the profession

Some MTRB participants liked the idea of RMTs earning a degree from a public university and others did not. Half of respondents were supportive of the idea, 3 respondents opposed the idea and 2 were undecided. Of those that were supportive, maintaining standards on par with other health professionals, increasing opportunities to transfer course credits and recognition for the amount of course work completed in the MT program were frequently cited reasons.

> "University degree status is unavoidable. We could create a working agreement between colleges and universities to make [the] TRU (Thompson Rivers University) agreement mandatory. Education may be better delivered at a public university than a private college [as we] dont need to raise the bar to get into university."

> "Yes – to remain viable as profession."

> "Yes . . . in order to remain competitive with other health professions."

> "Last time we had a stakeholders meeting people were not keen to mandate a degree, to allow laddering is good. Id be quite upset if this happened. In Ontario there is public education and it has created chaos."

In meeting with colleges of MT they too noted that they would like to see RMTs gaining a university degree but they would like to be granted the authority to grant degrees themselves. One of the colleges faculty members suggested that 3,000 hours of education was more than an undergraduate degree so it was only fair that RMTs should earn a degree and not a diploma.

> "What will it take [for us] to become a degree-granting institution? [Our graduates require] 3000 hours of training, [that is] more than university degree."

> "[We would like a] degree program [but] universities may not because private colleges [would be] offering it."

> "A local university/college was willing to partner with us [to obtain degree granting status for RMTs] but it didnt work after 3.5 years of trying. We spent approximately $100,000 trying to obtain such a status."

Baccalaureate status has helped advance the professions of physiotherapy and chiropractic, professions with similar "hands-on" approaches to healthcare [16]. To become a chiropractor in Canada, for example, one must complete undergraduate credits and then enrol in a postgraduate chiropractic college for 3–4 years [17]. Physiotherapists undergo a similar process with most students completing an undergraduate degree and then enrolling in a Masters of Physical Therapy program now available in many public universities across the country [18]. Increased educational requirements for both chiropractors and physiotherapists have meant, 1) graduates of these programs are more knowledgeable regarding clinical and research practice in their professions and, 2) exclusivity related to requiring a post-baccalaureate degree allows colleges to be highly selective in selecting their students for these programs, accepting only the most qualified and/or accomplished [16]. It is likely expected that a push for obtaining degree status for RMTs could facilitate their advancement in a similar way.

Insurance company participants express requirements for evidence-based practice

The top health issues that our insurance company participants address and stress and mental health issues, as well as soft tissue injuries – neck, back, shoulders and knees. All company representatives noted that RMTs effectively address these health issues and that MT provides positive health benefits. They also believed that MT successfully prevents disease and treats injury although some wanted more research-backed evidence regarding the effect on disease prevention. In terms of helping people get back to work, one insurer felt that RMT outcomes were good but not great, as the return to work (RTW) outcomes during 2000–2006 was, on average, 44.6%. The goal was to improve the RTW within 5 weeks of first visit to 50%.

Insurers also told us that their company would cover RMTs more widely for visits and larger maximum annual pay outs if there was proof of effectiveness, research and more endorsement from MDs. One said that they always gave approval to MT if doctors had recommended it. A review of massage therapy by a BC physician recommended that the physician who has referred a patient should ask the therapist to provide a progress note describing *measured* outcomes of the therapy [19].

One insurer felt that the perception of MT as a 'touchy/feely therapy had to change and that MT needs to be seen as an *active therapy* that shouldnt create dependency. The concept of active therapy came up in all interviews with insurance companies as they continuously compared exercises taught by physiotherapists to time on the table with RMTs. They encouraged the MTRB to make MT as 'active as possible.

Empirical evidence linking MT to benefit and outcomes would make RMT more appealing to all insurance company respondents we interviewed. All the insurance companies stated that they utilized research literature in determining the approval of claims and one even had an evidence-based practice group which did reviews of findings. All wanted to receive research literature on MT including information on return to work outcomes, new studies, emerging techniques and other focused information.

Concurring with the views expressed by the insurance companies, one member of an MT college stated:

> "The results speak for themselves. RMTs that do not keep up with best practice techniques may not get the results in their practice. Insurance companies see the poor results (and poor reporting of outcomes) by some therapists and generalize to all massage therapists. Published studies in peer-reviewed journals are what the insurance providers want to see. Even case reports and case series can be of benefit to the profession."

The MT-related organizations are keen to improve relations between RMTs and insurance providers. They hold information sessions for RMTs to learn about interacting with insurance companies effectively.

Abuse of claims

Another important issue insurance companies noted is the perceived abuse of claims, although they noted that these were not necessarily done deliberately. One private insurance company was concerned that some RMTs are billing for medically unnecessary MT. We repeatedly heard one example during an interview: a $300 receipt from a spa from an RMT. When the insurance company asked for an itemized receipt they saw that $300 included wine, chocolate covered strawberries and other items that were not legitimate. This company urged RMTs to be better informed about billing only for medically necessary MT. Currently, most RMTs use generic, non-specific receipts. They suggested that if RMTs had more official receipts they would be better able to judge the legitimacy of the claims. The other concern this private insurer had was that MT claims had substantially increased over the past 2 years. Participants were disturbed by this trend as they suspected part of the increase was due to illegitimate expenses.

Insurer respondents felt that there needed to be a clear distinction between medical massage and wellness massage. Within the MT profession there is a parallel discussion where some RMTs would like the profession to devote itself to rehabilitation and purely therapeutic practices whereas others believe MT better serves population health by being more comprehensive as a form of health promotion, disease prevention, rehabilitation and palliation. The latter group incorporate wellness massage into their practice. A third group, the spa practitioners, only practice relaxation massage. Insurers made it clear that they were interested in funding medical massage.

However, it was interesting to ask each participant about their own personal experience with MT. Those who had received regular MT stated that they were willing to pay out of pocket for relaxation massage and be covered for injuries only. The one participant who had never received the services of an RMT held the most negative views on MT. This suggests that personal experience with MT can have a significant influence on individuals professional views of it. Literature on holistic practices in general echo this idea. For example, physicians who have received MT treatment for their own healthcare services or have more knowledge regarding MT feel more comfortable discussing MT treatments with their patients [20].

Stakeholder dynamics

Each of these stakeholders has an agenda. The regulatory agencys agenda is related to their mandate of protecting the public. The agenda of the insurance companies is to protect their profits while assisting patients to improve their health. The agenda of the educational institutions is educating RMTs while maintaining profitability. Profit margins are important to at least two out of our three stakeholder groups and this is where conflict within the profession may exist. Furthermore, within each of these groups also lie many conflicts, partly based on personalities, egos and politics. The profession of MT in BC is fraught with internal struggles that impede its progress. It will not move forward until the agenda of all stakeholder groups are aligned and unity amongst groups and individuals is achieved.

Conclusion

This paper examined various factors in the development and enhancement of the profession of MT. Stakeholders of MT in British Columbia, Canada, identify research as a particularly important contributor. All stakeholders agree that more research would enhance the profession. Regulators specifically wanted more research on safety although no evidence currently exists to prove MT has serious adverse side effects. This emphasis on safety is understandable given that regulators main task is to protect the public. Other stakeholders, including RMTs themselves, are more interested in MT research that examines the efficacy of MT treatments.

Many MTRB participants were not satisfied with current curricula offered in MT colleges regarding research skills. Given the limited research training currently offered in MT colleges, many graduates of MT colleges are unable or unwilling to pursue MT research as a career option over or in combination with clinical practice. This is further exacerbated by the fact that limited funding opportunities for MT research exist across the country and since many RMTs graduate from college with large debts, engaging in clinical practice which is more profitable is often the priority. MT organizations, including colleges and the MTRB, are keen on collaborating with each other to increase the amount of MT research conducted.

Educators clearly stated that they saw research as an important way of advancing the profession but identified four main barriers: 1) faculty do not have the skills to teach research, 2) students are not keen to pursue research as a significant part of their studies, 3) there is very little room in a tight curriculum to incorporate research, 4) the MTRB board examination drives the current curriculum and research is not an important component of the board exam. Time, finances and motivation are additional barriers.

All stakeholders agreed that MT would move forward were their practitioners education validated by the conferral of baccalaureate status. Chiropractors and physiotherapists, professions with similar scopes of practice as RMTs, currently earn not only an undergraduate degree but postgraduate degrees which appear to have served them well. Currently MT colleges offer a 3,000 hour program which is more time than a standard university-level bachelors degree. If RMT colleges earn degree granting status, adding research to the curriculum will be a condition of this transition. There are two avenues to move toward this goal. The first would be to receive training entirely through a publicly funded university. Currently in British Columbia, trainees in MT at a private college can transfer three years of college credits to a public university towards a degree. However, no degree programs for MT exist and, therefore, individuals interested in pursuing a degree must study at private colleges beforehand. If students attend a public educational institution they are eligible for more loans and scholarships so they could potentially graduate with less debt. The second option would be for privately funded colleges to grant degrees themselves.

In addition to baccalaureate status, research has greatly impacted the advancement of nursing and other "hands-on" therapies such as physiotherapy and chiropractic. The combination of baccalaureate degree status and increased research into the efficacy of nursing, physiotherapy and chiropractic has increased the recognition of these professions as valuable components of healthcare by both their peers and various governments. A similar push is required, and is indeed occurring, in the profession of MT. However, obtaining undergraduate degree status for RMTs education has in itself been difficult, as indicated by some MT colleges actively engaged in the process.

MT is not understood by other healthcare professionals and there is an "identity crisis" within the profession. On the one hand, private funders interested primarily in profits, are willing to engage in the commercialization of MT. For example, connecting MT to aesthetic and cosmetic services and other beauty or fashion-oriented businesses is one way of increasing profits in this field. Indeed, one of the MT colleges we interviewed engages in such practices. Another "identity crisis" exists between MT as a medical or as a wellness profession. Insurance companies are keen to fund only medical MT and many RMTs are proponents of MT as a treatment-oriented medical practice. Others believe that MT ought to cover the complete spectrum of healthcare, incorporating wellness, disease prevention and rehabilitation. Agreement on the scope of MT practice has not been reached within or outside the profession. Further adding to this divide is the lack of unity between stakeholders of MT in the province. Acrimony and animosity between stakeholders characterize many relationships in BCs MT community. These divisions in the MT community have created a lack of leadership and common direction within the profession. The skeptical positions of other healthcare providers and governments towards MT create significant barriers to the advancement of this profession.

Besides the internal and external forces that prevent the advancement of this profession is the serious concern, on the part of insurers, that abusive claims occur. Insurers repeatedly noted that illegitimate charges were being made by RMTs.

In this paper we examined various issues related to the advancement of MT. MT is primarily a private healthcare service provided by practitioners who are largely outside the provincial healthcare system and it is misunderstood by other healthcare professionals. Despite these difficulties, British Columbians are increasingly accessing the services of RMTs and, therefore, the demand for RMTs has increased. Future research in this area should examine economic forces at play in the medical marketplace of BC. A study examining the financial and economic environment within which RMTs practice would be helpful to shed light on the larger context. When the profession is able to deal with the internal and external challenges we discuss here it will be able to move forward and be recognized as a significant player in healthcare in the province.

Additional file

Additional file 1: Appendix.1. MTRB Questionnaire. Insurance Company Questionnaire. Massage Therapy Schools Questionnaire.

Abbreviations

AMTA: American Massage Therapy Association; BC: British Columbia; MD: Medical Doctor; MT: Massage Therapy; MTA: Massage Therapists Association; MTRB: Massage Therapy Regulatory Board; RMT: Registered Massage Therapist.

Competing interests

The author(s) declared no potential conflicts of interest with respect to the research, authorship, and/or publication of this article.

Authors' contributions

FMS designed and conducted the study. FMS and ISS analyzed and interpreted the data and prepared the manuscript for publication. Both authors read and approved the final manuscript.

Authors' information

Farah M Shroff, PhD, is an Adjunct Professor in the Faculty of Medicine at the University of British Columbia in Vancouver, Canada. Inderjeet S Sahota, MSc, is a Research Associate in the Department of Biomedical Physiology and Kinesiology at Simon Fraser University in Vancouver, Canada.

Acknowledgements

The authors would like to thank the people who participated in this study. FMS received some financial support for the research from the Massage Therapists Association of British Columbia.

Author details

[1]Department of Family Practice and School of Population and Public Health, University of British Columbia, Third Floor David Strangway Bldg, 5950 University Blvd, Vancouver, BC V6T 1Z3, Canada. [2]Department of Biomedical Physiology and Kinesiology, Simon Fraser University, Simon Fraser, Canada.

References

1. BC Ministry of Health: **Health Professions Act [RSBC 1996] Chapter 183.** In *Book Health Professions Act [RSBC 1996] Chapter 183.* Queen's Printer 2011.
2. Shroff FM, Sahota IS: *How can massage therapy move forward? Registered Massage Therapists touch on key points shaping their profession in British Columbia.* Home Health Care Management and Practice: Canada; 2011.
3. *Massage therapy in Canada* http://www.rmtao.com/massage_therapy/regulation_of_mt/massage_therapy_in_canada.htm accessed April 2, 2011.
4. *Legislation & standards: overview* 2012. http://www.cmtbc.bc.ca/Legislation-and-Standards/Overview.aspx] accessed May 4, 2012.
5. *About the college - active registrants* 2011. http://www.cmtbc.bc.ca/About-The-College/active-registrants.aspx accessed January 3, 2011.
6. *Who We Are - education and training* 2012. http://www.massagetherapy.bc.ca/ accessed August 13, 2012.
7. *Medical and health care benefits* 2012. http://www.health.gov.bc.ca/msp/infoben/benefits.html accessed June 5, 2012.
8. College of Massage Therapists of British Columbia: *Brief for the BC Government's Conversation on Health. In Book Brief for the BC Government's Conversation on Health (Editor ed.)* 2007.
9. Oerton S: **Bodywork boundaries: Power, politics and professionalism in therapeutic massage.** *Gender Work Organ* 2004, **11**:544–565.
10. Shroff FM: *Hands on!: cultures of massage in global contex*, Presentation at 42nd annual meeting of the Canadian sociological association. Saskatoon, Canada 2007.
11. *Canada's health care system*2011. http://www.hc-sc.gc.ca/hcs-sss/pubs/system-regime/2011-hcs-sss/index-eng.php accessed July 5, 2011.
12. *National health expenditure database* 2012. www.cihi.ca accessed May 23, 2012.
13. *Exploring the 70/30 split: how Canada's health care system is financed* 2012. http://secure.cihi.ca/cihiweb/products/FundRep_EN.pdf accessed July 18, 2012.
14. Cherkin DC, Sherman KJ, Deyo RA, Shekelle PG: **A review of the evidence for the effectiveness, safety, and cost of acupuncture, massage therapy, and spinal manipulation for back pain.** *Ann Intern Med* 2003, **138**:898–906.
15. Shroff FM: *Massage therapy research plan phase 1 - ideas from stakeholders: RMTs, the CMT, MT colleges and insurance companies*, Massage therapy research plan phase 1 - ideas from stakeholders: RMTs, the CMT, MT colleges and insurance companies (shroff consulting 2007. Unpublished report.
16. Blood H: **Entry-level masters degree - a decade of experience.** *Phys Ther* 1984, **64**:208–212.
17. *Becoming a Chiropractor* 2011. http://www.chiropractic.on.ca/ChiropracticCare/WhoareChiropractors/BecomingaChiropractor.aspx accessed Oct 30, 2011.
18. *University education and registration* 2011. http://thesehands.ca/index.php/site/University_education_and_registration/ accessed November 18, 2011.
19. Sedergreen CJ: **Massage therapy-a review.** *B C Med J* 2000, **42**:342–344.
20. Verhoef MJ, Page SA: **Physicians' perspectives on massage therapy.** *Can Fam Physician* 1998, **44**:1018–1020. 1023–1014.

A survey of "mental hardiness" and "mental toughness" in professional male football players

Rainer Wieser[1*] and Haymo Thiel[2]

Abstract

Background: It is not uncommon for chiropractors to be associated with sports teams for injury prevention, treatment, or performance enhancement. There is increasing acceptance of the importance of sports psychology in the overall management of athletes. Recent findings indicate mental hardiness can be determined reliably using specific self-assessment questionnaires. This study set out to investigate the hardiness scores of professional footballers and examine the correlation between two questionnaires. It also included a mental hardiness rating of players by two coaches, and examined differences in hardiness and mental toughness between national and international players.

Methods: Two self-assessment questionnaires (modified Sports Mental Toughness Questionnaire [SMTQ-M] and Psychological Performance Inventory [PPI-A]) were completed by 20 male professional footballers. Two coaches, independently rated each player. A percentage score from each questionnaire was awarded each player and an average score was calculated ({SMTQ-M % + PPI-A %} ÷ 2). The PPI-A and SMTQ-M scores obtained for each player were analysed for correlation with Pearson's correlation coefficient. Cohen's kappa inter-reliability coefficient was used to determine agreement between coaches, and between the players' hardiness scores and coaches' ratings. The independent t-test was used to examine differences between national and international players.

Results: The players' scores obtained from PPI-A and SMTQ-M correlated well ($r = 0.709$, $p < 0.001$). The coaches ratings showed significant, weak to moderate agreement (Cohen's kappa = 0.33). No significant agreement was found between player self-assessments and coaches' ratings.
The average ({SMTQ-M % + PPI-A %} ÷ 2) mean score was 77% (SD = 7.98) with international players scoring 7.4% ($p = 0.04$) higher than non-international players.

Conclusions: The questionnaires (SMTQ-M and PPI-A) correlated well in their outcome scores. These findings suggest that coaches moderately agree when assessing the level of mental hardiness of football players. There was no agreement between player self-assessment and ratings by coaches. Footballers who play or had played for national teams achieved slightly higher mental hardiness scores.
Either questionnaire can offer the clinician a cost-effective, valuable measure of an individual's psychological attributes, which could be relevant within the wider context of bio-psycho-social model of care.

Keywords: Mental toughness, Mental hardiness, Survey, Male professional football players

Background

Optimal sports performance depends on physical and psychological components. Often, millimeters and microseconds are decisive factors between success or failure. When athletes, especially top performers of similar physical ability, have reached their optimal physical limits, the only difference for their success could depend on psychological components. One assumes that the competitor with greater control over his or her mind will emerge as the victor. In professional football over recent years, expectations of coaches and players have increased dramatically. Ever-growing demands to win, the fear of failure, and targets which are often set too high, are common causes to lead to psychological stress. However, it appears that some players or coaches are able to handle difficult

* Correspondence: rainer@c3chiropractic.co.uk
[1]C3 Chiropractic Clinic, 223-225 Pantbach Road, Rhiwbina, Cardiff, Wales CF14 6AE, UK
Full list of author information is available at the end of the article

and stressful situations better than others. Do they have certain characteristics or mental attributes which enable them to cope better with or even thrive under stress, and how can on measure these mental features?

Consequently, a deeper understanding of the contribution of certain elements of sports psychology in the overall treatment and management of athletes can be very beneficial for physiotherapists, chiropractors and other health care professionals who deal with sports injury management. One of the authors (RW) had been working with the local championship football team as a sports chiropractor for the past seven years, and during this period had come across the concept of "mental hardiness" and its possible relevance within the context of sports performance.

The concepts of mental hardiness [1,2] and mental toughness [3,4] are closely linked to the construct of what has been termed "positive psychology" by Seligman and Csikszentmihalyi [5]. A central tenet of the positive psychology paradigm is that stressors and other inordinate demands are inherent to the human condition. However, the paradigm also assumes that they can be sources of strength, through which adversity can be endured and even transcended. Physical, emotional, and social stressors can further personal development and enhance mental strength in some individuals. Such people are often able to tap into previously unknown capacities, perspectives, and virtues [6].

The concept of "hardiness" was first introduced by Kobasa [1] by trying to find a link between stressful life events and the onset of illness. The study reported on two groups of individuals who faced similar stressful life events, one group became ill after their stressful experience whilst the other remained healthy. It was proposed that the reason why individuals reacted differently to similar stressful events was a personality difference, best described as hardiness. The research found that the individuals who remained healthy showed more hardiness than the individuals who fell ill. The personality construct of hardiness emerged from existential psychology: a viewpoint that proposes that meaning in life is created through the decisions people make. It is composed of the "three C's - Commitment, Control and Challenge" [2]. Commitment is the predisposition to be involved with people and events, rather than to be isolated and detached [7,8]. Control is the belief that one can influence outcomes, rather than feeling powerless to change anything. Finally, Challenge is the attitude that change is not only inevitable, but beneficial, and that it offers incentives to learn and develop, rather than serving as a threat. Research conducted at the U.S. Military Academy at West Point found that mental hardiness protected Army reserve personnel mobilised for the Persian Gulf War [9]. In this study, the higher the hardiness level, the greater the ability of soldiers to experience life- and combat-related stress without apparent negative health consequences, such as post-traumatic stress disorder or depression.

The most important skills and techniques applied in contemporary sports psychology are: imagery, goal setting, self-talk, stress management, team building, efficacy management, attention control, emotion regulation and mental toughness [10]. A winning mentality and desire have been identified as key attributes of mentally tough soccer players in addition to other previously reported qualities such as self-belief, physical toughness, work ethic/ motivation, and resilience [11]. Key cognitions reported by mentally tough soccer players enable them to remain focused and competitive during training and matches, which reflects that positive self-talk can help some players in dealing with challenging situations [6].

Sheard and colleagues [4] identified mental toughness as a crucial attribute for success in sport. There are seven components to mental toughness, such as confidence, constancy, control, determination, self-belief, positive cognition and visualisation. These components can be measured with self-assessment questionnaires such as the Sports Mental Toughness Questionnaire (SMTQ) and the Psychological Performance Inventory (PPI-A) [12,13]. More specifically, the SMTQ measures confidence, constancy and control, whereas he PPI-A measures determination, self-belief, positive cognition and visualisation. Both questionnaires have been tried on larger sample sizes of athletes [4,14]. In answer to the question, "does a screening test accurately detect a hardiness score?" previous research has established that these tests are reliable and consistent instruments for self-assessment [14,15]. A cross-national analysis of mental toughness and hardiness in elite university rugby league teams revealed that Australian University players had significantly higher mean scores on positive cognition, visualisation, mental toughness and challenge than their opponents from Great Britain [13]. It has also been shown that individuals with greater hardiness scores are less likely to report injuries [2], and that players with higher mental toughness have "greater pain tolerance and therefore under-report injury and are often not compliant with their treatment" [16].

The first aim of the present study was to investigate the hardiness scores of professional footballers and examine the correlation between the outcome scores of a slightly modified SMTQ (SMTQ-M) and the PPI-A. As previous research has been primarily based on self-assessment scores provided by athletes only, the second aim of this study was to ask two coaches to independently assign a hardiness score to each player, and then to examine for the level of agreement between the coaches' and players' scores, and also between the two coaches themselves.

Methods

Study design

This study was a quantitative survey based on numerically derived data scores from two established psychology questionnaires adapted and slightly modified for professional footballers.

Ethical approval

Ethics approval was obtained through the Research and Ethics Sub-Committee of the Anglo-European College of Chiropractic, Bournemouth, United Kingdom.

Recruitment of subjects

The subjects were a convenience sample of football players. This consisted of 20 players of a local professional Welsh football team. RW had been the chiropractor to the football team for more than seven years.

Setting

The data collection took place at the training grounds of Cardiff City Football Club, South Glamorgan, Wales.

Data collection - players

A short player profile data collection tool captured details on a player's nationality, age, years of professional experience, highest level of performance and criteria for reporting an injury. The SMTQ and the PPI-A were slightly modified by removing numbers and letters across the options and replacing them with tick boxes so as not to influence the choice of response. A further alteration was made to the SMTQ, in that question one and five were made identical. This was done to assess for consistency of responses. The players were given an information sheet about the study and asked to complete a consent form. RW was on site to give further clarification on how to complete the questionnaires if required.

Data collection - coaches

Two experienced coaches, who had been with the club for more than five years were asked to independently rate all of the players for mental hardiness using the following scoring key: above average = 1, average = 2, below average = 3.

Data analysis

As the questionnaires were based on different scales, their overall numerical scores were converted into percentage scores to allow comparison between data sets. The average percentage score for each footballer ({SMTQ-M% + PPI-A%} ÷ 2) and a mean score for the whole sample of players was established. Pearson's correlation coefficient was used to determine the strength of linear dependence between the SMTQ-M and the PPI-A scores. Cohen's kappa inter-reliability coefficient was used to determine the level of agreement between the two football coaches. In order to assess the level of agreement between the players' self-ratings with the coaches' ratings, each individual player's score was converted into categorical data to be in line with the coaches scoring key. The independent t-test was used to examine differences in the average percentage scores between national and international players. PASW Statistics (version 18) software for apple mac computers was used for data analysis.

Results

The footballers' ages ranged from 18 to 33 years (mean = 24.8 years, SD = 4.63), and the length of their professional experience from one to 15 years (mean = 7.7 years, SD = 4.84). Eleven players (55%) responded that they report injury immediately after it had occurred, whilst six indicated that they report injury when they experience mild pain and three when they experience severe pain only. Three players were currently injured and were therefore not playing at the time of data collection. Six players had been playing for less than one year for the football club, 11 players for one to five years, and three players for more than five years. Eight players either had been or were members of a national team, two players had played in the Premier League in the past, and 10 played at Championship level. Two players were of foreign origin, and English was therefore their second language.

Figure 1 shows the mean group percentage scores of both questionnaires (PPI-A and SMTQ-M). There was a slightly overall higher score on the PPI-A questionnaire, with a mean of 78% (SD = 8.69) compared to the SMTQ-M with a mean of 75% (SD = 8.37), but this difference was not statistically significant. There was a significant difference (independent t-test, $p = 0.04$) in the average mean score between international and non-international players, with the international players scoring 7.4% higher (4.7% - 14.4%; 95% CI). The sub-group of eight international players achieved an average mean score of 81% (SD = 4.88) compared to the overall mean score of the 12 Non-Internationals, who had a lower mean score of 74% (SD = 8.41).

The Pearson's correlation revealed that there was a significant linear relationship between the SMTQ-M and the PPI-A scores ($r = 0.709$, $p < 0.001$) (Figure 2). Inter-reliability between the two coaches when rating the players was weak to moderate ($k = 0.33$), whilst there was no agreement between the coaches' ratings and the average player self-ratings (Coach A: $k = -0.17$, Coach B: $k = -0.07$).

Comparison of the sample's mean percentage scores for the seven hardiness components revealed high scores for control and determination, with confidence and visualisation achieving the lowest scores (Figure 3). The

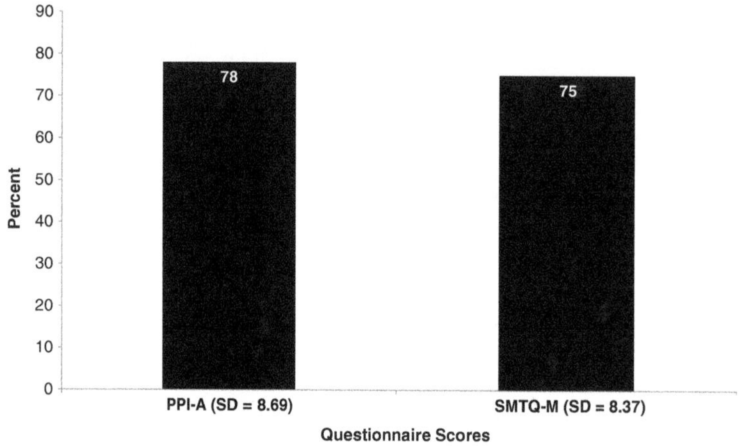

Figure 1 Mean group percentage scores for PPI-A and SMTQ-M.

analysis of the team's mean percentage scores of the 7 hardiness components revealed that at the time of the data collection the team scored well on the mean determination (88%, SD = 10.11) and constancy (88%, SD = 8.81) scores. However, the team's mean confidence (69%, SD = 12.36), self-belief (76%, SD = 10.24) and positive cognition (75%, SD = 9.30) scores were relatively low. The mean visualisation score was 71% (SD = 16.50) and the mean control score 72% (SD = 13.83).

Discussion

In contrast to most studies, which have focused on academy players, this study researched mental hardiness in professional footballers. An interesting finding of this study is that 45% of professional football players will report injury when they experience some form of pain, 30% will report when they experience mild pain, with 15% only reporting severe pain. One of the most likely reasons for being reluctant in reporting injuries could be a player's fear of losing his place in the first team. Delayed reporting makes it difficult for the team doctor and physiotherapist to deal with injuries effectively. Late diagnosis and delayed monitoring of a possible injury increases the chance of re-injury and could lead to more severe and chronic injuries. A self-centered mindset of a mentally tough performer could therefore be a disadvantage to the whole football team. The interest of the team should always take priority over personal achievement.

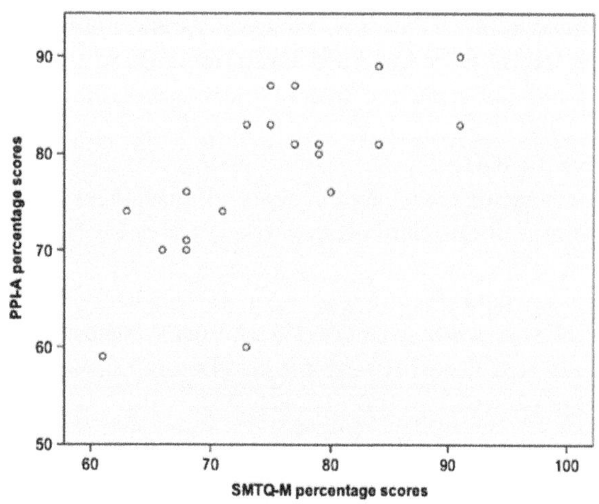

Figure 2 Scatter plot between SMTQ-M and PPI-A (r = 0.709, p <0.001).

Some of the other findings in this study, such as the correlation between SMTQ-M and PPI-A scores, the statistically significant higher hardiness scores of international football players concur with previous research [14,17]. However, to our best knowledge no previous study has utilised the two questionnaires in a combined fashion in order to arrive at one numerical score for mental hardiness. We feel that this approach provides for a good overall indicator of mental hardiness or toughness, as it combines most of the sub-components previously referred to within the literature.

Previous work had also found that athletes performing at an international level score higher in relation to mental hardiness [4,14]. Similar findings were demonstrated in this study, with the sub-group of eight international players achieving an average mean score which was 7% above that of non-internationals.

The analysis of the team's mean percentage scores of the seven hardiness components revealed that at the time of the data collection the team scored well on the mean determination score and constancy. However, the team's mean confidence, self-belief and positive cognition scores were relatively low and would therefore indicate room for improvement. The mean visualisation score was also low and as only certain players use this

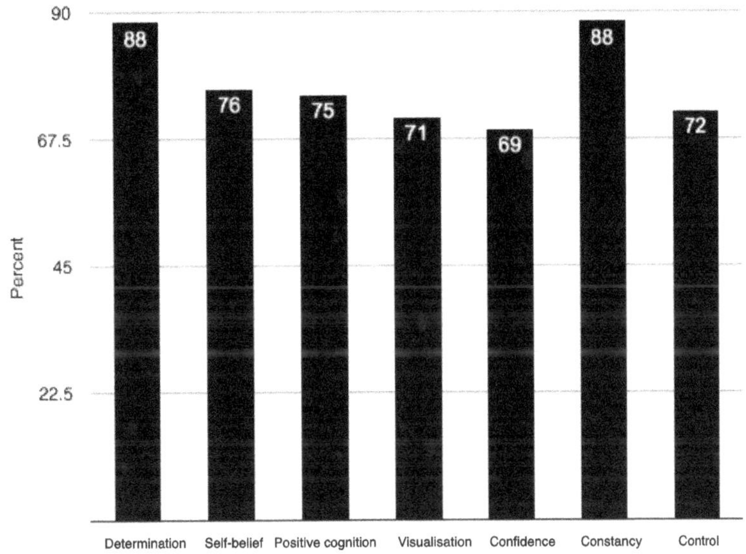

Figure 3 The teams mean percentage scores of the 7 hardiness components.

technique, there would be no need to address this issue for the benefit of the team.

This study also showed that there was a strong significant linear correlation between the SMTQ-M and the PPI-A questionnaires, which concurs with previous research by Sheard [11,15]. A recent paper by Crust and Swann [17] measured the correlation between the SMTQ and the Mental Toughness Questionnaire (MTQ 48) on a sample of 110 male athletes and also found that there was a significant positive correlation in higher order mental toughness scores ($r = 0.75$; $p < 0.001$). This compares well to the findings of the present study and shows that these tools produce consistent results even when slightly modified.

The ratings of the players by the two coaches showed weak to moderate agreement (Cohen's kappa = 0.33) and no agreement was found between player self-assessments and the ratings given by the coaches. These findings agree with those of another study [18] which also investigated the inter-rater agreement of two coaches, who took repetitive measurements on 21 professional academy players using two different questionnaires. This suggests that even amongst professional football coaches, there are considerable differences in interpreting the behaviours and characteristics of players and that their judgments are subjective. Individual coaches are likely to have their own interpretation of mental toughness as a common an agreed definition does not really exist [19]. Similarly the present study reflected the findings of previous work [18,20] in that there was no significant agreement between the coaches' scores and the player self-assessment scores. However, even though the results showed little agreement between the individual coaches, and between the coaches' and the player self-assessment scores, the scores provided for a good platform for player feedback and making individuals more self-aware of their various traits in relation to mental hardiness. The mean score was used as an indicator for overall team spirit. With this additional information, further options were now available to the coaches and players to either address weak areas, focus on strong psychological sub-components, or both, overall aiming for a more holistic player development. These outcomes could be very useful, as long as players are willing to adapt their behaviour, and coaches are willing to address and develop these components within their coaching methods.

Limitations of study and suggestions for further research

The data were collected on the basis of responses made at a single point in time. As such the results could have been strongly influenced by how the players were feeling at the time, especially as they had lost a number of preceding games. It was essential that the players answered the questions honestly, they may have over-estimated their abilities in their responses. Some played at several levels in different leagues during their career. However, the player's questionnaire only took into account the highest level of play throughout their career, even if they were not at this highest level currently. Although the sample represented a relatively homogenous group of professional footballers, it was of a small size and as such its findings cannot be generalised to other football teams. Furthermore, there is a risk of Type 1 and Type 2 errors. Although the coaches had been instructed to complete their questionnaires independently from each other, the researcher had no control over this to ensure that it actually happened. When the coaches considered a player they may have sub-consciously included in their assessment different components such as talent, skill and past performance.

Future research could include a more phenomenological approach to personality research. More longitudinal research into mental hardiness in contexts outside sports performance is required. Another interesting investigation could determine how intellectual skills influence the outcome scores on surveys, as it is possible that people with a better educational background will achieve higher hardiness scores.

Conclusion

Personality is a mixture of genetic predisposition and environmental influences. Individual traits and the environment can act as co-determinants of behaviour. Personality structure involves both a stable core of attitudes, values and beliefs about self, which remain relatively unchanged after early childhood. Exploring these characteristics through self and external assessment can be a valuable experience for a footballer, even if at present, there is no evidence upon which one can directly link mental hardiness with success in football.

The present study could only explore some components of the construct and was focused on the quantitative measurement of mental hardiness. There was good correlation between the two questionnaires and both are equally sufficient to measure characteristics of mental hardiness. The advantage of combining the questionnaires to achieve an overall mean score may lie in providing a more comprehensive assessment of an individual's mental hardiness. However, if due to practical or time saving reasons, one chooses to use only one of the questionnaires, the authors recommend the PPI-A as it measures slightly more components compared to the SMTQ-M.

The results showed that even amongst elite level professional soccer coaches, there is little agreement when judging the mental hardiness of their players and the players themselves have a different self-judgment compared with the coaches' ratings. However, through enhanced self-knowledge and feedback via the coach one could conceivably address certain weaknesses and build on strengths.

The understanding of the concept of mental hardiness is still evolving and the complexities of human psychology and its nature are such that it is difficult to condense them easily into discrete sub-components. However, in the present study the combination of these sub-components appeared to be a good indicator of an overall sense of the "team spirit".

"Knowing others is clever. Knowing yourself is enlightenment. Controlling others requires force. Controlling yourself requires strength" (Lao Tzu).

Competing interests

The authors declare that they have no competing interests.

Authors' contributions

RW: Concept and design of the study, collection and entry of data, analysis and interpretation of the manuscript, final approval of the manuscript. HT: Concept and design of the study, drafting and revising the manuscript and final approval of the manuscript. Both authors read and approved the final manuscript.

Acknowledgements

The authors thank the players and coaches of Cardiff City FC for participating in the study.

Author details

[1]C3 Chiropractic Clinic, 223-225 Pantbach Road, Rhiwbina, Cardiff, Wales CF14 6AE, UK. [2]Anglo-European College of Chiropractic, 13-15 Parkwood Road, Bournemouth, Dorset BH5 2DF, UK.

References

1. Kobasa S: **Stressful life events, personality and health: An inquiry into hardiness.** *J Pers Soc Psychol* 1979, **37**:1–11.
2. Kobasa S, Maddi S, Khan S: **Hardiness and health: A prospective study.** *J Pers Soc Psychol* 1982, **42**:168–177.
3. Golby J, Sheard M, Lavallee D: **A cognitive-behavioural analysis of mental toughness in national rugby league football teams.** *Percept Mot Skills* 2003, **96**(2):455–462.
4. Golby J, Sheard M, van Wersch A: **Evaluating the factor structure of the Psychological Performance Inventory.** *Percept Mot Skills* 2007, **105**(1):309–325.
5. Seligman M, Csikszentmihalyi M: **Positive psychology: An introduction.** *Am Psychol* 2000, **55**:5–14.
6. Coulter T, Mallett C, Gucciardi D: **Understanding mental toughness in Australian soccer: perceptions of players, parents, and coaches.** *J Sports Sci* 2010, **28**(7):699–716.
7. Maddi S: **The Story of hardiness: Twenty years of theorizing, research and practice.** *Consult Psychol J* 2002, **54**:173–185.
8. Maddi S: **Building an integrated positive psychology.** *J Posit Psychol* 2006, **1**:226–229.
9. Bartone P: **Hardiness protects against war-related stress in army reserve forces.** *Consult Psychol J* 1999, **51**:72–82.
10. Mellalieu S, Hanton S: *Advances in Applied Sport Psychology.* London: Routledge; 2009.
11. Sheard M: *Mental Toughness The Mindset Behind Sporting Achievement.* New York: Routledge; 2010.
12. Sheard M: **A cross-national analysis of mental toughness and hardiness in elite university rugby league teams.** *Percept Mot Skills* 2009, **109**(1):213–223.
13. Sheard M: **Hardiness commitment, gender, and age differentiate university academic performance.** *Br J Educ Psychol* 2009, **79**:189–204.
14. Sheard M, Golby J, Wersch A: **Progress Toward Construct Validation of the Sport Mental Toughness Questionnaire (SMTQ).** *Eur J Psychol Assess* 2009, **25**(3):186–193.
15. Sheard M: *Construct Validation of the Alternative Psychological Performance Inventory (PPi-A) and the Sports Mental Toughness Questionnaire (SMTQ).* Tartu; 2008. http://www.eapp.org/getmedia.php/_media/eapp/download/201012/1292449019-orig.pdf.
16. Ford IW, Eklund RC, Gordon S: **An examination of psychosocial variables moderating the relationship between life stress and injury time-loss among athletes of a high standard.** *J Sports Sci* 2000, **18**(5):301–312.
17. Crust L, Swann C: **Comparing two measures of mental toughnesss.** *Pers Indiv Differ* 2011, **50**:217–221.
18. Crust L, Nesti M, Littlewood M: **Player and coach ratings of mental toughness in an elite association football academy.** *Online J Sport Psychol* 2010, **12**(3):156–172.
19. Crust L: **A review and conceptual re-examination of mental toughness: Implications for future research.** *Pers Indiv Differ* 2008, **45**:576–583.
20. Crust L, Nesti M, Littlewood M: **A cross-sectional analysis of mental toughness in a professional football academy.** *Athletic Insight J* 2010, **2**(2). http://eprints.lincoln.ac.uk/2418/.

10

The effect of a lumbar support pillow on lumbar posture and comfort during a prolonged seated task

Diane E Grondin[*†], John J Triano[†], Steve Tran and David Soave

Abstract

Background: Several risk factors exist for the development of low back pain, including prolonged sitting and flexed spinal curvature. Several investigators have studied lumbar support devices and spinal curvatures in sitting, however few have investigated a pain population and reported a quantitative measure of comfort. The purpose of the current project was to determine whether a lumbar support pillow, outfitted with a cut-out to accommodate the bulk of posterior pelvic soft tissue volume, is more effective than a standard chair in promoting a neutral spinal posture and improving subjective and objective measures of comfort in healthy individuals and patients with low back pain.

Methods: Twenty eight male participants with and without a history of low back pain sat in a standard office chair and in a chair with the lumbar support pillow for 30 minutes. Lumbar and thoracolumbar postures were measured through electromagnetic markers. Comfort was determined based on the least squares radius of centre of pressure shifting, measured at the buttock-chair interface as well as reported discomfort through visual analog scales. Chair support effects were assessed through ANOVA methods. The study was approved by the Canadian Memorial Chiropractic College research ethics board.

Results: There was a main effect of condition on lumbar posture ($p = 0.006$) and thoracolumbar posture ($p = 0.014$). In the lumbar region, the support and standard chair differed by 2.88° (95% CI; 1.01-4.75), with the lumbar support being closer to neutral than the standard chair. In the thoracolumbar region, the support and standard chair differed by −2.42° (95% CI; -4.22 to −0.62), with the standard chair being closer to neutral than the support device. The centre of pressure measure was significantly improved with the pillow ($p = 0.017$), however there were no subjective changes in comfort.

Conclusions: A lumbar support pillow with a cut-out for the posterior pelvic tissues improved an objective measure of comfort in healthy individuals and patients with low back pain. Lumbar flattening was decreased and thoracolumbar curvature was increased. However, angular changes were small and future work is required to determine clinical relevance over the long term.

Trial registration: ClinicalTrials.gov, NCT00754585

Keywords: Posture, Low back pain, Sitting, Work

* Correspondence: dgrondin@cmcc.ca
[†]Equal contributors
Canadian Memorial Chiropractic College, 6100 Leslie Street, Toronto, ON M2H 3J1, Canada

Background

The interaction between the low back and chair support is an important health factor for employees using seated work stations. Canadian statistics indicate that back injuries make up 28.8% of the lost time claims and 7.0% occur in clerical jobs [1]. The result of the musculoskeletal conditions is a reduction in work attendance and performance. For instance, 19% of those with low back pain (LBP) lose 6.2 hours of work per month and those with severe pain lose 8.2 hours of work per month [2].

Several risk factors have been identified for the development of LBP in individuals who are required to sit throughout the majority of their work day. These include prolonged muscle contractions [3,4], vibration [5], and sustained body postures. Postures outside of neutral are particularly troublesome [3,6-9] as they lead to prolonged low level muscle contractions [6] and changes in intervertebral disc pressures [8,10]. During sitting, the lumbar spine flattens and there is posterior migration of the nucleus [11]. The pressure on the disc increases [8,10] and there is increased passive strain on the posterior spinal elements [12,13]. The seated lumbar pressures may be minimized by maintaining the natural lordotic curvature [8,14].

Health care practitioners rely on a variety of methods to improve the seated postures of their patients, and commonly lumbar support devices are prescribed. Numerous devices exist for use in office chairs or vehicles, including built-in static or variable controlled pads and lumbar support cushions [4,10,14-16]. A number of investigators have studied lumbar support pads and their effect on spinal posture and comfort [5,15,16].

De Carvalho and Callaghan [16] performed a radiological study on the effect of lumbar support prominences on spinal and pelvic postures in an automobile seat [16]. An increase in the depth of the support prominence was noted to significantly increase the extension of the intervertebral joints of the lumbar spine [16]. However, the investigators could not state whether comfort was affected over the long term and what changes could be expected in patients with LBP [16]. Moreover, Makhsous et al. [14] noted that a backrest fitted to the lower spine and reduced ischial support improved the position of the spine in healthy individuals. The total and segmental lumbar lordosis was maintained, the sacrum was rotated forward, and the lumbar intervertebral disc heights were increased. Again, any changes in patients with LBP could not be established.

While additional authors have investigated the effect of various support systems on bodily symptoms, much of this work has been performed on healthy individuals. Aota et al. [15] measured the biomechanical effects and comfort levels when using a lumbar support cushion that inflated from 0.5 to 8.0 cm thick in a continuous passive motion chair. They noted significant improvements in the subjective measures of LBP, stiffness and fatigue with use of the system in both static and dynamic states. Conversely, Carcone and Keir [17] noted that, while a lumbar pad measuring 9 cm thick best maintained the lumbar lordosis in sitting, participants tended to complain that it pushed their body forward, the result being a centre of pressure (CoP) that was more anteriorly located on the seat pan. In their study, participants also reported that configurations with less lordosis (i.e., less than 3 cm) were more comfortable [17]. Portable devices that do not account for the bulk of posterior pelvic soft tissue volume may push the lower body forward and distort the intended relationship between the seat pan features and the body [17]. The preferred degree of lordosis may be related to the pain state of the individual [17], in that comfort may be affected by the angular change as well as the interaction between the buttocks and the seat pan.

While past authors have commonly measured comfort through subjective means [17], objective measures such as changes in posture (or 'micro movements') may be good indicators of discomfort [18-21], as small movements are necessary to alleviate pain caused by static postures. While several past studies have examined the effects of various lumbar support pads, few have quantified the level of comfort through 'in chair movements', and most studies have been restricted to healthy individuals. The purpose of this study was to examine for differences in lordotic curvature and comfort between a support device that accounts for pelvic tissue bulk against a typical chair in healthy individuals and patients with LBP. Comfort was measured through subjective and objective means. The hypothesis underlying this work postulates that there will be differences in comfort and lordotic angulation for healthy individuals and patients with pain between the support conditions.

Methods

Participants

Twenty eight male participants (14 healthy individuals and 14 patients with LBP) between the ages of 21–50 were asked to participate in the study. Healthy individuals consisted of those who were free of LBP for the six months previous to the study, whereas patients with LBP had a history of LBP for at least three consecutive days over the last three consecutive weeks prior to testing. Individuals with a known neurological disorder, scoliosis or other deformity, inflammatory or degenerative arthropathy, connective tissue disease, or a history of spinal surgery were excluded from the study. Individuals with current or previous neck pain in the past three weeks were also excluded. Participants were asked to avoid engaging in any type of resistive exercise for the

48 hours prior to testing. All participants signed the informed consent form. The procedures used were in accordance with the institutional research ethics board. The clinical trial was registered at ClinicalTrials.gov (NCT00754585). Data were collected in the Biomechanics and Elastography laboratory at the Canadian Memorial Chiropractic College (CMCC).

Protocol and instrumentation

A Grahl Duo Back™ office chair (Rohde & Grahl, Steyerberg/Voigtei, Germany), fixed in position to prevent it from swivelling or rolling, was used for the study. The arm rests were lowered so that they were not used and to ensure the maximum amount of loading was transferred to the seat pan of the chair. The chair had all the features of a typical ergonomic office chair but it was unique in that the back rest did not provide any specific lordotic support and was split vertically, providing access to the midline for sensor attachment.

At the beginning of the data collection, participants were asked to stand in a neutral position "with their arms by their side, weight evenly balanced, and looking straight ahead". Kinematic data were collected over 30 seconds of neutral static stance for comparison against the seated conditions. Participants sat in the office chair and in the same seat pan but with a lumbar support pillow ("Logic Back™", Mediflow Inc., Toronto) to test the effect of the back rest profile on comfort and lumbar and thoracolumbar postures. The lumbar support is a portable device, convex in the anterior direction and contoured with an arched opening above the seat pan, that provides space for the bulk of the posterior pelvic tissues (Figure 1). The back frame of the device is constructed of a solid plastic, curved side-to-side and is relatively rigid. The frame acts as a bow which is strung anteriorly by four adjustable straps. These straps provide an elastic, anterior projection above the buttock tissues. A band affixes the device to the chair back. The lumbar support was "fitted" to each participant prior to testing by having the individual sit in the chair in a relaxed fashion, with the hips and knees flexed to 90°, feet flat and looking straight ahead. The pelvis was pushed all the way back into the aperture of the pillow, and the individual's lumbar spine rested against the back rest. The straps were tensioned to participant preference.

Study participants sat for 30 minutes in the regular chair with vertical (90°) back support and for 30 minutes in the chair with additional lumbar support while watching a video on a computer screen placed directly in front of them in the mid-sagittal plane. The angle of visual gaze was controlled by the height of the computer monitor which was placed 15 cm above waist height for each participant. The participants' feet rested on an adjustable foot rest such that their hips and knees were flexed to 90°. There were seven minutes of rest between conditions, whereby participants were asked to stand and move freely about. The order of conditions was randomized. All sources of metal (e.g., belts, keys in pockets, etc.) were removed prior to testing to minimize any interference with the electromagnetic equipment.

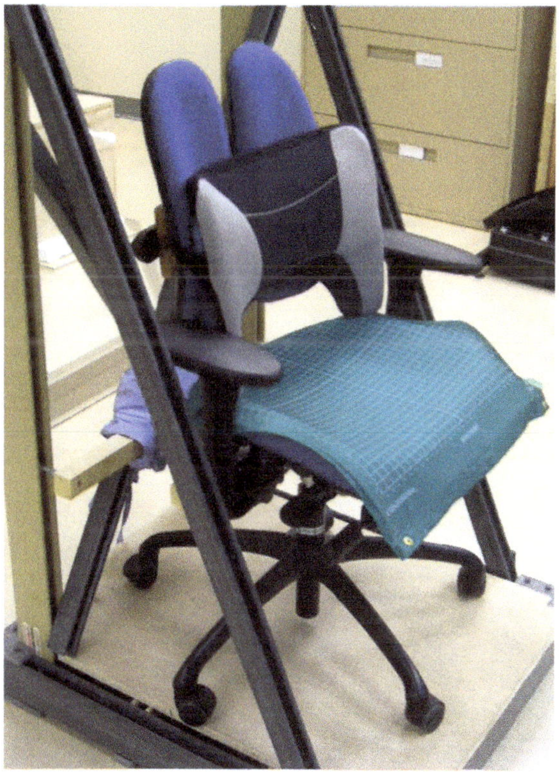

Figure 1 Photograph of the lumbar support pillow placed on the standard, split back office chair.

Postural measure

Electromagnetic sensors (Polhemus Liberty® system, Colchester, Vermont) were placed in the midline over the spinous processes at the junctions of the neck and upper back (T1), mid and lower back (T12), centre of the lower back (L3), and over the spinal base at the sacrum (S2). The spinal configuration was represented as a series of linkages connected by nodes that allowed for bending in the sagittal plane at the landmark pivots (Figures 2 and 3). The thoracic spine was treated as a single segment, rigid body, while the lumbar spine was modelled as a two segment linkage. The sensors were sampled at 240 Hz which allowed for the continuous and automatic monitoring of landmark positions and orientations in space. This system has an accuracy of 0.15° RMS. Difference in orientation between the thoracic link and the upper lumbar link were used as a surrogate for the thoracolumbar angle at T12 while the upper lumbar and lower lumbar links at L3 served to estimate the lumbar lordosis angle.

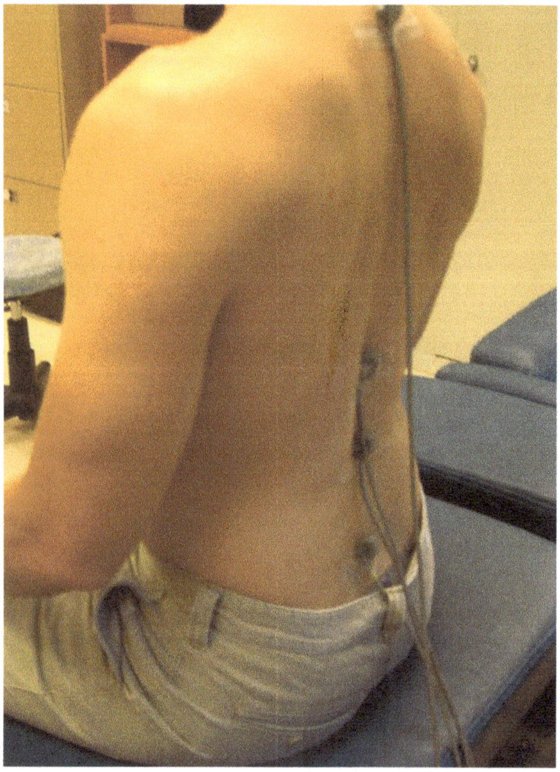

Figure 2 Sample view and placement of the kinematic electromagnetic sensors.

Comfort

Using methods inspired by Fenety et al. [22], the seat–user interface pressure distribution in the current study was measured using a pressure mapping system (CONFORMat®, Tekscan Incorporated, Boston). The sensor mat is an ultrathin (0.00400, 0.10 mm) flexible printed circuit with 1024 individual sensing elements or cells organized in a 32 × 32 array with a density of 0.5 sensels/cm^2. Before the study, the pressure mat sensels were preconditioned, equilibrated, and calibrated using the Tekscan Inc. uniform pressure vacuum pump and Tekscan Inc. user guide. During the collection, the pressure mat was placed only on the specific seat surface to measure the CoP at the buttock-chair interface. It was covered with a sheet that was fixed at the ends to prevent slipping of the mat and participant bias by observing the mat. Data were recorded at 60 Hz and fed into a PC computer. The first two minutes of data were removed from analysis to ensure that the individual was "settled" prior to calculation of the CoP.

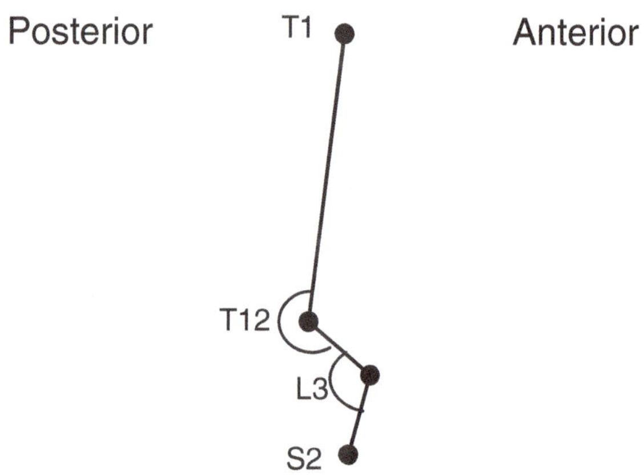

Figure 3 Sample demonstration of the thoracolumbar and lumbar angles (lateral view). The thoracolumbar and lumbar angles were calculated about T12 and L3, respectively.

Each trial was divided into three epochs of equal duration. Using MatLab 2007b (version 7.5.0.342, Mathworks Inc., Natick, MA), a circle of best fit was calculated for each epoch using a least squares method. The radius was of particular interest as it gave a measure of the overall CoP shifting, such that the larger the radius, the more the shift, and the greater the objective measure of discomfort. MatLab code inspired by Gander et al. [23] was used to calculate a best-fit circle that minimized algebraic error (Figure 4).

To obtain a subjective measure of comfort and to get an idea of how the pillow would affect comfort in other areas of the body, individuals were asked to complete a body map questionnaire [24]. They reported their level of discomfort in various areas of the body according to a visual analog scale (VAS) at baseline and after sitting in the chair with the lumbar support and without. Participants were asked to mark along a 100 mm line where their level of discomfort is "right now", 0 mm being "none" and 100 mm being the "worst possible". VAS measures were collected for the neck, upper back/back of shoulders, mid back, low back, buttocks, thighs and lower legs.

Data analyses

Data were selected for three distinct epochs (minutes 2–4; minutes 15–17; and minutes 27–29) for analysis to represent behaviour over the full 30-minute test interval. Significance in statistical comparisons was set at $p < 0.05$. To calculate the sample size for a three-factor repeated measures design, we used an approximate approach based on a paired t-test for the comparison between chair support. We set out to detect a large effect size ([25]; $d = 0.8$) with power of 0.8 and a significance level set at 0.05 within each group (healthy participants versus those with LBP). A sample size of 14 was required for each group.

Posture and objective measure of comfort

Three-factor repeated measures ANOVAs (with group, condition and epoch) were used to identify any significant main effects or their interactions on the lumbar and thoracolumbar angles. Similarly, a three-factor repeated measures ANOVA was used to identify any

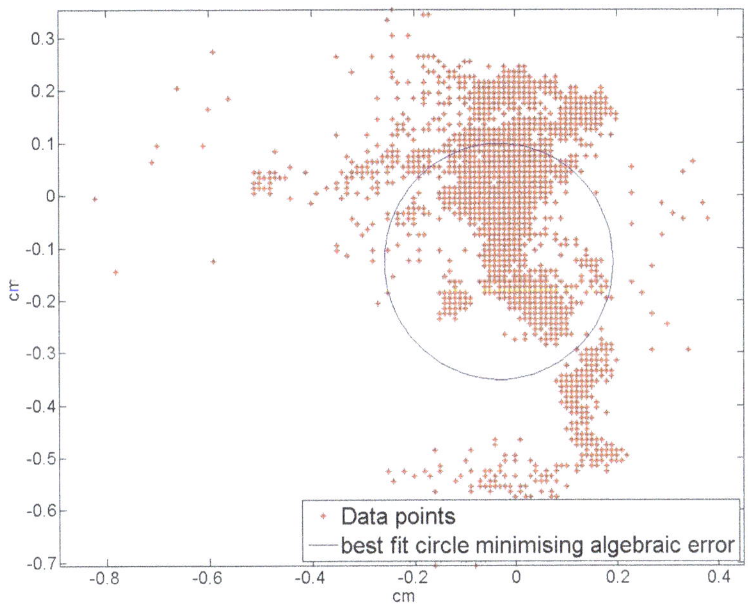

Figure 4 Sample MatLab output of the seated CoP tracing and best fit circle over time.

significant main effects or their interactions on the Least Squares Radius (LSR). There were two levels of group (healthy and LBP), three levels of condition (standing, lumbar support and standard chair), and three time intervals (epochs 1, 2 and 3).

Subjective measure of comfort: VAS

One-factor repeated measures ANCOVAs (baseline VAS measure as covariate) were used to identify any effect of condition (standing, lumbar support and standard chair) on VAS scores for each group separately (healthy individuals and patients with LBP).

T-tests (paired and unpaired where appropriate) employing Holm's method of p-value adjustment were used for all post-hoc pair-wise comparisons following significant ANOVA/ANCOVA results. The R-Project statistical software version 2.12.1 was used for all data analyses (The R Foundation for Statistical Computing, Institut für Statistik und Wahrscheinlichkeitstheorie, Vienna, Austria).

Results

The mean (SD) age for the healthy and LBP groups were 26.3 ± 2.1 years and 27.8 ± 6.1 years, respectively. The mean (SD) height and weight for the healthy and LBP groups were 174.6 ± 13.5 cm and 176.0 ± 9.7 cm (height) and 81.8 ± 11.8 kg and 80.7 ± 12.3 kg (weight), respectively. Furthermore, the mean (SD) of the intensity of the LBP in the patient group were 3.4 (1.6) out of 10 on the VAS. The posture data for only 25 participants were used (11 healthy individuals and 14 patients with LBP) as it was determined during data analysis that the markers had

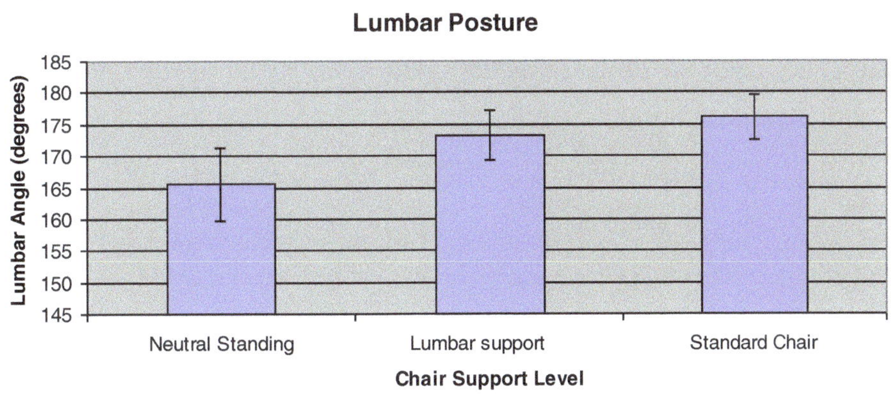

Figure 5 Mean lumbar angle across the standing, lumbar support and regular chair conditions. Error bars represent 95% confidence intervals. Each comparison between all three conditions was significant ($p < 0.05$).

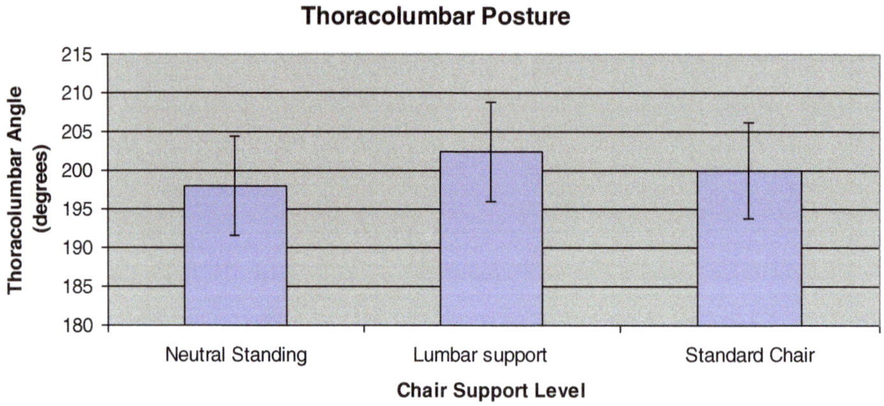

Figure 6 Mean thoracolumbar angle across the standing, lumbar support and regular chair conditions. Error bars represent 95% confidence intervals. Each comparison between all three conditions was significant ($p < 0.05$).

moved during collection for three participants and the data were not accurate. The comfort data from all 28 participants were used for analysis.

Posture

For lumbar angle, there were no significant interaction effects. The main effects of Group and Epoch were not significant. There was a significant main effect of Condition ($p = 0.006$), such that there were differences between each of the conditions. The mean lumbar angle was 7.73° greater with the lumbar support compared to standing (95% CI; 5.15-10.31). The mean lumbar angle was 10.61° greater with the standard chair compared to standing (95% CI; 8.28-12.94). The difference between the lumbar support and standard chair conditions was 2.88° (95% CI; 1.01-4.75). The lumbar support condition was closer to neutral standing than was the standard chair in the lumbar spine. When testing for a significant effect in static stance, the lumbar angle between healthy individuals and patients with LBP was not significantly different. See Figure 5 for a graphical representation of the angle means in the standing, lumbar support and regular chair conditions.

For thoracolumbar angle, there were no significant interaction effects. The main effects of Epoch and Group were not significant. The main effect of Condition was significant ($p = 0.014$), as each of the conditions were different from each other. The mean thoracolumbar angle was 4.39° greater with the lumbar support versus standing (95% CI; 2.21-6.57). The mean thoracolumbar angle was 1.97° greater with the standard chair compared to standing (95% CI; 0.35-3.59). The difference between the lumbar support and standard chair conditions was −2.42° (95% CI; -4.22 to −0.62). The standard chair was closer to neutral standing than was the lumbar support condition in the thoracolumbar spine. When testing for a significant effect in static stance, the thoracolumbar angle between healthy individuals and patients with LBP was not significantly different. Figure 6 illustrates the angle means for the standing, lumbar support and regular chair conditions.

A detailed review of the descriptive statistics for the lumbar and thoracolumbar angles can also be found in Table 1.

Comfort

LSR at buttock-chair interface

Table 2 provides details of the descriptive statistics for the CoP LSR. The results of the three-factor ANOVA for the entire sample of participants suggested that there was a significant effect of Condition ($p = 0.017$) and

Table 1 Means (standard deviations) of lumbar and thoracolumbar angles across condition, group and epoch

		Condition (lumbar support)			Condition (standard chair)		
	Standing	Epoch 1	Epoch 2	Epoch 3	Epoch 1	Epoch 2	Epoch 3
L Angle (°)							
Group (Healthy)	164.84(5.41)	174.23(3 35)	174.43(3.16)	174.54(2.45)	176.33(3.90)	177.07(2.67)	176.66(3.54)
Group (LBP)	166.01(6.15)	171.84(5.42)	172.54(4.11)	172.52(4.40)	176.34(3.97)	175.34(3.91)	175.26(3.44)
TL Angle (°)							
Group (Healthy)	196.08(6.04)	199.75(4.88)	200.52(6.40)	199.85(6.78)	198.27(6.56)	198.95(5.94)	199.01(5.69)
Group (LBP)	199.62(6.43)	204.35(6.33)	204.97(6.06)	203.72(6.66)	200.96(5.97)	200.96(6.45)	201.23(6.91)

Legend: L = lumbar and TL = thoracolumbar.

Table 2 Means (standard deviations) of CoP LSR across condition, group and epoch

	Groups pooled		LBP		Healthy	
Epoch	Condition (lumbar support)	Condition (standard chair)	Condition (lumbar support)	Condition (standard chair)	Condition (lumbar support)	Condition (standard chair)
1	0.305	0.475	0.314	0.510	0.296	0.440
	(0.228)	(0.267)	(0.284)	(0.323)	(0.164)	(0.204)
2	0.447	0.465	0.569	0.533	0.324	0.398
	(0.407)	(0.289)	(0.536)	(0.353)	(0.155)	(0.198)
3	0.468	0.555	0.506	0.720	0.423	0.389
	(0.287)	(0.494)	(0.280)	(0.637)	(0.298)	(0.202)

Epoch (0.028) but not Group ($p = 0.095$). The lack of any significant interaction effects, however, suggested that the effect of Condition was consistent over Epoch, in that the LSR was consistently lower in the lumbar support condition for both healthy and LBP groups than in the standard chair condition, suggesting greater comfort.

VAS scores

When comparing VAS scores between the lumbar support and standard chair conditions, a difference was seen only in the neck region in the LBP group ($p = 0.045$). The VAS was lower with the lumbar support than with the standard chair. However, due to the potential inflation of Type I error (falsely concluding a significant effect) due to the testing being done at seven different sites for each group, when proper adjustment is made for multiple testing using Holm's method, the neck region does not achieve statistical significance. The unadjusted means and standard deviations for the VAS scores for level of discomfort are summarized in Tables 3 and 4.

Discussion

Sitting has been shown to have a higher low back compressive load than standing [26] and deviation from the neutral posture has been linked with increased static muscular effort [3,4]. While past efforts have been made at designing back rest/seat pan combinations that promote a neutral spine [27], lumbar support pillows often do not account for the pelvis and may push the body forward on the seat pan [17]. While several investigators have studied the effect of various lumbar support pillows on asymptomatic individuals [15-17], the current study investigated the effect of a lumbar support pad that accounted for the posterior pelvic bulk on the posture and comfort of healthy individuals and patients with LBP.

Similar to previous studies investigating healthy individuals [15,16], the results of this study indicated that a lumbar support pad was better at increasing (or preserving) the natural lumbar lordosis in sitting in both healthy individuals and patients with LBP. However, the reverse was seen in the thoracolumbar spine, whereby the neutral curvature was increased with the support pad compared to the standard chair. This is not surprising given the closed-chain nature of the seated task. Changes in one region of the spine may be compensated for by changes in other regions along the linked kinetic chain [28]. Furthermore, use of the lumbar pillow often did not allow participants to make contact with the upper part of the back rest, which may account for the thoracolumbar change. Measures of comfort were not negatively affected, suggesting that any compensations that were employed may have been acceptable.

Table 3 Unadjusted mean (standard deviation) VAS scores for each body region in the healthy group

Healthy group (No LBP)	Discomfort VAS (out of 100 mm)		
Location	Baseline (mm)	Standard chair (mm)	Lumbar support (mm)
Neck	2.3 (5.5)	2.6 (4.7)	8.3 (18.0)
Upper Back	2.0 (4.1)	5.4 (7.0)	7.0 (15.0)
Mid Back	2.1 (4.2)	4.8 (7.4)	5.9 (9.8)
Low Back	2.9 (5.1)	4.5 (7.8)	4.5 (8.1)
Buttocks	1.4 (4.2)	4.5 (8.3)	4.2 (6.0)
Thighs	1.6 (4.8)	2.9 (7.1)	1.6 (2.9)
Lower Legs	0.8 (1.6)	1.5 (4.1)	1.4 (3.4)

Table 4 Unadjusted mean (standard deviation) VAS scores for each body region in the LBP group

LBP group	Discomfort VAS (out of 100 mm)		
Location	Baseline (mm)	Standard chair (mm)	Lumbar support (mm)
Neck	11.5 (19.1)	8.7 (10.4)	4.6 (7.0)
Upper Back	6.6 (10.1)	13.8 (20.4)	7.5 (10.7)
Mid Back	12.0 (11.0)	10.6 (9.7)	8.6 (8.1)
Low Back	25.0 (21.1)	19.7 (13.1)	17.7 (17.4)
Buttocks	6.6 (9.1)	10.2 (17.0)	5.3 (8.2)
Thighs	5.3 (13.6)	6.1 (17.5)	3.5 (8.1)
Lower Legs	2.1 (3.2)	6.5 (17.6)	6.1 (14.9)

The amplitude of the postural difference in the lumbar region was small, in the order of 2-3°, and it is unknown whether this degree of change is associated with clinical benefit. Although not directly applicable to the current study, small changes in the order of 2-3° may considerably influence the compressive load at L4-L5 [9], particularly when taking into account the cumulative effect of spinal loading throughout an entire work day. The effect of angular change in the low back, assuming erect seated posture, is multiplied by its action on the position of the center of upper body mass by means of a relatively long moment arm approximating 20% of body height [9]. While it has been shown that the longissimus/iliocostalis muscle fibre angles change when the lumbar spine flexes fully forward [29], the change in orientation with a small amount of flexion is unknown. A cadaveric study has shown that minimal amount of flexion removes the stress peaks in the posterior annulus but may increase stresses in the nucleus and anterior annulus [30].

In addition, the objective measure of comfort was improved in the current study with use of the pillow. The radius of the CoP shifting was lower for the lumbar support condition versus the standard chair in healthy individuals and in patients with LBP. However, the objective changes were not accompanied by subjective improvements, as the current study found no significant effects in reported comfort. While past studies have indicated that 30 minutes of sitting is adequate to determine comfort levels [22], it is possible that longer use of the device would have yielded more significant results. Carcone and Keir [17] noted subjective improvements in the middle lower back and upper back when using a lumbar support pillow for 15 minutes, however, the magnitude of the changes was small and clinical benefit is unknown.

While this study used a pain population and quantified the degree of discomfort in different seating systems, it has some limitations. Firstly, the sensors used for determining the thoracolumbar and lumbar postures were placed on the skin surface. While the electromagnetic equipment and methods used in the current study are commonly adopted in biomechanics research [9], it is possible that a more direct method, such as radiographic measurement, would have yielded more accurate angular changes of the vertebral column [16,31]. The benefit of using the current equipment, however, was that it posed little to no risk to the participants, and it avoided any harmful effects of radiation that are associated with radiographic investigation [16].

Furthermore, while the current authors tested participants with pain, the intensity of the patients' LBP was mild. While all participants with pain had experienced an episode of LBP for at least three consecutive days over the last three consecutive weeks, not all patients were symptomatic at the time of data collection.

This study did not include female participants as it has been shown that the female sitting posture is different from that of males [4]. While it would be interesting to study the effect of the lumbar support pillow on female participants, controlling for gender effects helped reduce the complexity of the analysis and the need for a much larger sample size. Moreover, the foundations of the chair were constrained, lowering arm rests and fixing the base to prevent rolling, to limit alternate strategies for changing comfort other than postural shifts with respect to the seat pan. Finally, while shorter term (30 minutes) static postural environments are reportedly adequate to determine comfort levels [22], the results may not generalize to longer seated exposure.

Future studies investigating the effect of different seating systems on patient postures and symptoms ought to include patients with higher pain levels, longer follow-up and female participants, so as to more realistically replicate the range of demographics and development of symptoms in those who work in seated environments.

While past authors have advocated the quantitative assessment of comfort through CoP shifting [22], the current study employed a novel method of determining CoP shift [23] and its potential to represent the full range relationship of comfort to posture remains to be explored.

Conclusions

Use of a lumbar support pillow that allows space for the posterior pelvic bulk significantly decreased lumbar flattening during sitting in healthy individuals and patients with LBP. However, thoracolumbar curvature was increased. The difference in angular change was small and further study is required to determine clinical relevance over the long term. Furthermore, an objective measure of comfort was improved with the pillow but subjective reports on comfort were not significantly affected. Future studies should investigate the long term clinical benefit of using a lumbar pillow in males and females with a higher intensity of LBP.

Abbreviations

LBP: Low back pain; CoP: Centre of pressure; CMCC: Canadian Memorial Chiropractic College; VAS: Visual analog scale; LSR: Least squares radius.

Competing interests

The authors declare that they have no competing interests.

Authors' contributions

DG participated in the study design, data collection, analysis and manuscript writing. JT participated in the study design, analysis and manuscript writing. ST carried out the data collections, processing and reviewed the manuscript. DS carried out the analysis and reviewed the manuscript. All authors read and approved the final manuscript.

Acknowledgements

All of the author contributions were funded by Mediflow Logic Back™ and CMCC. The funding body, Mediflow Logic Back™, had no direct role in the design, collection, analysis and interpretation of the data. They did not contribute to the writing of the manuscript, nor did they play a role in deciding to submit the manuscript.

Funding

This study was funded by Mediflow Logic Back™ and the Canadian Memorial Chiropractic College.

References

1. *Statistical Supplement to the 2007 Annual Report, Workplace Safety and Insurance Board of Ontario.* [http://www.wsib.on.ca/files/Content/Downloadable%20FileStatisticalSupplement07/2278A.pdf].
2. Lazarus H, Neumann CJ: **Assessing undertreatment of pain: the patient's perspectives.** *J of Pharmaceut Care Pain Symptom Contr* 2001, **9**:5–34.
3. Corlett N, Wilson J, Manenica I: *The Ergonomics of Working Postures.* London: Taylor & Francis; 1986.
4. Dunk NM, Callaghan JP: **Gender-based differences in postural responses to seated exposures.** *Clin Biomech (Bristol, Avon)* 2005, **20**:1101–1110.
5. M-Pranesh A, Rakheja S, Demont R: **Influence of support conditions on vertical whole-body vibration of the seated human body.** *Ind Health* 2010, **48**:682–697.
6. Hedman TP, Fernie GR: **Mechanical response of the lumbar spine to seated postural loads.** *Spine* 1997, **22**:734–743.
7. Nachemson AL: **The load on lumbar disks in different positions of the body.** *Clin Orthop Relat Res* 1966, **45**:107–122.
8. Wilder DG, Pope MH, Frymoyer JW: **The biomechanics of lumbar disc herniation and the effect of overload and instability.** *J Spinal Disord* 1988, **1**:16–32.
9. Chaffin DB, Andersson GBJ, Martin BJ: *Occupational Biomechanics.* 4th edition. New York: John Wiley and Sons; 2006.
10. Andersson BJ, Ortengren R, Nachemson AL, Elfström G, Broman H: **The sitting posture: an electromyographic and discometric study.** *Orthop Clin North Am* 1975, **6**:105–120.
11. Alexander LA, Hancock E, Agouris I, Smith FW, MacSween A: **The response of the nucleus pulposus of the lumbar intervertebral discs to functionally loaded positions.** *Spine* 2007, **32**:1508–1512.
12. Adams MA, Dolan P: **Time-dependent changes in the lumbar spine's resistance to bending.** *Clin Biomech* 1996, **11**:194–200.
13. McGill SM, Brown S: **Creep response of the lumbar spine to prolonged flexion.** *Clin Biomech* 1992, **7**:43–46.
14. Makhsous M, Lin F, Hendrix RW, Hepler M, Zhang L-Q: **Sitting with adjustable ischial and back supports: biomechanical changes.** *Spine* 2003, **28**:1113–1122.
15. Aota Y, Iizuka H, Ishige Y, Mochida T, Yoshihisa T, Uesugi M, Saito T: **The effectiveness of a lumbar support continuous passive motion device in the prevention of low back pain.** *Spine* 2007, **32**:E674–E677.
16. De Carvalho DE, Callaghan JP: **Influence of automobile seat lumbar support prominence on spine and pelvic postures: a radiological investigation.** *Appl Ergon* 2012, **43**:876–822.
17. Carcone SM, Keir PJ: **Effects of backrest design on biomechanics and comfort during seated work.** *Appl Ergon* 2007, **38**:755–764.
18. Alaranta H, Luoto S, Heliövaara M, Hurri H: **Static back endurance and the risk of low back pain.** *Clin Biomech (Bristol, Avon)* 1995, **10**:323–324.
19. Brereton L, McGill SM: **Effects of physical fatigue and cognitive challenges on the potential for low back injury.** *Hum Mov Sci* 1999, **18**:839–857.
20. Reenalda J, Van Geffen P, Nederhand M, Jannink M, IJzerman M, Rietman H: **Analysis of healthy sitting behavior: interface pressure distribution and subcutaneous tissue oxygenation.** *J Rehabil Res Dev* 2009, **46**:577–586.
21. Fenety A, Walker JM: **Short-term effects of workstation exercises on musculoskeletal discomfort and postural changes in seated video display unit workers.** *Phys Ther* 2002, **82**:578–589.
22. Fenety PA, Putnam C, Walker JM: **In-chair movement: validity, reliability and implications for measuring sitting discomfort.** *Appl Ergon* 2000, **31**:383–393.
23. Gander W, Golub GH, Strebel R: **Least-squares fitting of circles and ellipses.** *BIT* 1994, **34**:558–578.
24. Corlett EN, Bishop RP: **A technique for assessing postural discomfort.** *Ergonomics* 1976, **19**:175–182.
25. Cohen J: *Statistical Power Analysis for the Behavioral Sciences.* 2nd edition. Hillsdale, New Jersey: Lawrence Erlbaum Associates; 1988.
26. Callaghan JP, McGill SM: **Low back joint loading and kinematics during standing and unsupported sitting.** *Ergonomics* 2001, **44**:280–294.
27. Lengsfeld M, Frank A, Van Deursen DL, Griss P: **Lumbar spine curvature during office chair sitting.** *Med Eng Phys* 2000, **22**:665–669.
28. Oatis CA: *Kinesiology: The Mechanics & Pathomechanics of Human Movement.* 2nd edition. Baltimore: Lippincott Williams & Wilkins; 2009.
29. McGill SM, Hughson RL, Parks K: **Changes in lumbar lordosis modify the role of the extensor muscles.** *Clin Biomech* 2000, **15**:777–780.
30. Adams MA, McNally DS, Chinn H, Dolan P: **Posture and the compressive strength of the lumbar spine.** *Clin Biomech* 1994, **9**:5–14.
31. Vergara M, Page A, Sancho JL: **Analysis of lumbar flexion in sitting posture: location of lumbar vertebrae with relation to easily identifiable skin marks.** *Int J Ind Ergonom* 2006, **36**:937–942.

A pilot randomized controlled trial comparing the efficacy of exercise, spinal manipulation, and neuro emotional technique for the treatment of pregnancy-related low back pain

Caroline D Peterson[1*], Mitchell Haas[2] and W Thomas Gregory[3]

Abstract

Background: This pilot randomized controlled trial evaluated the feasibility of conducting a full scale study and compared the efficacy of exercise, spinal manipulation, and a mind-body therapy called Neuro Emotional Technique for the treatment of pregnancy-related low back pain, a common morbidity of pregnancy.

Methods: Healthy pregnant women with low back pain of insidious onset were eligible to enroll in the study at any point in their pregnancy. Once enrolled, they remained in the study until they had their babies. Women were randomly allocated into one of three treatment groups using opaque envelopes. The treatment schedule paralleled the prenatal care schedule and women received individualized intervention. Our null hypothesis was that spinal manipulation and Neuro Emotional Technique would perform no better than exercise in enhancing function and decreasing pain. Our primary outcome measure was the Roland Morris Disability Questionnaire and our secondary outcome measure was the Numeric Pain Rating Scale. Intention to treat analysis was conducted. For the primary analysis, regression was conducted to compare groups on the outcome measure scores. In a secondary responder analysis, difference in proportions of participants in attaining 30% and 50% improvement were calculated. Feasibility factors for conducting a future larger trial were also evaluated such as recruitment, compliance to study protocols, cost, and adverse events.

Results: Fifty-seven participants were randomized into the exercise (n = 22), spinal manipulation (n = 15), and Neuro Emotional Technique (n = 20) treatment arms. At least 50% of participants in each treatment group experienced clinically meaningful improvement in symptoms for the Roland Morris Disability Questionnaire. At least 50% of the exercise and spinal manipulation participants also experienced clinically meaningful improvement for the Numeric Pain Rating Scale. There were no clinically meaningful or statistically significant differences between groups in any analysis.

Conclusions: This pilot study demonstrated feasibility for recruitment, compliance, safety, and affordability for conducting a larger study in the future. Spinal manipulation and exercise generally performed slightly better than did Neuro Emotional Technique for improving function and decreasing pain, but the study was not powered to detect the between-group differences as statistically significant.

Trial registration: ClinicalTrials.gov (Identifier: NCT00937365).

* Correspondence: drcaroline@fertilegroundcenter.com
[1]Private Practice, Portland, OR, USA
Full list of author information is available at the end of the article

Background

Pregnancy-related low back pain (PRLBP) is pain of insidious onset in the lumbar or sacroiliac region that begins during pregnancy [1,2]. Over half of all pregnant women experience PRLBP [3,4] and the natural trajectory of the condition is intensification of pain over the course of pregnancy [2,5]. Low back pain experienced due to pregnancy is poorly understood and conjectured to result from suboptimal biomechanics [6], an increase in relaxin [7], or the evolution to bipedalism [8]. The literature on risk factors for PRLBP is inconsistent. In a summary review of 25 studies of risk factors for PRLBP the only consistent risk factor was a history of lumbar, pubic symphysis, or sacroiliac pain [9].

PRLBP is often (68%) unreported to health care providers [4], despite two thirds of pregnant women requiring sick leave secondary to PRLBP [10]. Of those mothers who report pain, only 25% are given recommendations for symptom management [4]. Over one third of untreated women continue to experience low back pain in the year after pregnancy [4,11,12]; this trend persists up to six years postpartum [13]. Those women who continue to experience low back pain in the postpartum are also more susceptible to concomitant morbidities such as postpartum depression [14]. For these reasons effective management of PRLBP is important to investigate.

Exercise [15], spinal manipulative therapy (SMT) [16,17], and a mind-body therapy called Neuro Emotional Technique (NET) that addresses the emotional component of a condition [18] have been demonstrated to be effective treatments for low back pain in non-pregnant populations. Exercise [19,20] and chiropractic SMT [21,22] have also been demonstrated to decrease PRLBP, however the quality of the chiropractic SMT studies is poor to moderate [23]. One pilot randomized controlled trial of osteopathic SMT for PRLBP was identified [24]. In that study no high velocity low amplitude thrusts were used. The study reported PRLBP did improve in the treatment group, but did not reach statistical significance when compared to the control group. Roland Morris disability scores worsened in all groups, although the control group worsened more than the treatment group. No studies were identified that evaluated NET for the treatment of PRLBP.

Our pilot study responded to the Cochrane Review's call for more research on the treatment of PRLBP [2]. In this study we evaluated the feasibility of conducting a larger randomized trial with consideration to recruitment, compliance to study protocols, cost, and adverse events. The pilot was also designed to compare the three treatment groups in order to estimate an effect size for disability and pain outcomes to inform the sample size of a future randomized controlled trial.

Methods

Design

This pilot parallel group design randomized controlled trial was conducted at Oregon Health & Science University through the Department of Obstetrics & Gynecology between August 2009 and April 2011. A total of 57 participants were enrolled. The trial evaluated the relative efficacy [25] of individualized treatment with exercise (control) (n = 22), SMT (n = 15), or NET (n = 20) for pregnancy-related low back pain. The intervention is discussed in detail below. Our primary null hypothesis was that SMT and NET performed no better than exercise for the treatment of PRLBP as measured by the Roland Morris Disability Questionnaire. Our secondary null hypothesis was that SMT and NET performed no better than exercise for the treatment of PRLBP as measured by an 11-point Numeric Pain Rating Scale.

All participants gave oral and written informed consent and received $20 for each study visit, which took about one hour to complete. The study was approved by Oregon Health & Science University's Institutional Review Board.

Study participants

Women were eligible for the study if they were pregnant with a singleton and had low back pain of unknown origin that began during pregnancy and was reproducible by manual palpation. Women with health conditions that contraindicated exercise (heart disease, diabetes, thyroid disease, hypertension, Body Mass Index greater than 40, infection, incompetent cervix, bleeding, ruptured membranes, severe anemia, intrauterine growth restriction, poorly controlled seizure disorder, thrombophlebitis, decreased fetal movement, amniotic fluid leakage) [26] or manipulation (unrelenting fever, unrelenting night pain, loss of bowel or bladder control, progressive neurological deficit, direct trauma, unexplained weight loss, radiating pain below the knee, cancer, spinal fracture or tumors, blood dyscrasias) [27] were excluded from consideration along with women who smoked, consumed alcohol, were medicated with anti-depressants, or had a Roland Morris score above 20 or below 4 [28]. Women were also excluded if they were planning to move during pregnancy, did not read and write English, were not willing to comply with the study visit schedule, or were not willing to be randomized into any of the treatment arms.

Before being randomized participants identified their treatment preference (*i.e.* exercise, SMT, NET, or none). Treatment preference is a well known predictor of outcomes and thus is a potential confounding variable [29-31]. The randomization schedule was completed prior to initiating the study and was concealed from all study staff by using consecutively numbered, sealed, opaque envelopes for each strata of preference group. Once a participant was found to be eligible, she would open the consecutive envelope in her preference strata in the presence of the researcher. Participants and the practitioner providing the intervention were not blinded to the intervention after randomization.

Study protocol

Study participants were recruited by fliers in prenatal clinics and by community, magazine, and internet announcements in the Portland, Oregon metropolitan area. Potential participants were first screened by phone and if study eligibility requirements were met, the initial study visit was scheduled. At the initial screening and prior to randomization each treatment group was described so all participants were familiar with all treatments. Participants could enter the study at any point in their pregnancy and remained in the study until they had their baby. All participants continued to receive their usual obstetric or midwifery prenatal care following randomization. The RCT treatment schedule paralleled the prenatal care schedule (once monthly until 28 weeks gestation, twice monthly until 36 weeks gestation, and weekly thereafter).

When the participant arrived for each study treatment visit she completed the primary and secondary outcome measures, drew a pain diagram, and responded to questions about adverse events, treatment by other practitioners, new injuries, and use of medication. After filling out the paperwork all participants were palpated and assessed with standard orthopedic and neurologic exams to ensure they were safe to treat. Each was also palpated to determine if intersegmental dysfunctions were present. Following the assessment each participant was treated in accordance with the protocol for their treatment arm, which is described below.

Intervention

The lead author served as the therapist and has practiced chiropractic medicine for 15 years. At the baseline visit she screened volunteers for study eligibility through case history and standard orthopedic and neurologic tests. Participants in all three treatment groups were advised to use ice after each treatment since a little soreness is commonly experienced after treatment.

Exercise

Exercise participants were given a booklet and enthusiastically instructed on pelvic tilts, pelvic floor, gluteus maximus, latissimus dorsi, and hip adductor strengthening exercises to promote low back stability and flexibility. The specific exercises in the booklet have been shown to decrease PRLBP [32]. The booklet also instructed exercise participants on recommendations for postural and movement patterns that help alleviate low back pain. Finally, warnings in the booklet about when to stop exercising were reviewed with the participant. At each study visit exercises and lifestyle suggestions were reviewed and practiced with participants. Additional individualized stretching or strengthening exercises were prescribed, demonstrated, and practiced at each study visit based on muscle strength and flexibility assessment. Exercises took about 15 min to perform at home and participants were requested to exercise five times weekly.

Spinal Manipulative Therapy

Participants in the SMT group were palpated to determine if each had intersegmental dysfunction prior to manipulating [33]. Hypomobile joints were isolated through positioning, then a slow force was applied to preload the joint at the physiological end range. After loading the joint, a high velocity, low amplitude thrust was applied to the isolated joint to move it just past the physiological end range in the side posture position for lumbar and sacroiliac lesions. The thrust was applied in the direction, velocity, and amplitude as determined by the clinician from the palpation exam findings [33]. A hypermobile joint or region was stabilized by creating a fulcrum at a specific joint by the participant lying on padded blocks [34]. The blocks were always used to adjust a Sacro Occipital Technique Category II pelvis, and the Activator was always used to adjust the pubic symphysis [35].

Neuro emotional technique

Neuro Emotional Technique (NET) is a chiropractic mind-body technique that combines desensitization procedures (such as relaxed breathing and visualization) with elements of Five Element Chinese medicine (such as the association of emotions with certain organs or meridians) and chiropractic medicine (the adjustment of the spinal levels that innervate the organ in question) in an attempt to address cognitive distortions through the use of a semantic algorithm [36]. The reliability and validity of the manual muscle testing used to guide the technique are unknown [37], but muscle testing is considered to be part of the treatment package of NET. The NET standard protocol was followed [38].

Outcomes

At each assessment visit, each participant completed a form indicating if she was following the study protocol, was taking any pain medication, had been injured outside of the study, or had experienced any adverse effects as a result of the intervention. Participants were asked to rate their low back function and pain "today" as measured by the Roland Morris Disability Questionnaire (primary outcome) and an 11-point Numeric Pain Rating Scale (secondary outcome). The Roland Morris Disability Questionnaire is a 24-item index of activities of daily living related to low back function that has been shown to be valid, reliable, and sensitive for measuring changes in mild to moderate disability [39,40]. The 11-point Numeric Pain Rating Scale (0–10) has been shown to be valid [41]. A four point change on the Roland Morris Disability Questionnaire, a two point change on the Numeric Pain Rating Scale, or a 30% change in either from the baseline is considered to be clinically meaningful within-persons [41-44].

Statistical analysis

Intention-to-treat analysis was conducted with participants included in the original assigned group. In the primary analysis, linear regression was used to compare the three groups with follow-up disability and pain scores as continuous dependent variables. The covariates included in all between group models were gestational age at entrance into the study, baseline score of the outcome measure, maternal age, and history of low back pain. The endpoint was the eighth study visit assessment or the last study visit if the participant did not complete eight visits.

A secondary responder analysis was conducted for the Roland Morris Disability Questionnaire and Numeric Pain Rating Scale. Two categorical outcome variables were created to reflect a minimum of 50% improvement (yes/no), and a minimum of 30% improvement (yes/no). Differences in the proportion of responders between groups were then calculated. Thirty percent improvement is considered to be the minimal change needed to identify clinically meaningful improvement [44,45]. However, 50% improvement is typically the standard used in responder analysis [46,47].

Missing data were imputed using the last observation carried forward [48,49]. Although last observation carried forward method of controlling for missingness is biased toward participants not worsening over the remaining segment of the study, we elected to use this method so our results could be compared with a similarly designed osteopathic trial of treatment for pregnancy related low back pain [24]. To determine if this approach was appropriate for our data, we also conducted a sensitivity analysis excluding participants with only baseline data.

Statistical significance was set at 0.05 for all tests with no correction for multiple group comparisons. Sample size was limited by available funds and the enrollment window established for this pilot; it was not determined by *a priori* power analysis. A post hoc power analysis was conducted to identify what effect sizes were detectable with 80% power at the 0.05 level of significance. A study is said to be adequately powered if the detectable effect size is no larger than a clinically important difference between groups. Statistical analysis was performed with SPSS v18.0 (SPSS, Inc, Chicago, IL).

Results

We screened 138 pregnant women (approximately 10 per month) for eligibility and 57 were randomized (Figure 1). Twenty-two participants were randomized into the exercise group, 20 were randomized into the NET group, and 15 were randomized into the SMT group. Six exercise participants and one NET participant discontinued the study after the first visit for reasons listed in Figure 1.

Participant baseline characteristics

Baseline health characteristics and demographics were somewhat balanced across groups (Tables 1, 2 and 3). Women in the exercise group were less likely to be married, to work during pregnancy, and to have good or quite good self-perceived general health status prior to pregnancy. Additionally, their low back pain began earlier in pregnancy and they were more likely to be taking medication for pain, and to have missed work because of the pain than were the women in the other treatment groups. Finally, women in the exercise group also entered the study earlier in their pregnancies than those in the NET or SMT groups, and perhaps because of this had a lower BMI at their first study visit. If the seven women who withdrew from the study immediately upon randomization were not included in the descriptive analysis, the study groups were balanced across all variables except women in the exercise group were less likely to have good or quite good health prior to pregnancy.

Outcomes data

The majority in all three groups had clinically meaningful improvement in function (4 point or 30% improvement on the Roland-Morris), and the majority of participants in the exercise and SMT groups also had clinically meaningful improvement in pain (2 point or 30% improvement on the numeric rating scale) (Tables 4 & 5). The SMT group attained a minimal clinical important improvement in 80% of the participants for function and 67% for pain. Smaller proportions were observed in the other two groups.

Between-groups comparisons

No statistically significant differences between groups were noted in either the Roland Morris Disability Questionnaire or Numeric Pain Rating Scale scores in the pair-wise comparison of treatment groups in either the

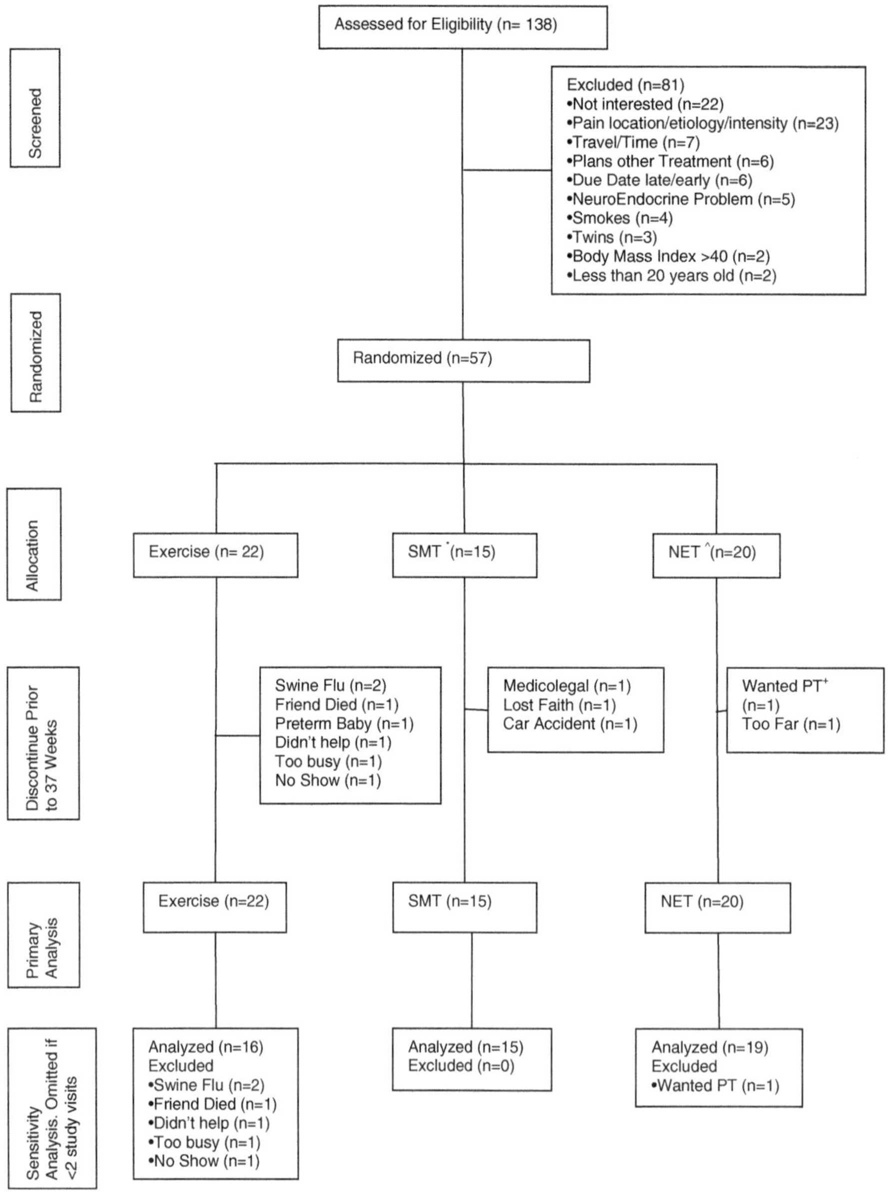

Figure 1 Flow of Participants Through the Trial.

primary or secondary analyses (Tables 6 & 7). All confidence intervals were wide for the between-groups comparisons, demonstrating imprecision in the treatment effect point estimates and lack of power to detect differences between groups.

Sensitivity analysis

The results of the sensitivity analysis were consistent with the primary analysis when the seven individuals with only baseline data were excluded. One comparison (Exercise *vs.* NET) became statistically significant for the Numeric Pain Rating Scale. The primary analysis was the most conservative analysis performed. This suggests that our method of imputing missing data using last observation carried forward did not bias our results toward the group with more dropouts, as is sometimes the case.

Post hoc power analysis

The study had 80% power to detect mean between-group differences of approximately 4.7 points on the Roland-Morris and 1.8 points on the Numeric Pain Rating Scale at the .05 level of significance. The study was not powered to detect a minimal clinically important differences between groups [50,51].

Table 1 Baseline demographics of participants by treatment group and total

Variable	Exercise (n = 22)	NET (n = 20)	SMT (n = 15)	Total (n = 57)
	Mean (SD) or n (%)	Mean (SD) or n (%)	Mean (SD) or n (%)	Mean (SD) or n (%)
Age, years	28.7 (5.1)	29.7 (5.5)	31.1 (4.2)	29.7 (5.0)
Race/ethnicity				
White	17 (77.3%)	17 (65.0%)	10 (66.7%)	44 (77.2%)
Black	0	0	2 (13.3%)	2 (3.5%)
Asian	1 (4.5%)	0	1 (6.7%)	2 (3.5%)
Hispanic	4 (18.2%)	3 (15.0%)	2 (13.3%)	9 (15.8%)
Education				
High School or Less	5 (22.7%)	2 (10.0%)	2 (13.3%)	9 (16.3%)
Some College or Tech/Trade School	7 (31.8%)	9 (45.0%)	5 (33.3%)	21 (36.8%)
4 Year College	6 (27.3%)	2 (10.0%)	6 (40.0%)	14 (24.6%)
Graduate School	4 (18.2%)	7 (35.0%)	2 (7.4%)	13 (22.8%)
Married	13 (59.1%)	17 (85.0%)	11 (73.3%)	41 (71.9%)
Work During Pregnancy	15 (68.2%)	17 (85.0%)	12 (80.0%)	44 (77.2%)

*SMT = Spinal Manipulative Therapy, ^NET = Neuro Emotional Technique, +PT = Physical Therapy.

Feasibility evaluation

Adherence to care

Three of the 16 exercise participants who had more than one study visit did not follow the prescribed study visit schedule. Because study participants could enter the study at any point in their pregnancy, 5 (23%) exercise participants, 6 (30%) NET participants, and 3 (20%) SMT participants completed eight study visits. Seven (38%) of the exercise participants who had more than one study visit reported that they did not perform their exercises at least five times a week. However, all seven reported between 40% - 100% improvement in function. Five of the seven reported 50%-75% improvement in pain intensity; pain intensity did not change for one participant and worsened for another who did not perform her exercises regularly.

Table 2 Baseline health characteristics of participants by treatment group and total

Variable	Exercise (n = 22)	NET (n = 20)	SMT (n = 15)	Total (n = 57)
	Mean (SD) or n (%)	Mean (SD) or n (%)	Mean (SD) or n (%)	Mean (SD) or n (%)
Gravida	3* (1.8)	2* (2.3)	3* (2.7)	3* (1.9)
Para	0* (1.2)	1* (1.3)	1* (0.9)	1* (1.1)
Body Mass Index at study start	26.9 (3.9)	28.2 (4.4)	29.3 (4.4)	27.9 (4.3)
Took Medication for Pain at Study Start	4 (18.2%)	2 (10.0%)	1 (6.7%)	7 (12.3%)
Very Good or Quite Good Health Prior to Pregnancy	18 (81.8%)	20 (100.0%)	15 (100.0%)	53 (93%)
Exercised Prior to Pregnancy				
Daily	4 (18.2%)	5 (25.0%)	2 (13.3%)	11 (19.3%)
Weekly	9 (40.9%)	8 (40.0%)	7 (46.7%)	24 (42.1%)
Occasional	6 (27.3%)	6 (30.0%)	6 (40.0%)	18 (31.6%)
Never	3 (13.6%)	1 (5.0%)	0	4 (7.0%)
History of low back pain	10 (45%)	13 (65%)	8 (53%)	31 (54%)
Gestational age at onset of this episode	11.7 (6.1)	13.9 (6.6)	16.1 (5.8)	25.4 (6.4)
Sick Leave due to PRLBP	5 (33%)	4 (24%)	2 (17%)	11 (25%)
Pain Location				
Lumbosacral	10 (45.5%)	12 (60.0%)	7 (46.7%)	29 (50.9%)
Pelvis	6 (27.3%)	4 (20.0%)	2 (13.3%)	12 (21.0%)
Lumbar	3 (13.6%)	3 (15.0%)	2 (13.3%)	8 (14.0%)
Composite	3 (13.6%)	1 (5.0%)	2 (13.3%)	6 (10.5%)

*Median.

Table 3 Treatment and gestational age

Variable	Exercise (n = 22)	NET (n = 20)	SMT (n = 15)	Total (n = 57)
	Mean (SD) or n (%)	Mean (SD) or n (%)	Mean (SD) or n (%)	Mean (SD) or n (%)
Gestational age				
Baseline	23.7 (7.5)	27.0 (5.8)	25.7 (5.3)	25.4 (6.4)
Follow-up*	33.0 (8.0)	35.9 (4.8)	36.2 (4.5)	34.8 (6.3)
Treatment Preference at baseline.				
No Preference	6 (27.3%)	5 (25.0%)	4 (26.7%)	15 (26.3%)
Exercise	2 (9.1%)	2 (10.0%)	2 (13.3%)	6 (10.5%)
NET	7 (31.8%)	6 (30.0%)	3 (20.0%)	16 (28.1%)
SMT	7 (31.8%)	7 (35.0%)	6 (40.0%)	20 (35.1%)
Total number of treatments	5.4 (0.7%)	7.8 (0.9%)	7.5 (0.6%)	6.8 (3.5%)

* Gestational Age at the last visit (for which outcomes were used in the analysis).

Study costs

The study cost for recruitment, participation, software, and supplies was approximately $210 per participant. A subsample also participated in more extensive data collection and a three month postpartum follow-up that will be reported in a future article. The subsample's additional expense for participation, lab work, and maternal-infant attachment assessment were approximately $250 for each person.

Care outside the study

Only two NET study participants reported accessing care for their low back pain outside of the study. One of these NET participants did so after she injured her back lifting a box and required care while the study clinician was out of town. A third exercise participant failed to report whether she had sought care for her low back pain outside of the study at one of the study visits.

Adverse outcomes

No adverse events were reported by study participants in any group. However, 6% of exercise and SMT study visits produced soreness, while 18% of NET study visits produced soreness.

Participant feedback

Study participants were asked for feedback about the study when they reached 37 weeks gestation. All women reported enjoying participating in the study. All but one mother surveyed reported satisfaction with the improvement she experienced in symptoms or in stabilization of symptoms. Because pregnancy-related low back pain worsens over the course of pregnancy, women were satisfied with their outcome even if symptoms did not improve because they compared their pain and disability for this pregnancy with those from a previous pregnancy.

I found the study very helpful in getting rid of a large amount of pain I have been experiencing since the beginning of my pregnancy. The exercise allowed me to do activities that otherwise would have been too painful to participate in, and I believe it has helped prepare my body for labor and after the baby arrives (EX19).

I noticed a dramatic decrease in the amount and intensity of the low back pain I experienced. I also was able to become aware of some issues regarding this pregnancy and my past that I wasn't aware of consciously. That was helpful because it made me make more of an effort to bond with this baby when sometimes I would feel distracted (*i.e.* when work/family responsibilities would take over) (NET05).

Table 4 Roland morris disability questionnaire within-group continuous and categorical comparisons for pre- and post-intervention

	Continuous data		Categorical data		
	Baseline	Endpoint	4+ Point Improve	30% Improve	50% Improve
	Mean (SD)	Mean (SD)			
Exercise (n = 22)	10.7 (4.9)	6.1 (5.9)	60%	68%	55%
NET (n = 20)	9.3 (3.7)	5.7 (4.7)	60%	60%	50%
SMT (n = 15)	8.7 (4.1)	4.1 (4.3)	50%	80%	67%

* Significance of raw score change using a repeated-measures *t*-test.

Table 5 Numeric pain rating scale within-group continuous and categorical comparisons for pre- and post-intervention

	Continuous data		Categorical data		
	Baseline	Endpoint	2+ Point improve	30% Improve	50% Improve
	Mean (SD)	Mean (SD)			
Exercise (n = 22)	3.9 (1.5)	2.4 (1.8)	55%	64%	55%
NET (n = 20)	3.2 (1.4)	2.4 (1.6)	35%	45%	35%
SMT (n = 15)	3.5 (1.1)	1.9 (1.7)	60%	67%	53%

* Significance of raw score change using a repeated measures *t*-test.

I think the study was really good for me. I feel much better, the pain decreased a lot. I also think that my baby liked it. I really enjoy being on this study and I definitely recommend it for all pregnant women. It also helped me to feel more relaxed (SMT05).

Discussion

This was the first identified RCT to compare the relative efficacy of three conservative interventions for the treatment of PRLBP and to show improvement in pain and function with care. The function and pain improvement within the SMT and exercise groups were clinically meaningful (dependent *t*-test $p < 0.002$)). This is important because the only other RCT identified to use manual medicine intervention for the treatment of PRLBP was an osteopathic pilot study that found Roland Morris Disability scores worsened over time in all groups, but function deteriorated less in the osteopathic manipulation group than in the placebo or control group. They also found pain intensity improved by less than half a point on a 11-point pain scale in the osteopathic manipulation group, and there was no statistically significant difference from the placebo or control groups [24]. In the osteopathic pilot RCT [24], our pilot RCT, and other studies [4] PRLBP was mild to moderate in severity and provoked mild to moderate disability. Participants in our study had Roland Morris scores that were approximately 2 points worse at study entrance than those in the osteopathic study. Our participants experienced Numeric Pain Rating Scale scores that were about 1 point less intense than in the osteopathic study. In contrast to the osteopathic PRLBP pilot our participants experienced more improvement in their Roland Morris scores than in their pain scores. This could be due to a floor effect for the pain score since our baseline pain measures were lower than in the osteopathic study.

We have demonstrated the feasibility of recruiting a sufficient sample in a reasonable time for a future full-scale RCT and that there is reasonable adherence to treatment and compliance with follow-up. We found that only 11% of our study participants preferred to be randomized into the exercise group while 28% preferred NET and 35% preferred SMT. This could explain, in part, why we had 27% attrition from the exercise group immediately following randomization while only one participant (5%) in the NET arm withdrew immediately following randomization, and no SMT participants withdrew immediately following randomization. Exercise appears to appeal to only a sub-group of women. Thus, because all treatments were associated with some improvement, a future large randomized controlled trial for the conservative treatment of pregnancy-related low back pain might consider comparing SMT, which performed better than other treatment interventions and was preferred by participants, to a standard of care control group so the number of participants in each study arm would be reasonable to recruit and retain.

It is important to further investigate conservative intervention options such as manual medicine, exercise, and mind-body therapy for the treatment of PRLBP, since pharmaceutical management of pain during pregnancy has been poorly researched and the short- and long-term consequences of pharmaceutical management during pregnancy are largely unknown for the mother and the fetus [52]. Additionally, passive intervention for the treatment of PRLBP using support belts is not well substantiated by the literature [53]. In non-pregnant populations the use of support belts promotes deconditioning and the possibility of injury [54]. The potential safety of exercise, SMT, and NET for a pregnant population with low back pain was demonstrated in this pilot study and paralleled the safety demonstrated for SMT in non-pregnant populations [17,23,55-58]. If safety and effectiveness can be demonstrated in a larger study of conservative intervention for PRLBP, chiropractic care for PRLPB might be a valuable option since chiropractic low back pain management is approximately 60% more cost effective in a non-pregnant population than traditional biomedical care after controlling for case complexity [59]. Finally, although this pilot study was not powered for generalizability, it did substantiate other reports that exercise and manual medicine care for PRLBP are beneficial with low associated risk [21,23,60].

Another reason it is important to further investigate the treatment of PRLBP is because it appears to signify an underlying weakness in the musculoskeletal system

Table 6 Roland morris disability questionnaire between-group comparisons

Comparison groups	Outcome score			30% Improvement		50% Improvement	
	Crude mean difference (95% CI)	Adjusted mean difference[1] (95% CI)	P	Crude proportional difference (95% CI)	P	Crude proportional difference (95% CI)	P
Ex[2] vs NET	−0.3 (−3.7, 3.0)	0.7 (−2.9, 4.2)	.712	0.08 (−0.21, 0.37)	.530	0.05 (−0.26, 0.36)	.760
Ex[2] vs SMT	−2.0 (−5.6, 1.6)	0.01 (−3.2, 3.2)	.995	−0.12 (−0.41, 0.17)	.420	−0.12 (−0,45, 0.21)	.239
SMT[2] vs NET	1.6 (−1.5, 4.8)	1.2 (−2.1, 4.5)	.453	0.2 (−0.13, 0.53)	.881	0.18 (−0.06, 0.42)	.841

[1] Adjusted for Gestational Age at entrance into the study, Outcome Measure score at baseline, Maternal age, and history of low back pain using linear regression for testing adjusted mean differences of outcome scores.

[2] Reference Category: A positive mean difference favors the reference category.

Table 7 Numeric pain rating scale between-group comparisons

Comparison groups	Outcome score			30% Improvement		50% Improvement	
	Crude mean difference (95% CI)	Adjusted mean difference[1] (95% CI)	P	Crude proportional difference (95% CI)	P	Crude proportional difference (95% CI)	P
Ex[2] vs NET	−0.1 (−1.1, 1.0)	0.1 (−1.0, 1.3)	.818	0.19 (−0.12, 0.50)	.898	0.20 (−0.11, 0.51	.894
Ex[2] vs SMT	−0.5 (−1.8, 0.7)	−0.3 (−1.5, 1.0)	.656	−0.03 (−0.34, 0.28)	.425	0.02 (−0.29, 0.33)	.552
SMT[2] vs NET	0.5 (−0.7, 1.6)	0.5 (−0.8, 1.7)	.442	0.22 (−0.09, 0.53)	.916	0.18 (−0.13, 0.49)	.871

[1] Adjusted for Gestational Age at entrance into the study, Outcome Measure score at baseline, Maternal age, and history of low back pain using linear regression for testing adjusted mean differences of outcome scores[2] Reference Category: A positive mean difference favors the reference category.

that, if not addressed during pregnancy, portends future suffering. Women who experience PRLBP and are not treated during pregnancy are at increased risk of experiencing back pain at 3, 6, and 12 months postpartum, and at 3 and 6 years postpartum when compared with women who did not have back pain during pregnancy and women who had back pain during pregnancy and received treatment [13,61,62]. Treatment of PRLBP might not only alleviate low back pain during pregnancy, but could prevent future episodes of low back pain thus saving the health care system unnecessary expenditures [63]. Pregnancy is widely conceptualized as a testing ground for unmasking weaknesses in organ systems that would not appear until later life but for pregnancy [64]. Pregnancy disorders predicting later related health problems have been best established for gestational diabetes predicting diabetes type II [65] and for preeclampsia predicting chronic hypertension [66]. Biomechanical evidence suggests that the female lumbar spine is well designed to respond to fetal load [8], thus PRLBP is not necessarily an inherent morbidity of pregnancy, but might be another warning sign of future ill health just as are gestational diabetes and preeclampsia.

Limitations and future directions

This feasibility study was designed to inform the construction of a future sufficiently powered RCT of PRLBP. Several limitations flawed this study. One major limitation was that the first author conducted all aspects of the trail including provision of care to all study participants. As a result, she was not blinded to intervention during the analysis phase, insufficient time was available for satisfactory recruiting, and treatment effects could be related to investigator proclivities rather than to the modalities themselves. In a future well funded study separate individuals will randomize participants, treat participants, and analyze the data. Also, more active engagement of prenatal care practitioners can be ensured to enhance recruitment by building on the relationships that were formed during this study.

Another limitation was that allowing women to enter the study at any point in their pregnancy made it difficult for latecomers to complete the treatment protocols before birth and also complicated the analysis. We suggest the next trial should be designed so women enter the study at approximately the same point in pregnancy (*e.g.* 28–32 weeks) and complete the eight study visits by 37 weeks gestation. Toward the beginning of the study we also had difficulty retaining the first women who were randomized into the exercise treatment arm. By mid-study we had resolved that issue by strenuous vetting of potential participants to be certain they were willing to participate in the exercise arm of the study.

Finally, the imputation method of last observation carried forward could bias the outcome in favor of the treatment group that had more people who withdrew early in the study or for the group with more women who arrived at their 8th study visit earlier in pregnancy. This is so because low back pain tends to intensify throughout pregnancy. However, we found that the results for the exercise group and NET group were worse when the seven participants who only had baseline measures were included. This suggests imputation by last observation carried forward was a conservative means of inferring outcome and did not prejudicially preference the group with early withdrawals in our study.

Conclusion

This pilot RCT demonstrated that a larger study is feasible in terms of recruitment in a reasonable timeframe, adequate adherence to care, compliance with follow-up, and safety. All three interventions appear to provide clinically meaningful improvement in function and pain intensity. However, although no between-groups differences were noted in function and pain intensity following treatment, exercise and SMT might have larger treatment effect sizes than does NET. All three interventions merit further investigation.

Competing interests

This study was funded in part by The ONE Foundation, the research division of the Neuro Emotional Technique. The ONE Foundation did not contribute to the study in any other way. The authors declare that they have no competing interests.

Authors' contributions

CDP was responsible for all aspects of the study including study design, recruitment, randomization, treatment, analysis and interpretation of findings, and manuscript preparation. MH was involved in study design, logistics, interpretation of findings, and manuscript preparation. WTG was involved in study design, acquisition of funding, logistics, and manuscript preparation. All authors read and approved the final manuscript.

Acknowledgements

This study was funded by The ONE Foundation and The Tartar Foundation. CDP was funded by the National Center for Complementary & Alternative Medicine/National Institutes of Health T32AT0026888. MH was funded by the University of Western States. WTG was funded by National Institute of Child Health & Human Development/National Institutes of Health RO1 HD049541.

Author details

[1]Private Practice, Portland, OR, USA. [2]Division of Research, University of Western States, Portland, OR, USA. [3]Department of Obstetrics & Gynecology, Oregon Health & Science University, Portland, OR, USA.

References

1. Vleeming A, Albert HB, Ostgaard HC, Sturesson B, Stuge B: **European guidelines for the diagnosis and treatment of pelvic girdle pain.** *Eur Spine J* 2008, **17**:794–819.
2. Pennick V, Young G: **Interventions for preventing and treating pelvic and back pain in pregnancy.** *Cochrane Database Syst Rev* 2007, doi:10.1002/14651858.CD001139.pub2.

3. Gutke A, Ostgaard HC, Oberg B: **Association between muscle function and low back pain in relation to pregnancy.** *J Rehabil Med* 2008, **40**(4):304–311.
4. Wang S-M, Dezinno P, Maranets I, Berman MR, Caldwell-Andrews AA, Kain ZN: **Low back pain during pregnancy: prevalence, risk factors, and outcomes.** *Obstet Gynecol* 2004, **104**:65–70.
5. van de Pol G, van Brummen HJ, Bruinse HW, Heintz APM, van der Vaart CH: **Pregnancy-related pelvic girdle pain in The Netherlands.** *Acta Obstetricia et Gynecologica* 2007, **86**:416–422.
6. Borg-Stein J, Dugan S, Gruber J: **Musculoskeletal aspects of pregnancy.** *Am J Phys Med Rehabil* 2005, **84**(3):180–192.
7. Kristiansson P, Svardsudd K, von Schoultz B: **Serum relaxin, symphyseal pain, and back pain during pregnancy.** *Am J Obstet Gynecol* 1996, **175**:1343–1347.
8. Whitcome KK, Shapiro LJ, Lieberman DE: **Fetal load and the evolution of lumbar lordosis in bipedal hominins.** *Nature* 2007, **450**:1075–1080.
9. Bastiaanssen JM, de Bie RA, Bastiaenen CHG, Essed GGM, van den Brandt PA: **A historical perspective on pregnancy-related low back and/or pelvic girdle pain.** *Eur J Obstet Gynecol Reprod Biol* 2005, **120**:3–14.
10. Mogren I: **Perceived health, sick leave, psychosocial situation, and sexual life in women with low-back pain and pelvic pain during pregnancy.** *Acta Obstet Gynecol Scand* 2006, **85**:647–656.
11. To WWK, Wong MWN: **Factors associated with back pain symptoms in pregnancy and the persistence of pain 2 years after pregnancy.** *Acta Obstet Gynecol Scand* 2003, **82**:1086–1091.
12. Mogren I: **BMI, pain and hyper-mobility are determinants of long-term outcome for women with low back pain and pelvic pain during pregnancy.** *Eur Spine J* 2006, **15**:1093–1102.
13. Ostgaard HC, Zetherstrom G, Roos-Hansson E: **Back pain in relation to pregnancy: a 6-year follow-up.** *Spine* 1997, **22**(24):2945–2950.
14. Gutke A, Josefsson A, Oberg B: **Pelvic girdle pain and lumbar pain in relation to postpartum depressive symptoms.** *Spine* 2007, **32**:1430–1436.
15. Hayden JA, van Tulder MW, Tomlinson G: **Systematic review: strategies for using exercise therapy to improve outcomes in chronic low back pain.** *Ann Intern Med* 2005, **142**(5):776–785.
16. Assendelft WJJ, Morton SC, Yu EI, Suttorp MJ, Shekelle PG: **Spinal manipulative therapy for low back pain.** *Ann Intern Med* 2003, **138**:871–881.
17. Bronfort G, Haas M, Evans RL, Bouter LM: **Efficacy of spinal manipulation and mobilization for low back pain and neck pain: a systematic review and best evidence synthesis.** *Spine J* 2004, **4**:335–356.
18. Bablis P, Pollard H: **A randomized controlled trial of neuro-emotional technique for low back pain. Proceedings of the World Federation of Chiropractic 11th Biennial Congress, Rio de Janeiro, April 6–9, 2011.** *Clinical Chiropractic* 2011, **14**(4):168–169.
19. Garshasbi A, Zadeh SF: **The effect of exercise on the intensity of low back pain in pregnant women.** *Int J Gynecol Obstet* 2005, **88**:271–275.
20. Morkved S, Salvesen KA, Schei B, Lydersen S, Bo K: **Does group training during pregnancy prevent lumbopelvic pain? a randomized clinical trial.** *Acta Obstetrica et Gynecologica* 2007, **86**:276–282.
21. Khorsan R, Hawk C, Lisi AJ, Kizhakkeveettil A: **Manipulative therapy for pregnancy and related conditions.** *Obstet Gynecol Surv* 2009, **64**(6):416–427.
22. Lisi AJ: **Chiropractic spinal manipulation for low back pain of pregnancy: a retrospective case series.** *J Midwifery Womens Health* 2006, **51**(1):e7–e10.
23. Stuber KJ, Smith DL: **Chiropractic treatment of pregnancy-related low back pain: a systematic review of the evidence.** *J Manipulative Physiol Ther* 2008, **31**(6):447–454.
24. Licciardone JC, Buchanan S, Hensel KL, Kind HH, Fulda KG, Stoll ST: **Osteopathic manipulative treatment of back pain and related symptoms during pregnancy: a randomized controlled trial.** *Am J Obstet Gynecol* 2010, **202**(43):e41–e48.
25. Eichler H-G, Bloechl-Daum B, Abadie E, Barnett D, Konig F, Pearson S: **Relative efficacy of drugs: an emerging issue between regulatory agencies and third-party payers.** *Nat Rev Drug Discov* 2010, **9**:277–291.
26. Gynecologists. ACoOa: **Exercise during pregnancy and the postpartum period.** *Clin Obstet Gynecol* 2003, **46**(2):496–499.
27. Bigos S, Bowyer O, Braen G, Brown K, Deyo R, Haldeman S: *Acute low back problems in adults. Clinical Practice Guideline, Quick Reference Guide Number 14.* Rockville, MD: U.S. Department of Health and Human Services, Public Health Service, Agency for Health Care Policy and Research, AHCPR Pub. No. 95–0642; 1994.
28. Stratford PW, Binkley J, Solomon P, Finch E, Gill C, Moreland J: **Defining the minimum level of detectable change for the Roland-Morris questionnaire.** *Physical Therapy* 1996, **76**(4):359–365.
29. Iacoviello BM, McCarthy KS, Barrett MS, Rynn M, Gallop R, Barber JP: **Treatment preferences affect the therapeutic alliance: implications for randomized controlled trials.** *Journal of Consulting and Clinical Psychology* 2007, **75**(1):194–198.
30. McPherson K, Britton AR, Wennberg JE: **Are randomized controlled trials controlled? patient preferences and unblind trials.** *Journal of the Royal Society of Medicine* 1997, **90**:652–656.
31. Corrigan PW, Salzer MS: **The conflict between random assignment and treatment preference: implications for internal validity.** *Evaluation and Program Planning* 2003, **26**(2):109–121.
32. Depledge J, McNair PJ, Keal-Smith C, Williams M: **Management of symphysis pubis dysfunction during pregnancy using exercise and pelvic support belts.** *Physical Therapy* 2005, **85**:1290–1300.
33. Bergmann T, Peterson D: *Chiropractic Technique: Principles and Procedures.* St. Louis, MI: Elsevier Mosby; 2011.
34. Hochman JI: **The effect of sacro occipital technique category II blocking on spinal range of motion: a case series.** *Journal of Manipulative and Physiological Therapeutics* 2005, **28**(9):719–723.
35. Shearar KA, Colloca CJ, White HL: **A randomized clinical trial of manual versus mechanical force manipulation in the treatment of sacroiliac joint syndrome.** *Journal of Manipulative and Physiological Therapeutics* 2005, **28**(7):493–501.
36. Monti DA, Sufian M, Peterson C: **Potential role of mind-body therapies in cancer survivorship.** *Cancer* 2008, **112**(11Supplement):2607–2616.
37. Peterson K, Peterson C: **A case series evaluating the accuracy of manual muscle testing for predicting fetal sex.** *The Journal of Chiropractic Medicine* 2012, **11**:1–6.
38. Bablis P, Pollard H, Bonello R: **Neuro Emotional Technique for the treatment of trigger point sensitivity in chronic neck pain sufferers: a controlled clinical trial.** *Chiropractic & Osteopathy* 2008, **16**:4.
39. Roland M, Morris R: **A study of the natural history of back pain: Part I: development of a reliable and sensitive measure of disability in low-back pain.** *Spine* 1983, **8**(2):141–144.
40. Roland M, Fairbank J: **The Roland-Morris Disability Questionnaire and the Oswestry Disability Questionnaire.** *Spine* 2000, **25**(24):3115–3124.
41. Childs JD, Piva SR, Fritz JM: **Responsiveness of the Numeric Pain Rating Scale in patients with low back pain.** *Spine* 2005, **30**(11):1331–1334.
42. Bombardier C, Hayden J, Beaton DE: **Minimal clinically important difference. Low back pain: outcome measures.** *The Journal of Rheumatology* 2001, **28**(2):431–438.
43. Hurley DA, McDonough SM, Martin D, Moore AP, Baxter GD: **A randomized clinical trial of manipulative therapy and interferential therapy for acute low back pain.** *Spine* 2004, **29**(20):2207–2216.
44. Jordan K, Dunn KM, Lewis M, Croft P: **A minimal clinically important difference was derived for the Roland-Morris Disability Questionnaire for low back pain.** *Journal of Clinical Epidemiology* 2006, **59**(1):45–52.
45. Farrar JT, Young JP, LaMoreaux L, Werth JL, Poole RM: **Clinical importance of changes in chronic pain intensity Numerical Pain Rating Scale.** *Pain* 2001, **94**(2):149–158.
46. Straube S, Derry S, Moore RA, Paine J, McQuay HJ: **Pregabalin in fibromyalgia - responder analysis from individual patient data.** *BMC Musculoskeletal Disorders* 2010, **11**:150.
47. Food and Drug Administration: **Draft Guidance for Industry: Patient-Reported Outcome Measures: Use in Medical Product Development to Support Labeling Claims.** In Edited by US Department of Health & Human Services. Rockville, MD: Office of Communications, Division of Drug Information; 2006.
48. Wood AM, White IR, Thompson SG: **Are missing outcome data adequately handled? a review of published randomized controlled trials in major medical journals.** *Clinical Trials* 2004, **1**:368–376.
49. Hamer RM, Simpson PM: **Last observation carried forward versus mixed models in the analysis of psychiatric clinical trials.** *American Journal of Psychiatry* 2009, **166**(6):639–641.
50. Gallagher EJ, Liebman M, Bijur PE: **Prospective validation of clinically important changes in pain severity measured on a visual analog scale.** *Annals of Emergency Medicine* 2001, **38**(6):633–638.

51. Salaffi F, Stancati A, Silvestri CA, Ciapetti A, Grass W: **Minimal clinically important changes in chronic musculoskeletal pain intensity measured on a numerical rating scale.** *European Journal of Pain* 2003, **8**(4):283–291.
52. Koren G, Sakaguchi S, Klieger C, Kazmin A, Osadchy A, Yazdani-Brojeni P, Matok I: **Toward improved pregnancy labelling.** *Journal of Population Therapeutics and Clinical Pharmacology* 2010, **17**(3):e349–e357.
53. Ho SSM, Yu WWM, Lao TT, Chow DHK, Chung JWY, Li Y: **Effectiveness of maternity support belts in reducing low back pain during pregnancy: a review.** *Journal of Clinical Nursing* 2009, **18**:1523–1532.
54. van Duijvenbode I, Jellema P, van Poppel M, van Tulder MW: **Lumbar supports for prevention and treatment of low back pain.** *Cochrane Database of Systematic Reviews* 2008, **16**(2):CD001823.
55. Hurwitz EL, Morgenstern H, Kominski GF, Yu F, Chiang L-M: **A randomized trial of chiropractic and medical care for patients with low back pain.** *Spine* 2006, **31**(6):611–621.
56. UK BEAM Trial Team: **United Kingdom back pain, exercise and manipulation (UK BEAM) randomized trial: effectiveness of physical treatments for back pain in primary care.** *British Medical Journal* 2004, **329**:1377–1381.
57. King HH, Tettambel MA, Lockwood MD, Johnson KH, Arsenault DA, Quist R: **Osteopathic manipulative treatment in prenatal care: a retrospective case control design study.** *Journal of American Osteopathic Association* 2003, **103**(12):577–582.
58. Hertzman-Miller RP, Morgenstern H, Hurwitz EL, Fei Y, Adams AH, Harber P, Kominski GF: **Comparing the satisfaction of low-back pain patients randomized to receive medical or chiropractic care: Results from the UCLA Low-Back Pain Study.** *American Journal of Public Health* 2002, **92**:1628–1633.
59. Grieves B, Menke JM, Pursel KJ: **Cost minimization analysis of low back pain claims data for chiropractic vs medicine in a managed care organization.** *Journal of Manipulative and Physiological Therapeutics* 2009, **32**(9):734–739.
60. Murphy DR, Hurwitz EL, McGovern EE: **Outcome of pregnancy-related lumbopelvic pain treated according to a diagnosis-based decision rule: a prospective observational cohort study.** *Journal of Manipulative and Physiological Therapeutics* 2009, **32**(8):616–624.
61. Noren L, Ostgaard S, Johansson G, Ostgaard HC: **Lumbar back and posterior pelvic pain during pregnancy: a 3-year follow-up.** *European Spine Journal* 2002, **11**:267–271.
62. Nilsson-Wikmar L, Holm K, Oijerstedt R, Harms-Ringdahl K: **Effect of three different physical therapy treatments on pain and activity in pregnant women with pelvic girdle pain: a randomized clinical trial with 3, 6, and 12 months follow-up postpartum.** *Spine* 2005, **30**(8):850–856.
63. Becker A, Held H, Redaelli M, Strauch K, Chenot JF, Leonhardt C, Keller S, Baum E, Pfingsten M, Hildebrandt J, *et al:* **Low back pain in primary care: costs of care and prediction of future health care utilization.** *Spine* 2010, **35**(18):1714–1720.
64. Williams D: **Pregnancy: a stress test for life.** *Current Opinions in Obstetrics & Gynecology* 2003, **15**:465–471.
65. Chodick G, Elchalal U, Sella T, Heymann AD, Porath A, Kokia E, Shalev V: **The risk of overt diabetes mellitus among women with gestational diabetes: a population-based study.** *Diabetic Medicine* 2010, **27**(7):779–785.
66. Drost JT, Maas AHEM, van Eyck J, van der Schouw YT: **Preeclampsia as a female-specific risk factor for chronic hypertension.** *Maturitas* 2010, **67**:321–326.

A biopsychosocial approach to primary hypothyroidism: treatment and harms data from a randomized controlled trial

Benjamin T. Brown[1*], Petra L. Graham[2], Rod Bonello[3] and Henry Pollard[4]

Abstract

Background: Hypothyroidism is a common endocrine condition. There is evidence to suggest that, for a proportion of sufferers, the standard medical treatment does not completely reverse the constitutional and neuropsychiatric symptoms brought about by this condition. The management of hypothyroidism follows a biomedical model with little consideration given to alternative management approaches. There exists anecdotal evidence and case reports supporting the use of a biopsychosocial-based intervention called Neuro-Emotional Technique (NET) for this population. The aim of this study was to explore the potential short-medium term clinical efficacy and safety of NET for individuals with primary hypothyroidism.

Design

Placebo-controlled, blinded, parallel groups, randomized trial.

Methods: Ninety adults with a diagnosis of primary hypothyroidism were recruited from Sydney, Australia. Blinded participants were randomized to either the NET or placebo group and received ten intervention sessions over a six week period. The primary outcome involved the measurement of states of depression using the DASS-42 questionnaire. Secondary outcomes included thyroid function, thyroid autoimmunity testing, SF-36v2 questionnaire, resting heart rate and temperature measurement. Outcomes were obtained at baseline, seven weeks and six months. Questionnaires were completed at the private clinics, and serum measures were obtained and analysed at commercial pathology company locations. Heart rate and temperature were also measured daily by participants. Linear mixed-effects models were used to analyse the continuous outcomes. Unadjusted odds ratios with 95% confidence intervals were calculated for the binary outcomes.

Results: Participants were randomly allocated to the NET (n=44) and placebo (n=46) groups. A proportion of the sample displayed neuropsychiatric disturbances and alterations in quality of life measures at baseline. There were no statistically significant or clinically relevant changes in the primary or secondary outcomes between the NET and placebo groups at time seven weeks or six months. There were a few short-lived minor adverse events reported in both the NET and placebo groups that coincided with the application of the intervention.

Conclusions: The application of the NET intervention appears to be safe, but did not confer any clinical benefit to the participants in this study and is unlikely to be of therapeutic use in a hypothyroid population.

Clinical trials registration number: Australian and New Zealand Clinical Trials Registry Number: 12607000040460.

Keywords: Chiropractic, Hypothyroidism, Randomized controlled trial, Therapeutics, Neuro-emotional technique

* Correspondence: benjamin.brown@mq.edu.au
[1]Department of Chiropractic, Macquarie University, Balaclava Road, North Ryde 2109NSW, Australia
Full list of author information is available at the end of the article

Background

Hypothyroidism is a common endocrine condition that affects a significant proportion of individuals worldwide. Using data from a community-based sample from an iodine-replete region in Western Australia, it is estimated 0.54 % of Australians suffer from this condition [1]. Females are more likely to develop hypothyroidism compared to males (Prevalence - women 1–2 % and men 0.1 %) [1–3]. The primary variant of this disease accounts for the vast majority (99 %) of cases. Primary hypothyroidism is due to a failure of the thyroid gland and results in a deficient concentration of thyroid hormones in the serum. The most common cause of this glandular failure is an autoimmune condition called Hashimoto's thyroiditis [4, 5]. The symptoms of overt hypothyroidism are based on deficits in energy metabolism and thermogenesis. Consequently, patients present with a constellation of physical and neuropsychiatric findings (i.e. musculoskeletal complaints, depression, free-floating anxiety, memory deficits) [6, 7], and in cases of thyroid autoimmunity, formation of antibodies to thyroglobulin (Tg) and thyroid peroxidase (TPO) [4]. The gold-standard treatment for primary hypothyroidism is relatively straightforward and involves supplementation of one of the deficient hormones using a synthetic version of the thyroid hormone - thyroxine. This synthetic analogue is called levothyroxine (LT4). The treatment dosage of thyroid hormone is gradually titrated upwards until an individual displays normal physiological concentrations of free-thyroxine (FT4) and thyroid stimulating hormone (TSH) in the serum. Put simply, the product of the dysfunctional gland is 'topped up' using an exogenous source of thyroid hormone, with the required dose being modified according to the patient's FT4 and TSH assay results. The patient continues with this program, combined with regular check-ups, either for the rest of their lives or until some event occurs (e.g. pregnancy) that warrants a change in the patient's thyroxine dosage. The normal reference range for TSH is 0.4–3.5 mIU/L. Patients receiving thyroid hormone replacement are given sufficient quantities of thyroxine to maintain their serum TSH concentrations within an ideal range (0.5–2.0 mIU/L) [8].

While the treatment regimen for primary hypothyroidism is regarded by many as one of the major 'success stories' of medicine [9], there is evidence to suggest that a small proportion of individuals with managed-hypothyroidism continue to display the overt manifestations of the disease despite normalised blood test results - indicating a euthyroid state [10–12]. Furthermore, the decreased quality of life (QOL) that is observed in hypothyroid individuals does not always improve with the appropriate treatment [10, 13–15]. Large community-based studies [14, 16, 17] demonstrate that there is neurocognitive and psychological impairment in individuals with hypothyroidism. Unfortunately, in some patients, the restoration of normal thyroid hormone levels through thyroxine supplementation only partially ameliorates these impairments.

One of the main reasons for the persistence of symptoms in euthyroid patients with hypothyroidism is the underlying autoimmune process. Patients with Hashimoto's thyroiditis are more likely to experience higher symptom loads with reference to mood and quality of life, despite being euthryoid [18]. Furthermore, it is not uncommon for patients with Hashimoto's thyroiditis to have other comorbid autoimmune conditions e.g. rheumatoid arthritis [19]. The presence of these additional conditions contributes to an increased symptom load that is unaltered by the restoration of normal thyroid hormone concentrations in the serum. McDermott [20] suggests that a complete blood count, serum 25-hydroxyvitamin D, erythyrocyte sedimentation rate, sleep apnoea testing, celiac disease testing as well as a metabolic, hormonal, psychological, and lifestyle assessment should be performed in euthyroid patients with persistent symptoms. This strategy can be used to rule out comorbid medical conditions and/or to identify modifiable risk factors.

Researchers [21, 22] have identified polymorphisms in genes that encode for the deiodinase enzymes in patients with hypothyroidism. There is preliminary evidence to suggest [23] that patients with polymorphisms in the Deiodinase Type II gene may display poorer outcomes on levothyroxine therapy compared with patients receiving preparations containing both levothyroxine and liothyronine (synthetic T3). However, this combination therapy has not proven superior to standard monotherapy [24–27].

With respect to therapeutic intervention, very little attention has been given to the main cause of primary hypothyroidism – thyroid autoimmunity [28]. The main reason for this is that the pathogenesis of thyroid autoimmunity is not fully understood [28]. Current research suggests that autoimmune thyroid disease may result from complex interactions between environmental triggers and genetic susceptibilities [29–32]. The purported environmental triggers include: iodine excess [33, 34], selenium deficiency [35], fetal microchimerism [36, 37], infections [38, 39], and stress [40]. With regard to stress as an environmental trigger, associations have been reported most frequently with Graves' disease [41–46].

Psychological stress, via alterations in the sympathetic-adrenal-medullary (SAM) axis and the hypothalamic-pituitary-adrenal (HPA) axis, can have deleterious effects on the endocrine and immune systems [47–49]. With respect to the immune system, chronic stress shifts the balance of the cell-mediated immune response, specifically suppressing the subset of T-helper lymphocytes called the Th1 cells [49]. This suppression has a permissive effect on the production of another subset of T-helper cells called Th2 cells [50]. This shift in the Th1/Th2 balance has been observed in certain autoimmune diseases such as Systemic Lupus Erythematosus and Graves' disease [50, 51]. As a hyperactivation of the HPA axis is a common response to most forms of stress [52], it would be logical to expect a shift to Th2 dominance and a resultant increase in cases of Graves' disease in genetically susceptible individuals who are stressed. The contribution of stress to Hashimoto's thyroiditis however is less intuitive. There is some research to suggest that there is HPA axis hypoactivation in patients with hypothyroidism [53, 54]. While hyperactivation of the HPA axis leads to a suppression of Th1 dominant states, a hypoactivation of the HPA axis promotes Th1 dominant states [50]. Autoimmune conditions such as rheumatoid arthritis, Hashimoto's thyroiditis, multiple sclerosis and diabetes type I are T-cell mediated diseases, however they are thought to occur due to these Th1 dominant states [50, 55, 56]. Hypoactivation of the HPA axis has also been observed in patients with a history of childhood abuse [57] and post-traumatic stress disorder [58], which may be an adaptive response to intense or prolonged psychological stress. The role of stress in Hashimoto's thyroiditis has received far less attention compared to the role of stress in Graves' disease [59]. While it is biologically plausible that stress could play an etiological role in genetically susceptible individuals, there are no reported positive associations between stress and autoimmune induced hypothyroidism in the current literature [60–62].

Anecdotal evidence and case reports [63, 64] exist that suggest that a biopsychosocial-based intervention called Neuro-Emotional Technique (NET), which is described as a mind-body stress reduction intervention [65, 66], may be useful in the treatment of hypothyroidism. This technique has been taught and used by practitioners of varying backgrounds since the late 1980s [66], however there is very little quality evidence regarding its therapeutic utility and safety in a primary care setting.

The aim of this manuscript is to outline and discuss the results from a randomized controlled trial of the biopsychosocial-based intervention, NET, for individuals with primary hypothyroidism. This document has been prepared using the CONSORT 2010 guide for the reporting of parallel group randomized trials [67, 68], as well as the associated documents for randomized trials of non-pharmacological treatments [69], and the guide to harms reporting [70].

Methods

The research presented in this manuscript was approved by the Macquarie University Ethics Review Committee (Reference no.: HE-27AUG2004-MO3136).

Design

Parallel, blinded, multi-centre (11 sites), randomized, placebo-controlled, trial conducted from August 2006 – March 2010. The study was designed to align with quality recommendations set out in the PEDro scale [71] and The Delphi list [72] as well as with the relevant CONSORT guidelines available at the time of trial design [67, 69, 70, 73, 74].

Participants

The study team sought to recruit participants from the Sydney Metropolitan area of Australia using advertisements in a variety of hardcopy and electronic media. Participants were randomized into either the NET group or the placebo group after being screened for eligibility by the chief investigator.

Inclusion criteria - participants

For inclusion, participants had to be ≥18 years of age and have received a diagnosis of primary overt hypothyroidism from a qualified medical practitioner or specialist. In long-standing hypothyroidism there is pituitary thyrotroph hyperplasia [75]. For this reason, it can take up to six months for TSH levels to fall into normal ranges after the initiation of LT4 therapy [76]. Based on this information, if a respondent was taking medication, e.g. levothyroxine, it was stipulated that they be on a stable dose of this medication for at least six months before enrolment into the trial. Acknowledging that treatment is commonly initiated promptly after diagnosis, participants were only included in the trial if they had received their diagnosis more than six months prior to enrolment. Participants were not asked by the research team to alter or cease their thyroid medication at any point during the trial as this would be deemed unethical given the experimental nature of the intervention. However, participants were asked to immediately report any such changes to the chief investigator so that this information could be incorporated into the interpretation of the final results.

Exclusion criteria – participants

Participants who were <18 years of age were excluded. Individuals with variants of hypothyroidism other than primary overt hypothyroidism, such as hypopituitarism, were excluded. This also included iatrogenic forms of hypothyroidism. Individuals who were on medications that could potentially impair thyroid function e.g. Lithium were excluded. Participants who reported a history of significant head or neck trauma/surgery/radiotherapy were excluded, as were individuals with diagnosed serious psychological or physical co-morbidities. Females who were pregnant or looking to conceive within the trial period were excluded. As participants were required to interact mentally and physically with the practitioner during the intervention phase of the trial, those with cognitive or physical disabilities e.g. individuals who are hard of hearing were excluded from the trial.

Inclusion criteria – practitioners

It was necessary that the practitioners applying the intervention were well-versed with the NET procedure. Consequently, practitioners were only included if they had attained the maximum qualification available at the time ('Certification' in NET) [77] and a minimum experience of two years with the procedure. This ensured a high degree of competency and also acted as a means of standardising the intervention. Practitioners were required to be available for the full duration of the intervention phase for each participant. Practitioners had to agree to treat within the confines of the research methodology and comply with the study protocol, which included the application of a placebo intervention to the relevant participants. The treating practitioners were asked to make times available in their normal practice hours for the treatment of the trial participants. There was no remuneration offered to the practitioners involved in the trial.

Inclusion criteria – research centres

The research was conducted at 11 private practices. To be included as a research venue, the practice had to fulfil several criteria: be located in the Sydney Metropolitan area, have practitioners with the relevant training and clinical expertise in NET, and be open at least two days per week with capacity for both during and after-hours business operations.

Intervention

The NET and placebo procedures have been described in depth by several authors [63, 64, 78–84] and it is not within the scope of this article to replicate this discussion. A detailed version of the NET and placebo protocols used in this trial was published in an open-access journal in 2010 [85]. The treatment protocol used in this study was also similar to that employed by Karpouzis *et al.* [78] and Karpouzis [79].

The placebo treatment was developed by a panel that included experts in NET and members of the research team. The placebo intervention was designed to closely mimic the NET intervention protocol but with the purported therapeutic components removed and replaced with innocuous steps.

Participants who were randomized to the intervention group received ten NET treatments over a six week period. Similarly, participants in the placebo group received ten placebo treatments over the same period. Two treatments per week were scheduled in the initial four weeks and one treatment per week in the final two weeks of the intervention phase. There was no further intervention after this point. Each treatment, NET or placebo, went for 5–20 min in duration. Participants attended the same clinic and saw the same practitioner for all of their treatments, all participants attended clinics that were closest to their place of work or residence.

All practitioners involved in the trial were given a training session by the chief investigator, and issued with an information booklet detailing the steps involved with the application of each individual arm of the intervention (NET and Placebo). Practitioners were instructed to deliver the placebo treatment with the same vigour and enthusiasm as the NET treatment. Both practitioners and participants had 24-hour access to the chief investigator at all times during the trial via a toll-free telephone number.

Outcomes

Several outcome variables were used to capture potential psychological and/or physiological changes that may have coincided with the application of therapy.

Primary outcome

The primary outcome was the change in depressive states at 7 weeks and 6 months using the Depression, Anxiety, Stress Scale (DASS-42) [86]. The normal range for states of depression is between zero and nine points, with scores greater than nine indicating high states of depression. States of depression was chosen as the primary outcome as it is one of the most common neuropsychiatric symptoms observed in primary overt hypothyroidism, and it is a commonly reported symptom in individuals with continued symptomatology despite normalised thyroid function tests.

Secondary outcomes

Although it was anticipated that many of the participants would be entering into the trial with pre-existing management plans, i.e. thyroid hormone replacement schedules, it was prudent that thyroid function tests be added to the list of outcomes. The thyroid function tests included the serum measurement of thyroid stimulating hormone (TSH), free-thyroxine (FT4) and free-triiodothyronine (FT3) concentrations. The normal reference range used in this research for TSH was 0.40–3.50 mIU/L and the assay calibration range was 0.00–100.00 mIU/L [87]. The normal reference range used in this research for FT4 and FT3 was 9.0–19.0 pmol/L and 2.6–6.0 pmol/L respectively. The calibration range for the FT3 and FT4 assays was 0.000–9.216 pmol/L and 0.00–77.22 pmol/L respectively [88, 89].

In addition to the thyroid function tests, serum concentrations of antibodies to thyroid peroxidase (TPO-Ab) and thyroglobulin (Tg-Ab) were also measured. The normal reference range for TPO-Ab was 0–35 mIU/L, and the normal reference range for Tg-Ab was 0–40 mIU/L. The calibration range for the TPO-Ab and the TG-Ab assays was 0.0–1000.0 mIU/L and 0.0–3000.0 mIU/L respectively [90, 91].

The remaining items on the DASS-42 questionnaire, states of anxiety and stress, were assessed (Normal Range: Anxiety 0–7, and Stress 0–14). Scores outside of the normal reference range indicate abnormal states.

The Short Form-36 version two (SF-36v2) questionnaire [92] was also included in the list of secondary outcomes. The mean score for a normal population for the domains and component summary scores is 50 norm-based scoring points with a standard deviation of 10 points. High scores on the SF-36v2 represent high functioning whereas scores below the normal mean indicate poorer function.

In addition to the DASS and SF-36v2 questionnaires, participants were instructed to measure their resting heart rate (RHR) (radial pulse method) and resting temperature (RT) at a set time each day and record this data in a diary provided by the researchers. The normal ranges for RHR used for this trial were 75–85 bpm. Participants measured their RT by placing a digital thermometer in their axilla for approximately one minute. The normal reference range for resting temperature used in this research was 35.5–37 °C.

The aim with each of these primary and secondary outcomes measures was to examine the change in each measure at 7 weeks and 6 months to determine whether there was evidence that NET was different (efficacious) compared to placebo. This schedule would allow for the detection of any slow adaptations of the Hypothalamic Pituitary Thyroid axis in response to any short term (7 weeks) and medium term (6 months) benefit derived from the NET intervention.

Schedule of assessments

Baseline measurements were taken for both the primary and secondary outcomes. Thyroid function tests and thyroid auto-antibody measurements were performed at commercial pathology facilities approximately one week before the commencement of the intervention. The DASS, SF-36v2, and a demographic questionnaire were issued and completed by participants at the respective clinic just prior to the initial treatment. The first follow-up assessment was performed at seven weeks which included; a thyroid function test, serum thyroid auto-antibody measurements, and the DASS and SF-36v2 questionnaires. A second follow-up assessment was performed at six months which was identical to the one performed at seven weeks only with the addition of a health update questionnaire (HUQ) (Appendix). The HUQ was designed by the research team to capture any changes in a participant's health status, i.e. changes in medication, lifestyle, or major life events in the previous six months that may have influenced the final results and the associated interpretation. The daily home recording of RT and RHR commenced one week before the intervention phase and continued for the full duration of a participant's enrolment in the trial.

Blinding survey

The chief investigator contacted each participant by phone after the participant's final results had been received. The chief investigator thanked the participant for their involvement in the trial and asked them to identify which group, NET or placebo, they felt that they had been allocated to. The participant's response was recorded and used to assess the adequacy of the blinding process.

Harms data

A combination of active and passive harms surveillance was used in this study. Practitioners were required to maintain clinical records for each participant visit during the intervention phase. At the beginning of each intervention session participants were asked by the treating practitioner if they had experienced any adverse events in the period that followed the last intervention. Participants were also asked how they felt directly after each intervention. Any responses to these questions were detailed in the participants' records. In addition to the active harms surveillance participants were also asked to contact the chief investigator if any problems or difficulties arose using the toll free telephone number. These two strategies, combined with information from the HUQ, were used to capture any adverse events that may have coincided with the application of the intervention. These data were compiled and used in the final interpretation of technique safety by the chief investigator. *Adverse events* were defined as an adverse consequence of the intervention (placebo or NET) that occurred any time after the first intervention. Classification of the event as being an 'adverse event' was determined by either the participant and/or members of the research team.

Modifications to the trial protocol

There were several modifications made to the trial protocol between August 2006 and March 2010. In 2007, the pathology company commissioned to analyse the serum measures changed the methodology for analysing the thyroid auto-antibody concentrations. This resulted in the early auto-antibody measures being incompatible/non-comparable to the newer measures. This change prompted the research team to change the TPO-Ab and the Tg-Ab from being continuous variables to dichotomous variables (i.e. either 'within' the normal reference range or 'outside' of normal reference range) in the final analysis. This resulted in a loss of sensitivity with respect to the minimal clinically important difference detectable for this particular measure.

As the measurement of TSH and FT4 is the standard 'first-line' test for individuals with thyroid dysfunction, there were several instances in which the pathology company, due to internal protocols, did not measure the FT3 or thyroid auto-antibody concentrations. Many of these cases were picked up by the chief investigator, however there were instances in which the participant's sample was destroyed before the chief investigator was able to notify the pathology company of the omission. This resulted in six participants having only partial data for certain variables. This remains a limitation of the study.

As the trial was run over a four year period, there were several changes in the line-up of treating practitioners. Four practitioners started out in 2006. Eight more practitioners were recruited between 2006 and 2010, and four practitioners ceased their involvement in the study during this period due to personal reasons. Despite these changes, each participant received their intervention from a single practitioner.

Sample size

A two-sided, power-analysis indicated that 51 participants per group would yield a greater than 80 % chance of detecting a difference in depression scores of at least four points in the NET group compared to placebo group using a standard deviation of 6.97 based on normative data [86, 93]. A four point reduction in depression scores, as defined by the DASS-42, would represent a clinically meaningful reduction in states of depression. The ranges for the depression scale are: normal 0–4, mild 5–6, moderate 7–10, severe 11–13 and extremely severe 14+ [86].

Stopping guidelines

Guidelines were set that dictated that the trial would be stopped in the event of serious adverse events occurring in participants during their participation in the trial.

Randomization

A simple randomization technique was employed. A random sequence generator [94] was used to produce a random sequence with no repeats. These numbers were then recorded on individual pieces of paper and placed into opaque envelopes which were then sealed. After each consenting participant completed their initial blood test an envelope was selected for that participant by the chief investigator. Participants allocated an even number were assigned to the NET group, and those receiving an odd number were assigned to the placebo group. The chief investigator, practitioners and other researchers remained naive to a participant's group allocation until just before the application of the intervention.

Blinding

Pathology company staff and any primary care provider/s involved in the participant's non-trial management (e.g. the participant's general practitioner or endocrinologist) were blinded to the group allocations. The allocation of individual participants to treatment groups was concealed to the chief investigator up until the point of a participant commencing treatment. Practitioners were notified of each participant's group allocation prior to performing the intervention and were instructed not to reveal the allocation to the participant. Individual participants were not told their group allocation until the end of their involvement in the trial and after the completion of the blinding survey (Table 1).

Statistical procedures

The R software program [95] was used to conduct all the analyses. Linear mixed-effects (LME) models were employed for all continuous outcome measures except for the thyroid antibody concentrations. Linear mixed-effects models utilise all available data to provide unbiased estimates of the mean difference between groups in the presence of missing at random data and hence form an intention to treat (ITT) analysis [96]. Since these are more widely used methods, the imputation techniques and statistical methods described in the original protocol were not conducted. The thyroid antibody measures had been dichotomised and logistic mixed-effects models were the planned analysis technique. However model convergence issues meant that it was necessary to calculate unadjusted odds ratios with 95 % confidence intervals for each time point instead. The final data set was screened for errors prior to all analyses. P-values for the interaction and pairwise difference at each time point have been presented for each outcome measure together with 95 % confidence intervals (CI). All participants were analysed according to their initial group allocation. A sensitivity analysis was conducted by adjusting for baseline differences between groups by using baseline data as a covariate in the mixed-effects model. However, the effect of this was that

Table 1 Trial timeline. The trial timeline depicts the timing of all interventions and outcomes measured during the trial

Event	Week 1	Weeks 2-7	Week 8	Week 26	Week 27
Intervention					
Thyroid function tests					
DASS questionnaire					
SF-36v2 questionnaire					
Demographic questionnaire					
Basal temperature recording					
Basal heart rate recording					
Health update questionnaire					
Blinding survey					

Shaded Area = Event occurrence, *DASS* depression anxiety stress scale, *SF-36v2* short form 36 version 2 cases with missing baseline data were excluded from the analysis and the analysis may no longer be considered ITT. Demographic characteristics of participants were summarised using frequency tables. Summary values (mean, median, minimum, maximum, and standard deviation) for each group were used for the discussion of baseline group equivalence. Fisher's exact test was used to analyse the results of the blinding survey. Two-sided tests with a significance level of 5 % were used throughout all analyses. No corrections (e.g. Bonferroni method) were made to the significance level to adjust for multiple testing due to the exploratory nature of the secondary analyses.

Results

Post-randomization losses to follow-Up and protocol deviations

The dropouts and protocol deviations that occurred at various phases of the trial are detailed in Fig. 1.

Not all participants in the NET group received the full ten treatments. The reasons for these protocol deviations were either: personal reasons (1/44), administrative error (5/44), the deterioration of a pre-existing medical condition (1/44), minor reaction to treatment (1/44), other time commitments (1/44), and undisclosed reason/s (2/44). With regards to outcome measures, the main reasons for missing data were administrative errors at the private clinics or the pathology company. Several participants in the NET and placebo groups found the daily recording of heart rate and temperature inconvenient and cumbersome. As a result, there was incomplete compliance with the recording of these outcomes.

Not all participants in the placebo group received the full schedule of interventions or completed the full complement of outcomes. The reasons for these deviations were: work issues (1/46), expenses associated with travel to the clinic location (1/46), undisclosed reason/s (5/46), dissatisfaction with the placebo intervention (3/46), other time commitments (1/46), non-compliance with the trial protocol (5/46), and administrative error (4/46).

Dates of recruitment

Recruitment for the clinical trial took place between August 2006 and March 2010. Two hundred and forty five individuals responded to the advertisements for participation. Eligible consenting participants were followed for six months after randomization.

Trial closure

A strict external schedule (stopping rule) was imposed that meant that the trial must be commenced and completed between August 2006 and October 2010 due to the length of the chief investigator's PhD candidature. No interim analyses were performed and hence the decision to close the trial was independent of the trial outcomes. The prescribed schedule meant that no further participants could be recruited after March 2010 despite needing additional participants to fulfil the sample size target.

Baseline participant data

The demographic information and the mean baseline clinical characteristics for participants are presented in Tables 2 and 3 respectively. The two groups were very similar with respect to demographic data. A comparison of the baseline clinical data is presented below.

Primary outcome - baseline

Boxplots of baseline depression scores are depicted in Fig. 2. The mean and median depression scores for the placebo group were within normal range, however the mean score for the NET group fell just outside of the normal range. A large proportion (19/44) of participants in the NET group and 15/46 participants in the placebo group reported states of depression that fell outside of the normal range at the time of initial testing.

Secondary outcomes and clinical data - baseline

With respect to baseline clinical data, the mean TSH scores for the NET group were skewed by one individual with an extremely high TSH value that remained high at the subsequent seven week and six month reassessments. With reference to thyroid autoimmunity, 30/44 participants in the NET group demonstrated higher than the normal concentrations of TPO-Ab and 12/44 demonstrated higher than normal concentrations of Tg-Ab. Similar results were seen in the placebo group with 30/46 and 14/46 of participants demonstrating abnormally high TPO-Ab and Tg-Ab concentrations respectively.

With respect to the additional DASS items, 17/44 of the NET group and 10/44 of the placebo group reported anxiety scores in the mild to severe range. A considerable proportion of the trial participants also reported mild to extremely severe stress scores (NET 19/44, Placebo 13/44).

The mean baseline scores for the SF-36v2 questionnaire revealed that the trial participants had lower mean self-reported general health (NET 11/44, Placebo 9/46), vitality (NET = 21/44, Placebo 23/46) social functioning (NET 9/44, Placebo 11/46) and mental health (NET 8/44, Placebo 10/46) compared to normative data.

Resting temperature was comparable and within normal range at baseline for both the NET and placebo groups. The data regarding heart rate highlight that the majority of participants in both the NET and placebo groups had

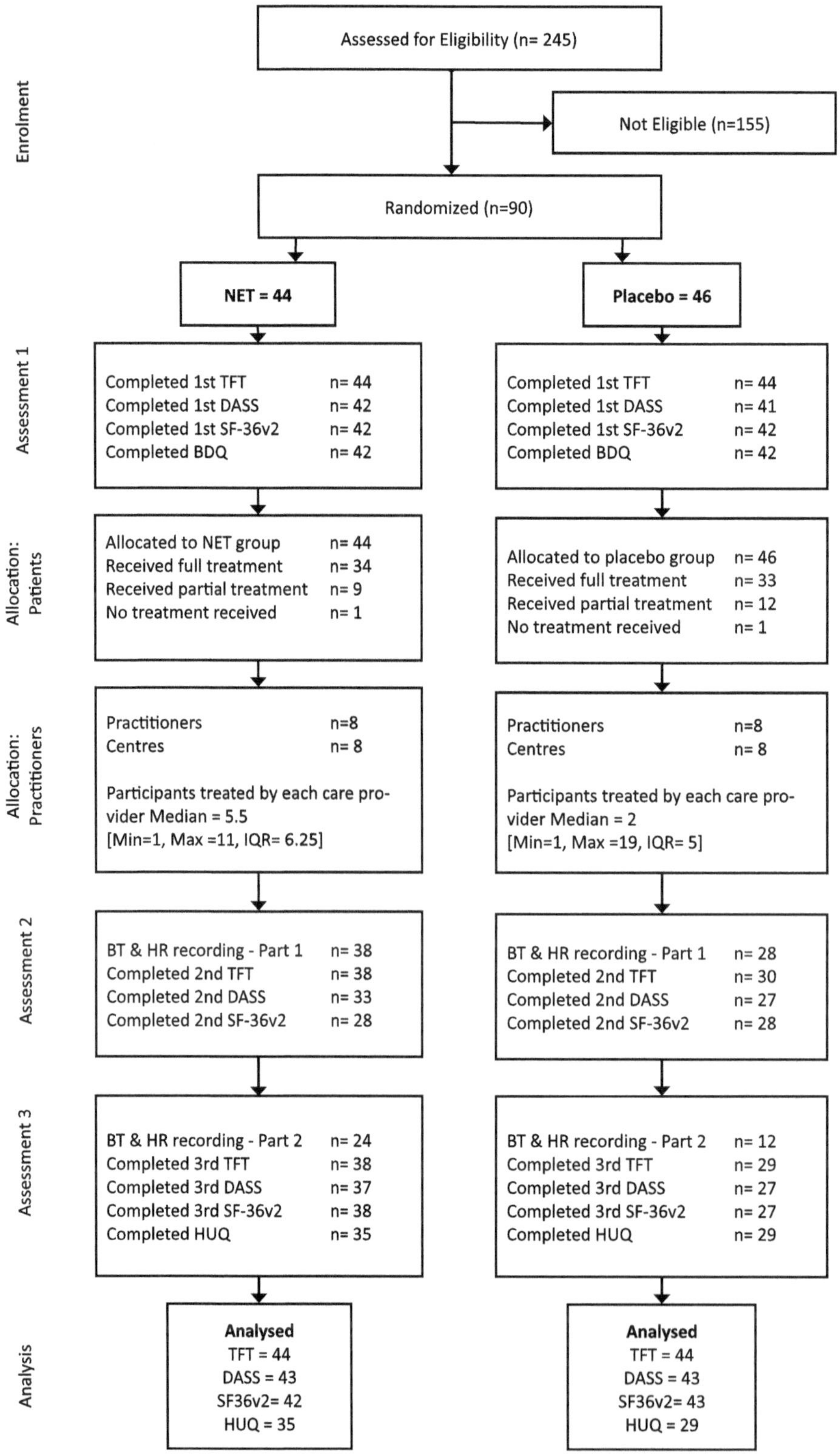

Fig. 1 Participant flow diagram. DASS = Depression Anxiety Stress Scale, HUQ = Health Update Questionnaire, NET = Neuro-Emotional Technique, SF-36v2 = Short Form 36 Version 2, TFT = Thyroid Function Test, Min = Minimum, Max = Maximum, IQR = Interquartile Range

Table 2 Demographic information

		Treatment ($n = 44$)	Placebo ($n = 46$)
Age	Median	46	43
	Minimum	20	20
	Maximum	72	75
	Mean	45.55	44.61
	Standard Deviation	11.21	11.32
Number of children	Mean	1.51	1.81
	Standard Deviation	1.30	1.20
Gender	Female	43	40
Ethnicity	Caucasian	40	38
	Asian	2	2
	Arab	1	0
	Aboriginal/Torres Strait Islander	0	1
	Unknown	1	5
Birthplace	Australia	26	29
Highest level of education	School Certificate	5	0
	HSC	3	10
	TAFE	13	8
	Undergraduate	13	15
	Postgraduate	8	11
	Unknown	2	2
Marital status	Married	20	27
	Separated	6	5
	Single	14	8
	Widowed	1	0
	Defacto	2	3
	Unknown	1	3
Employment	Full-Time	17	16
	Part-Time	11	13
	Retired	13	11
	Not Working	2	4
	Unknown	1	2

HSC higher school certificate, *TAFE* technical and further education

lower than normal heart rate compared to the normal range (NET = 37/44, Placebo 44/46).

In addition to the primary and secondary outcomes researchers also gathered data on the previous use of psychological services and concurrent use of medications and/or nutritional supplements. Thirty four percent (15/44) of the NET group and 37 % (17/46) of the placebo group reported that they had used support services (e.g. counselling service) in the past for emotional, psychological or lifestyle problems. At baseline, the vast majority of participants (NET 40/44, Placebo 43/46) reported currently using some form of thyroid medication for the treatment of their condition. With respect to additional medication use, 21/44 of participants in the NET group and 20/46 of participants the placebo group reported using medications other than those prescribed for their thyroid condition. A substantial proportion of trial participants (NET 28/44, Placebo 27/46) reported taking nutritional products or supplements.

Analysis

The results from the linear mixed-effects modelling for the primary outcome may be seen in Table 4 and Fig. 3. Secondary outcomes that comprised of continuous data are presented in the remaining rows of Table 4. There was no significant interaction between time and treatment group for any of the outcome variables included in the study (final column of Table 4) indicating that there was no evidence of a difference between groups over time (Fig. 3 Primary outcome). There were no significant differences, at the 5 % significance level, between the NET and placebo groups at time seven weeks or six months (see the 3rd and 6th columns of Table 4) for any of the primary or secondary outcomes.

There were no significant differences between the NET and placebo groups for either RHR ($p = 0.20$) and RT ($p = 0.18$) readings over time.

The odds ratios and 95 % confidence intervals indicated no significant differences, at the 5 % significance level, between groups in the odds of demonstrating Tg-Ab concentrations outside of reference range at the seven weeks (OR: 0.65, 95 % CI: 0.24 to 1.73, $p = 0.38$) or the six month (OR: 1.24, 95 % CI: 0.45 to 3.38, $p = 0.68$) time points. Similar outcomes were observed with TPO-Ab concentrations (7 week OR: 0.94, 95 % CI: 0.32 to 2.74, $p = 0.90$; 6 month OR: 0.69, 95 % CI: 0.25 to 1.92, $p = 0.48$).

Sensitivity analysis was undertaken by using baseline outcome as a covariate in each of the continuous outcome models shown in Table 4. While the baseline value was consistently a highly significant factor ($p < 0.0001$), the interaction between time and group remained non-significant for all outcomes ($p > 0.3$). In other words, the only differences between groups, were those differences observed at baseline with no significant change over time.

Harms/adverse events

The harms/adverse events section has been written in accordance with the CONSORT document for the better reporting of harms in randomized trials [70]. No validated harms recording instruments were used.

Adverse events - NET group

Six (14 %) participants in the NET group reported adverse events that coincided with the application of intervention. One participant in the NET group reported feeling "sad" after the fifth treatment session. This same

Table 3 Mean baseline clinical characteristics

Outcome measure		Treatment		Placebo	
	Normal range	Median (Min, Max)	Mean (SD)	Median (Min, Max)	Mean (SD)
Thyroid function tests:					
TSH (mIU/L)	0.40–3.50	0.96 (0.00, 55.77)	2.98 (8.39)[a]	1.34 (0.01, 7.30)	1.85 (1.76)
FT4 (pmol/L)	9.0–19.0	15.00 (7.00, 26.00)	15.09 (3.22)	14.20 (3.80, 24.50)	14.51 (3.91
FT3 (pmol/L)	2.6–6.0	4.06 (2.80, 7.45)	4.13 (0.80)	3.80 (3.00, 5.73)	3.95 (0.64)
DASS Scores:					
Depression	0–9	6.50 (0.00, 29.00)	9.43 (8.60)	6.00 (0.00, 41.00)	7.85 (8.52)
Anxiety	0–7	6.00 (0.00, 19.00)	6.79 (5.13)	4.00 (0.00, 30.00)	6.27 (7.73)
Stress	0–14	13.00 (3.00, 35.00)	13.71 (8.28)	11.00 (2.00, 38.00)	12.76 (8.53)
SF-36v2 Scores:	Normal Mean (SD)	Median (Min, Max)	Mean (SD)	Median (Min, Max)	Mean (SD)
Physical functioning	50 ± 3 (10)	52.82 (25.46, 57.03)	48.06 (8.36)	50.72 (29.68, 57.03)	48.66 (7.72)
Role physical	50 ± 3 (10)	49.51 (22.57, 56.85)	48.85 (8.60)	51.96 (17.67, 56.85)	46.32 (11.25)
Bodily pain	50 ± 3 (10)	46.06 (24.08, 62.12)	49.97 (9.87)	46.06 (24.08, 62.12)	46.53 (9.43)
General health	50 ± 3 (10)	45.31 (23.38, 57.70)	43.72 (11.26)	45.78 (23.78, 62.47)	45.16 (9.71)
Vitality	50 ± 3 (10)	39.60 (23.99, 58.33)	40.15 (8.88)	41.16 (20.87, 58.33)	41.68 (10.33)
Social functioning	50 ± 3 (10)	45.94 (13.22, 56.86)	42.09 (12.49)	45.94 (13.22, 56.85)	41.12 (12.82)
Role emotional	50 ± 3 (10)	48.10 (20.89, 55.88)	44.78 (10.71)	44.22 (20.89, 55.88)	43.58 (10.96)
Mental health	50 ± 3 (10)	44.38 (21.85, 61.27)	43.79 (11.04)	47.19 (16.22, 58.46)	43.03 (11.62)
Physical component summary	50 ± 3 (10)	50.46 (30.08, 61.73)	48.27 (7.76)	51.39 (16.70, 59.78)	48.45 (9.54)
Mental component summary	50 ± 3 (10)	42.59 (16.70, 60.18)	41.10 (11.49)	41.59 (16.40, 61.35)	40.79 (12.71)
	Normal Range	Median (Min, Max)	Mean (SD)	Median (Min, Max)	Mean (SD)
Resting temperature (°C)	35.5–37.03	35.8 (32.8, 37.0)	35.6 (0.9)	35.6 (33.4, 36.6)	35.6 (0.7)
Resting heart rate (bpm)	75–85	64 (30, 86)	65.7 (9.6)	64 (44, 86)	63.9 (11.3)

The SF-36v2 scores are based on the norm based scoring system (NBS) which is based on a mean score with a normal range between 47 and 53 NBS points. Resting temperature and resting heart rate data were analysed based on 'Day 1' dairy entries

[a]Strongly influenced by one person with very high TSH

DASS Depression, Anxiety, Stress Score, *NET* Neuro-Emotional Technique, *TSH* Serum thyroid stimulating hormone, *FT4* Free thyroxine, *FT3* Free triiodothyronine, *SF-36v2* Short Form-36 Version 2, *Min* minimum, *Max* Maximum, *SD* standard deviation

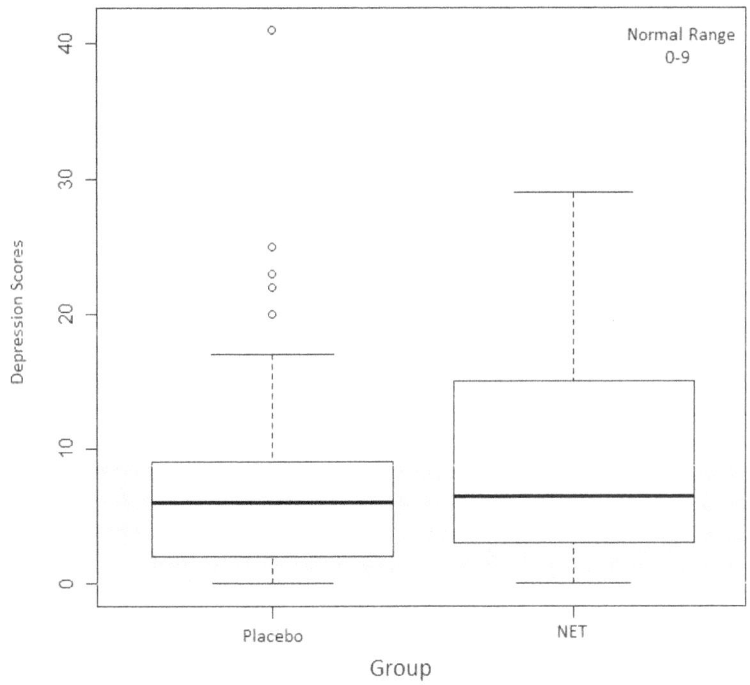

Fig. 2 Baseline depression scores

participant also described feeling "light-headed" after the sixth treatment session. One participant described feeling "drained" after the ninth treatment session. One participant described the sensation of her "head spinning" after the first treatment session. This same participant reported "pain in the lower neck" after the second session and reported a "light headed" feeling after treatments three, four, six and nine. On treatment number nine the participant reported "Always feeling a bit light headed". On visits seven and eight this same participant reported feeling "tired". One participant in the NET group developed a sore throat during the middle of the treatment phase which abated after two weeks. One participant reported feeling "a bit sad" after the ninth treatment session. One participant reported feeling "depressed" after the first and second treatment sessions. During the second treatment session, the participant felt uncomfortable while discussing a memory from her past that was prompted by the questioning associated with the intervention. The participant reported that a couple of hours after this treatment that she experienced a migraine headache that lasted for several hours. The participant was unhappy with the nature of treatment and withdrew herself from the trial. The vast majority of adverse events observed in the NET group occurred directly after the application of the intervention and were not reported at the time of subsequent interventions indicating that these events were of a limited duration. The participants who did experience adverse events did not require any treatment aside from reassurance from the associated practitioner. No adverse events were reported in the NET group during the post-intervention phase of the clinical trial.

Adverse events - placebo group

Six (13 %) participants reported adverse events that coincided with the application of the placebo intervention. Five of the six described feeling "tired" directly after one or more of the placebo intervention sessions. One participant described feeling "sore" after the tapping applied by the treating practitioner to the right inferior angle of the scapula. No adverse events or harms were reported in the placebo group during or after the post-intervention phase of the clinical trial.

Blinding survey

Of the total number of participants that undertook the blinding survey ($n = 81$), 10/41 (24 %) of placebo participants correctly assumed that they were allocated to the placebo group. Two out of 40 (5 %) participants in the NET group correctly assumed their assignment to the NET group. There was a statistically significant difference between these two proportions (Fisher's exact test, $p = 0.025$). Based on these results, participants in the placebo group appeared more likely to correctly guess their group allocation compared to individuals in the NET group.

Table 4 Analysis of primary and secondary outcomes

Outcome	MCID (±)	Difference between groups 7 weeks (NET-Placebo)		Difference between groups 6 months (NET-Placebo)		Time x group interaction
		Mean difference (95 % CI)	P-value	Mean difference (95 % CI)	P-value	P-value
Depression	4	−0.58 (−4.62, 3.45)	0.78	−0.04 (−4.04, 3.96)	0.98	0.60
Anxiety	5	0.63 (−2.19, 3.46)	0.66	0.36 (−2.44, 3.16)	0.80	0.98
Stress	4	0.29 (−3.63, 4.21)	0.88	1.47 (−2.42, 5.35)	0.46	0.86
TSH	0.75	0.11 (−2.64, 2.88)	0.93	1.01 (−1.76, 3.77)	0.47	0.49
FT4	6.0	0.67 (−0.81, 2.15)	0.37	0.33 (−1.14, 1.80)	0.66	0.85
FT3	1.5	0.29 (−0.24, 0.83)	0.28	0.15 (−0.38, 0.68)	0.58	0.82
Physical functioning	3.5	−0.76 (−9.07, 7.56)	0.86	1.75 (−6.41, 9.91)	0.67	0.35
Role physical	3.2	4.25 (−7.31, 15.81)	0.47	4.35 (−6.93, 15.63)	0.45	0.99
Bodily pain	4.5	3.56 (−7.62, 14.73)	0.53	2.35 (−8.43, 13.13)	0.67	0.76
General health	5.7	2.11 (−8.20, 12.43)	0.69	3.35 (−6.78, 13.47)	0.52	0.28
Vitality	5.5	0.27 (−9.76, 10.30)	0.96	−0.10 (−9.84, 9.65)	0.98	0.76
Social functioning	5.0	9.05 (−4.55, 22.66)	0.19	5.58 (−7.54, 18.69)	0.40	0.65
Role emotional	3.8	2.12 (−8.72, 12.96)	0.70	1.13 (−9.36, 11.61)	0.83	0.86
Mental health	5.5	4.73 (−5.23, 14.72)	0.35	4.83 (−4.84, 14.49)	0.33	0.65
Mental component summary	3.1	4.11 (−1.58, 9.79)	0.16	0.22 (−5.25, 5.69)	0.94	0.36
Physical component summary	3.8	1.02 (−3.14, 5.18)	0.63	0.97 (−3.10, 5.03)	0.64	0.50

MCID minimal clinically important difference, *TSH* thyroid stimulating hormone (mIU/L), *FT4* free thyroxine (pmol/L), *FT3* Free triiodothyronine (pmol/L)

Discussion

This is the first randomized controlled trial investigating the short-medium term effects of NET treatment on individuals with primary hypothyroidism. Both treatment effects and harms data were captured in this study with the major findings presented below.

The NET and placebo groups were comparable with respect to clinical and demographic data at baseline. The vast majority of the study population were taking some form of thyroid medication, most commonly LT4, for their condition. The mean and median serum TSH, FT3, and FT4 concentrations were within the normal range. The

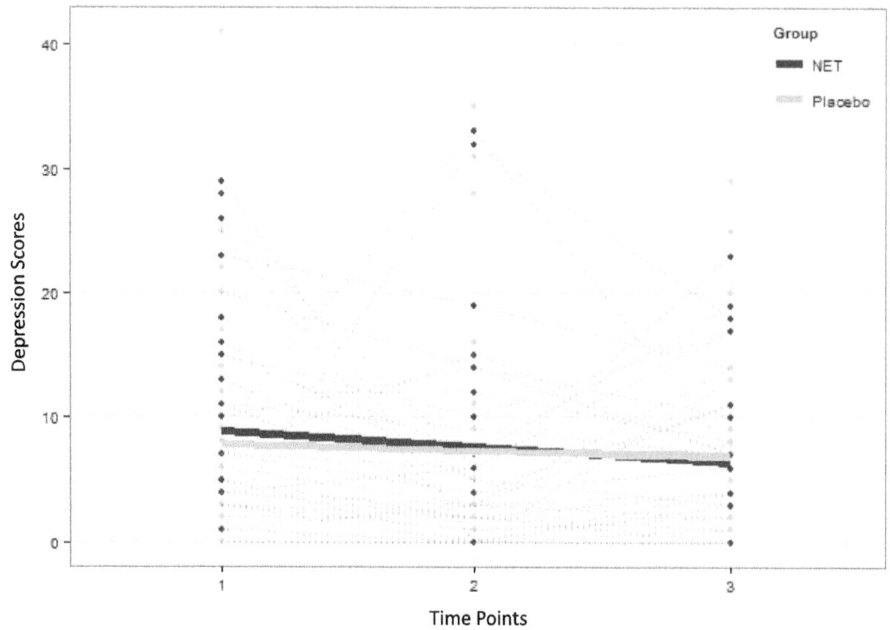

Fig. 3 Depression scores over time

majority of participants displayed abnormal TPO-Ab concentrations at baseline indicating the presence of thyroid autoimmunity. The mean and median depression scores were within normal range however, a substantial proportion of participants displayed abnormal depression scores at baseline. A similar scenario was observed with respect to the anxiety and stress scores at the time of the initial assessment. For the SF-36v2 data, mean self-reported general health, vitality, social functioning, and mental health scores were lower in the study population compared to normative data. These baseline neuropsychiatric findings were expected given the continued symptomatology reported large community based samples of patients with treated hypothyroidism [14, 16, 23].

The results of the analyses revealed that there were no significant differences, at the 5 % significance level, between the NET and placebo groups at time seven weeks or six months for any of the trial outcomes.

If NET has a stress-reducing effect, either; this has not been demonstrated in this particular study; or stress may not be a salient factor in onset and/or progression of this chronic disease. Further research, with much larger sample sizes, is required to ascertain the exact role of stress in the pathogenesis and progression of primary hypothyroidism.

With respect to harms, the way in which the NET treatment was applied, including the dosage, was well-tolerated by the study participants. There were some minor, short-lived adverse-events that followed the application of both the NET and placebo interventions.

Strengths of the study

This is the first RCT investigating the short-medium term treatment effects of NET in participants with primary hypothyroidism. Practitioners of varying backgrounds with similar clinical expertise in NET applied the intervention to the cohort. The approach to delivery, as well as the dosage of the intervention was based on a private practice model of care. The typical participant in the trial was a Caucasian female with a mean age of 45 years, with evidence of thyroid autoimmunity. This profile aligns strongly with epidemiological data regarding patients with primary hypothyroidism [3, 8, 97]. Due to the systemic influence of the thyroid hormones a wide selection of outcome measures were employed that would have captured any short-medium term physiological and psychological changes that coincided with the application of the intervention.

Limitations

Designing placebo interventions can be difficult in research when the underlying biological mechanism behind the therapy is unknown [98]. For this reason, designing a placebo in complementary and alternative medicine research is often dependent on unsubstantiated assumptions about the specificity of the intervention [99]. With this in mind, the placebo was designed via the collaboration of a group of NET certified practitioners, and members of the research team. The aim was to create a placebo intervention that would: closely mimic the NET intervention; would not provide any therapeutic benefit; would be considered credible by the participants; and would be of comparable duration to the NET procedure. The results from the analysis of the blinding survey results would suggest that the placebo intervention was more likely to be viewed as a 'sham' procedure compared to the NET treatment. As the practitioners were involved in the administration of both the NET and placebo interventions, it was not possible to blind these individuals to group allocation. However, to reduce the problem of non-blinding, practitioners were under strict instruction not to reveal group allocation to participants during the trial, and also to refrain from discussing any of the procedures in detail. Furthermore, as the treatment being provided by the practitioners in their private clinics was not recorded or monitored it was not possible to guarantee the fidelity of either of the treatment arms. Slight differences in the delivery of the NET and placebo intervention may account for the results observed in the blinding survey.

The participant's subjective report regarding reactions or adverse events associated with the intervention had the potential to be selectively-filtered by the treating practitioners. The majority of practitioners involved in the trial regularly use NET in their private clinics. These practitioners would presumably want to demonstrate the efficacy and safety of the intervention which may have introduced performance and/or reporting bias.

The study was designed to explore the influence of a biopsychosocial-based treatment approach on the clinical manifestations of primary hypothyroidism. The approach involved a diverse number of outcome measures, and multi-centre format in order to make use of all available resources. This scenario can be problematic in that it introduces the statistical problem of multiple comparisons in which the chances of obtaining a false positive result are increased [100]. While no corrections for multiple testing were used given the exploratory nature of the secondary outcomes this type of correction would not have changed the results obtained in this study.

A power analysis indicated that 51 participants per group would yield a more than 80 % chance of detecting a difference in depression scores of at least four points in NET group compared to the placebo group using a standard deviation of 6.97 based on normative data. The fact that the recruitment of participants fell short of the desired sample size means that there is reduced power to find a difference between groups. If we examine how many participants in each group achieved a four point decrease in depression scores at 7 weeks (11/22 for NET vs 7/18 for placebo) then a 95 % confidence interval for the number needed to treat before a positive treatment outcome occurred would be (−19 to 29). This wide interval indicates anything from no benefit to benefit for 1 in 29 participants and reflects the uncertainty in the data collected.

The sample that was obtained aligns well with profiles from large population studies regarding patients with primary hypothyroidism. There is however the potential that a specific type of participant responded to the recruitment advertisements. As the advertisements were calling for participation in research investigating a new, drug-free treatment for hypothyroidism, it is possible that individuals who were either: not taking medication; opposed to the concept of taking medication; poorly compliant with their current medication regimens; or dissatisfied with their current management regimens were more likely to respond. Furthermore, the advertisements made reference to the Department of Chiropractic at Macquarie University, as the host of this research. Proponents of chiropractic/complementary and alternative medicine, or individuals with positive past experiences with chiropractic treatment may therefore have been over represented in the sample population.

Both the DASS-42 and the SF-36v2 have recall periods of less than one month. For this reason, treatment effects with long latency periods may have been missed in between the seven-week and six-month assessments.

Dr Scott Walker [101], the creator of NET, originally designed the technique to be an adjunct to the usual manual therapy procedures he was using in his private practice. Walker deemed psychosomatic stress to be an important factor contributing to continued or cyclical symptomatology in his patients and designed NET to tackle this problem. The technique represented an additional tool that a practitioner could use if the standard manual procedures alone were not having a longstanding therapeutic effect in patients with musculoskeletal conditions [102]. Later on in the development of NET, Walker added nutritional elements and aspects of homeopathy to the NET procedure. In an attempt to make the investigation of NET more manageable, and the results from the study more comprehensible, the research team restricted the intervention to only the component of NET that deals with psychosocial stress. Based on reviews of homeopathy trials, the magnitude and plausibility of treatment effects of homeopathy for specific medical conditions remains poorly defined [103–105]. In a recent report from the National Health and Medical Research Council of Australia a working committee concluded that there were no health conditions for which there is reliable evidence that homeopathy is effective [106]. In the latest guidelines for the management of hypothyroidism, produced by the American Thyroid Association Taskforce, strong recommendations were made against the use of dietary supplements and nutraceuticals [12]. The main reasons for these recommendations were A) the lack of evidence regarding the efficacy of these products and B) the potential risks associated with the use of these products for individuals with thyroid conditions. There is a dearth of high quality evidence regarding manual therapy for the treatment of hypothyroidism and a limited evidence-base for homeopathy and nutrition in this role. It is therefore difficult to ascertain what effect removing these components may have had on the overall efficacy of the NET procedure.

As stress is a potential environmental risk factor for the development of primary hypothyroidism, it is possible that NET treatment, a purported stress reduction technique, may function better in a preventative role. In cases of long standing autoimmune thyroid disease there is inflammation and subsequent destruction of the thyroid follicles. This results in the replacement of the thyroid parenchymal tissue with non-functional fibrous tissue [107]. In this scenario, the pathophysiological consequences of autoimmune thyroid disease have resulted in tissue that no longer has an endocrine function. While the disease process and the associated symptomatology continues, the damaged tissue is unlikely to respond, from an endocrine perspective, to any therapeutic intervention. To determine the preventative effect of NET treatment would require a large scale preventative trial which currently lacks evidential support and is beyond the scope of this discussion.

In obtaining ethics approval for this study researchers were required to outline the foreseeable risks associated with participation in the study. At the time of the trial design there were no published harms data regarding NET. As a result, an information and consent form was drafted that included likely potential adverse events such as muscle soreness, tiredness, and an uncomfortable recall of past events. These events were suggested as potential outcomes during consultation with experts in NET. While there were some minor adverse events that coincided with the intervention in both the NET and placebo groups, there is the possibility that participants were primed [108] to report certain events due to the content of this information and consent form.

Conclusions

In this study, NET intervention was not found to confer any clinical benefit to the participants in the short or medium term.

The data recorded on harms suggest that there are some minor, short-term, adverse events associated with the application of this procedure. These events however were predictable, relatively innocuous and did not require further intervention to remedy.

Appendix

Health update questionnaire

Name: ________________________ Date: ____________

There are events and situations that occur in our lives that can influence our health and well-being. When running a clinical trial it is important for researchers to be aware of any events or situations that may influence the findings of the trial.

This questionnaire is designed to identify any factors that may influence the findings of the trial, and hence influence the final interpretation of results.

We ask that you fill out the questionnaire as accurately as possible. This information, when combined with the data obtained from initial and subsequent assessments, will help researchers accurately interpret the findings at the end of the trial.

Q1) Have you changed your medication or changed the way in which you are managing your condition (Hypothyroidism) in the last 6 months since beginning the trial? (Please circle one)

Yes No

If so, what have you changed?

____

____

Q2) Have you tried any other forms of treatment for your condition in the last 6 months since beginning the trial? (Please circle one)

Yes No

If so, what have you tried?

____

____

Q3) Have there been any major stressful situations or events in the last 6 months that may have influenced you general health and well-being? (Please circle one)

Yes No

If so, what were these situations or events? (Optional)

____

____

Q4) Have you made any significant alterations to your life or your lifestyle in the last 6 months since beginning the trial? (Please circle one)

Yes No

If so, what alterations have you made? (Optional)

____

____

Thank you for taking the time to fill out this questionnaire

Abbreviations

DASS-42: Depression anxiety stress scale-42 item; DQ: Demographic questionnaire; FT4: Free-Thyroxine; HPA: Hypothalamic-pituitary-adrenal; HUQ: Health update questionnaire; LT4: Levothyroxine; QOL: Quality of life; RCT: Randomized control trial; RHR: Resting Heart Rate; RT: Resting Temperature; SF-36v2: Short form 36 version 2; TFT: Thyroid function test; Tg-Ab: Thyroglobulin antibody; Tg: Thyroglobulin protein; TPO-Ab: Thyroid peroxidase antibody; TPO: Thyroid peroxidase enzyme; TSH: Thyroid stimulating hormone.

Competing interests

BTB is a chiropractor who works part-time in private practice. BTB has received training in NET and uses this technique in his private practice. HP was an employee of the ONE Research Foundation from 2002–2011. RB and PLG have no conflicts of interest to declare.

Authors' contributions

BTB wrote and compiled the manuscript. PLG, RB and HP were involved with the data collection and analysis and helped edit and review the final manuscript. BTB, RB and HP designed the trial. All authors read and approved the final manuscript.

Acknowledgements

The research project was funded (AUD $28,000) by the Australian Spinal Research Foundation (ASRF), as well as smaller ongoing contributions from the Macquarie University Postgraduate Research Fund (PGRF). The ASRF had no input into the design, conduct and publication of the study results.
The authors would like to thank the individual practitioners who donated their time and expertise: Gerald Vargas, Bill Stathoulis, Nicholas Kovacs, Alison Griffiths, Luke Rossmanith, Peter O'Dwyer, Jackie Castell, Suzanne Labrie, Walter Kiris, and Alex McLennan.
The authors would like to thank Peter Bablis for his advice and assistance in the design of the clinical trial.

Author details

[1]Department of Chiropractic, Macquarie University, Balaclava Road, North Ryde 2109NSW, Australia. [2]Department of Statistics, Macquarie University, Balaclava Road, North Ryde 2109NSW, Australia. [3]School of Health Professions - Murdoch University, 90 South Street, Murdoch 6150WA, Australia. [4]Private Practice, 84 Kingsway, Cronulla 2230NSW, Australia.

References

1. O'Leary PC, Feddema PH, Michelangeli VP, Leedman PJ, Chew GT, Knuiman M, et al. Investigations of thyroid hormones and antibodies based on a community health survey: the Busselton thyroid study. Clin Endocrinol (Oxf). 2006;64(1):97–104.
2. Vanderpump MP, Tunbridge WM, French JM, Appleton D, Bates D, Clark F, et al. The incidence of thyroid disorders in the community: a twenty year follow-up of the Wickham Survey. Clin Endocrinol. 1995;43(1):55–68.
3. Canaris GJ, Manowitz MR, Mayor G, Ridgway EC. The Colorado thyroid disease prevalence study. Arch Intern Med. 2000;160(4):526–34.
4. McLeod DSA, Cooper DS. The incidence and prevalence of thyroid autoimmunity. Endocrine. 2012;42(2):252–65.
5. McDermott MT. In the clinic. Hypothyroidism. Ann Intern Med. 2009;151(11):ITC61.
6. Monzani F, Del Guerra P, Carraccio N, Pruneti CA, Pucci E, Luisi M, et al. Subclinical hypothyroidism: neurobehavioural features and beneficial effect of L-thyroxine treatment. Clin Invest. 1993;71:367–71.
7. Roberts CGP, Ladenson PW. Hypothyroidism. Lancet. 2004;363(9411):793–831.
8. Hollowell JG, Staehling NW, Flanders WD, Hannon WH, Gunter EW, Spencer CA, et al. Serum TSH, T(4), and thyroid antibodies in the United States population (1988 to 1994): National Health and Nutrition Examination Survey (NHANES III). J Clin Endocrinol Metab. 2002;87(2):489–99.
9. O'Reilly DSJ. Thyroid hormone replacement: An iatrogenic problem. Int J Clin Pract. 2010;64:991–4.
10. Romijn JA, Lamberts JW, Smit SW. Intrinsic imperfections of endocrine replacement therapy. Eur J Endocrinol. 2003;149(2):91–7.

11. Fava GA, Sonino N, Morphy MA. Psychosomatic view of endocrine disorders. Psychother Psychosom. 1993;59(1):20–33.
12. Jonklaas J, Bianco AC, Bauer AJ, Burman KD, Cappola AR, Celi FS, et al. Guidelines for the treatment of hypothyroidism. Thyroid. 2014;24(12):1670–751. doi:10.1089/thy.2014.0028.
13. Saravanan P, Visser TJ, Dayan CM. Psychological well-being correlates with free thyroxine but not free 3,5,3'-triiodothyronine levels in patients on thyroid hormone replacement. J Clin Endocrinol Metab. 2006;91(9):3389–93.
14. Saravanan P, Chaut WF, Roberts N, Vedharas K, Greenwood R, Dayan CM. Psychological well-being in patients on adequate doses of L-thyroxine: results of a large, controlled community based questionnaire study. Clin Endocrinol. 2002;57:577–85.
15. Samuels MH, Schuff KG, Carlson NE, Carello P, Janowsky JS. Health status, psychological symptoms, mood, and cognition in L-thyroxine-treated hypothyroid subjects. Thyroid. 2007;17(3):249–58.
16. Wekking EM, Appelhof BC, Fliers E, Schene AH, Huyser J, Tijssen JG, et al. Cognitive functioning and well-being in euthyroid patients on thyroxine replacement therapy for primary hypothyroidism. Eur J Endocrinol. 2005;153(6):747–53.
17. Panicker VEJ, Bjøro T, Asvold BO, Dayan CM, Bjerkeset O. A paradoxical difference in relationship between anxiety, depression and thyroid function in subjects on and not on T4: findings from the HUNT study. Clin Endocrinol. 2009;71:574–80.
18. Ott J, Promberger R, Kober F, Neuhold N, Tea M, Huber JC, et al. Hashimoto's thyroiditis affects symptom load and quality of life unrelated to hypothyroidism: A prospective case–control study in women undergoing thyroidectomy for benign goiter. Thyroid. 2011;21(2):161–7.
19. Boelaert K, Newby PR, Simmonds MJ, Holder RL, Carr-Smith JD, Heward JM, et al. Prevalence and relative risk of other autoimmune diseases in subjects with autoimmune thyroid disease. Am J Med. 2010;123(2):183.e1–e9.
20. McDermott MT. Does combination T4 and T3 therapy make sense? Endocr Pract. 2012;18(5):750–7.
21. Peeters RP, van Toor H, Klootwijk W, de Rijke YB, Kuiper GG, Uitterlinden AG, et al. Polymorphisms in thyroid hormone pathway genes are associated with plasma TSH and iodothyronine levels in healthy subjects. J Clin Endocrinol Metab. 2003;88(6):2880–8.
22. Peeters RP, Attalki H, Toor H, de Rijke YB, Kuiper GG, Lamberts SW, et al. A new polymorphism in the type II deiodinase gene is associated with circulating thyroid hormone parameters. Am J Physiol Endocrinol Metab. 2005;289:E75–81.
23. Panicker V, Saravanan P, Vaidya B, Evans J, Hattersley AT, Frayling TM, et al. Common variation in the DIO2 gene predicts baseline psychological well-being and response to combination thyroxine plus triiodothyronine therapy in hypothyroid patients. J Clin Endocrinol Metab. 2009;94(5):1623–9.
24. Walsh JP, Ward LC, Burke V, Bhagat CI, Shiels L, Henley D, et al. Small changes in thyroxine dosage do not produce measurable changes in hypothyroid symptoms, well-being, or quality of life: Results of a double-blind, randomized clinical trial. J Clin Endocrinol Metab. 2006;91(7):2624–30.
25. Grozinsky-Glasberg S, Fraser A, Nahshoni E, Weizman A, Leibovici L. Thyroxine-Triiodothyronine combination therapy versus thyroxine monotherapy for clinical hypothyroidism: meta-analysis of randomized controlled trials. J Clin Endocrinol Metab. 2006;91:2592–9.
26. Wojcicka A, Bassett JHD, Williams GR. Mechanisms of action of thyroid hormones in the skeleton. Biochim Biophys Acta Gen Subj. 2013;1830(7):3979–86.
27. Joffe RT, Brimacombe M, Levitt AJ, Stagnaro-Green A. Treatment of clinical hypothyroidism with thyroxine and triiodothyronine: A literature review and metaanalysis. Psychosomatics. 2007;48(5):379–84.
28. Caturegli P, De Remigis A, Rose NR. Hashimoto thyroiditis: Clinical and diagnostic criteria. Autoimmun Rev. 2014;13(4–5):391–7.
29. Quaratino S. Models of autoimmune thyroiditis. Drug Discov Today. 2004;1(4):417–23.
30. Prummel MF, Strieder T, Wiersinga WM. The environment and autoimmune thyroid diseases. Eur J Endocrinol. 2004;150(5):605–18.
31. Tomer Y, Huber A. The etiology of autoimmune thyroid disease: A story of genes and environment. J Autoimmun. 2009;32:231–9.
32. Wasserman EE, Nelson K, Rose NR, Rhode C, Pillion JP, Seaberg E, et al. Infection and thyroid autoimmunity: A seroepidemiologic study of TPOaAb. Autoimmunity. 2009;42(5):439–46.
33. Oddie TH, Fisher DA, McConahey WM, Thompson CS. Iodine intake in the United States: a reassessment. J Clin Endocrinol Metab. 1970;30(5):659–65.
34. Hay ID. Thyroiditis: a clinical update. Mayo Clin Proc. 1985;60:836–43.
35. Krassas GE, Pontikides N, Tziomalos K, Tzotzas T, Zosin I, Vlad M, et al. Selenium status in patients with autoimmune and non-autoimmune thyroid diseases from four European countries. Expert Rev Endocrinol Metab. 2014;9(6):685–92.
36. Srivatsa B, Srivatsa S, Johnson KL, Samura O, Lee SL, Bianchi DW. Microchimerism of presumed fetal origin in thyroid specimens from women: a case–control study. Lancet. 2001;358(9298):2034–8.
37. Klintschar M, Schwaiger P, Mannweiler S, Regauer S, Kleiber M. Evidence of fetal microchimerism in Hashimoto's thyroiditis. J Clin Endocrinol Metab. 2001;86(6):2494–8.
38. Wang J, Zhang W, Liu H, Wang D, Wang W, Li Y, et al. Parvovirus B19 infection associated with Hashimoto's thyroiditis in adults. J Infect. 2010;60(5):360–70.
39. Antonelli A, Ferri C, Fallahi P, Ferrari SM, Ghinoi A, Rotondi M, et al. Thyroid disorders in chronic hepatitis C virus infection. Thyroid. 2006;16(6):563–72.
40. Winsa B, Karlsson A, Bergstrom R, Adami HO, Gamstedt A, Jansson R, et al. Stressful life events and Graves' disease. Lancet. 1991;338(8781):1475–9.
41. Gibson JG. Emotions and the thyroid gland: A critical appraisal. Psychosom Res. 1962;6:93–116.
42. Winsa B, Adami H, Bergström R, Gamstedt A, Dahlberg PA, Adamson U, et al. Stressful life events and Graves' disease. Lancet. 1991;338:1475–9.
43. Matos-Santos A, Lacerda Nobre E, Garcia E, Costa J, Nogueira PJ, Macedo A, et al. Relationship between the number and impact of stressful life events and the onset of Graves' Disease and toxic nodular goitre. Clin Endocrinol. 2001;55(1):15–9.
44. Boscarino JA. Posttraumatic stress disorder and physical illness: Results from clinical and epidemiologic studies. Ann N Y Acad Sci. 2004;1032:141–53.
45. Ferguson-Raypoht SM. The relation of emotional factors to recurrence of thyrotoxicosis. Can Med Assoc J. 1956;75:993–9.
46. Graves RJ. Newly observed affection of the thyroid gland in females. London Med Surg. 1835;7:516–7.
47. Glaser R, Kiecolt-Glaser JK. Stress-induced immune dysfunction: Implications for health. Nat Rev Immunol. 2005;5:243–51.
48. Juster R-P, McEwen BS, Lupien SJ. Allostatic load biomarkers of chronic stress and impact on health and cognition. Neurosci Biobehav Rev. 2010;35(1):2–16.
49. Segerstrom SC, Miller GE. Psychological stress and the human immune system: A meta-analytic study of 30 years of inquiry. Psychol Bull. 2004;130(4):601–30.
50. Elenkov IJ, Chrousos GP. Stress hormones, Th1/Th2 patterns, pro/anti-inflammatory cytokines and susceptibility to disease. Trends Endocrinol Metab. 1999;10(9):359–68.
51. Elenkov IJ. Glucocorticoids and the Th1/Th2 balance. Ann N Y Acad Sci. 2004;1024:138–46.
52. Chrousos GP. Stressors, stress, and neuroendocrine integration of the adaptive response - The 1997 Hans Seyle memorial lecture. Ann N Y Acad Sci. 1998;851:311–35.
53. Chrousos GP, Gold PW. The concepts of stress and stress system disorders: Overview of physical and behavioral homeostasis. JAMA. 1992;267(9):1244–52.
54. Wilder RL. Neuroendocrine-immune system interactions and autoimmunity. Ann Rev Immunol. 1995;13:307–38.
55. Ganesh BB, Bhattacharya P, Gopisetty A, Prabhakar BS. Role of cytokines in the pathogenesis and suppression of thyroid autoimmunity. J Interferon Cytokine Res. 2011;31(10):721–31.
56. Parish NM, Cooke A. Mechanisms of autoimmune thyroid disease. Drug Discov Today Dis Mech. 2004;1(3):337–44.
57. Trickett PK, Noll JG, Susman EJ, Shenk CE, Putnam FW. Attenuation of cortisol across development for victims of sexual abuse. Dev Psychopathol. 2010;22(1):165–75.
58. Danielson CK, Hankin BL, Badanes LS. Youth offspring of mothers with posttraumatic stress disorder have altered stress reactivity in response to a laboratory stressor. Psychoneuroendocrinology. 2015;53:170–8.
59. Bagnasco M, Bossert I, Pesce G. Stress and autoimmune thyroid diseases. Neuroimmunomodulation. 2007;13(5–6):309–17.

60. Strieder TGPM, Tijssen JG, Brosschot JF, Wiersinga WM. Stress is not associated with thyroid peroxidase autoantibodies in euthyroid women. Brain Behav Immun. 2005;19:203–6.
61. Strieder TG, Prummel MF, Tijssen JG, Endert E, Wiersinga WM. Risk factors for and prevalence of thyroid disorders in a cross-sectional study among healthy female relatives of patients with autoimmune thyroid disease. Clin Endocrinol. 2003;59(3):396–401.
62. Oretti RG, Harris B, Lazarus JH, Parkes AB, Crownshaw T. Is there an association between life events, postnatal depression and thyroid dysfunction in thyroid antibody positive women? Int J Soc Psych. 2003;49(1):70–6.
63. Bablis P, Pollard H. Hypothyroidism: A new model for conservative management in two cases. Chiropr J Aust. 2004;34:11–8.
64. Bablis P, Pollard H. A mind-body treatment for hypothyroid dysfunction: A report of two cases. Complement Ther Clin Pract. 2009;15:67–71.
65. Touzard JB, Busch-Pate T, Busch J. Thinking about a problem while getting adjusted? Dr Scott Walker may have the answer? The American Chiropractor. 2008.
66. Walker D, Walker S. Chiropractic technique summary: Neuro Emotional Technique (NET) 2010. http://www.chiroaccess.com/Articles/Chiropractic-Technique-Summary-Neuro-Emotional-Technique-NET.aspx?id=0000185. Last accessed 6th of May 2015.
67. Moher D, Hopewellb S, Schulzc FS, Montorid V, Gøtzschee PC, Devereauxf PJ, et al. CONSORT 2010 explanation and elaboration: updated guidelines for reporting parallel group randomized trials. BMJ. 2010;63:1–37.
68. Schulz KF, Altman DG, Moher D. Consort 2010 statement: updated guidelines for reporting parallel group randomized trials. Ann Intern Med. 2010;152(11):1–7.
69. Boutron I, Moher D, Altman DG, Schulz KF, Ravaud P. Extending the CONSORT statement to randomized trials of nonpharmacologic treatment: explanation and elaboration. Ann Intern Med. 2008;148:295–309.
70. Ioannidis JPA, Evans SJW, Gøtzsche PC, O'Neill RT, Altman DG, Schulz K, et al. Better reporting of harms in randomized trials: an extension of the CONSORT statement. Ann Intern Med. 2004;141:781–8.
71. The George Institute for Global Health. PEDro scale: The George Institute; 1999. http://www.pedro.org.au/english/downloads/pedro-scale/. Last accessed 6th May 2015.
72. Verhagen AP, de Vet HC, de Bie R, Kessels AG, Boers M, Bouter LM, et al. The Delphi list: a criteria list for quality assessment of randomized clinical trials for conducting systematic reviews developed by Delphi consensus. J Clin Epidemiol. 1998;51(12):1235–41.
73. Altman DG, Schulz KF, Moher D, Egger M, Davidoff F, Elbourne D, et al. The Revised CONSORT statement for reporting randomized trials: explanation and elaboration. Ann Intern Med. 2001;134(8):663–94.
74. Boutron I, Moher D, Altman DG, Schulz KF, Ravaud P. Methods and processes of the CONSORT group: example of an extension for trials assessing nonpharmacologic treatments. Ann Intern Med. 2008;148:60–6.
75. Horvath E, Kovacs K, Scheithauer BW. Pituitary hyperplasia. Pituitary. 1999;1(3–4):169–80.
76. Alkhani AM, Cusimano M, Kovacs K, Bilbao JM, Horvath E, Singer W. Cytology of pituitary thyrotroph hyperplasia in protracted primary hypothyroidism. Pituitary. 1999;1(3–4):291–5.
77. NET Inc. Seminar Information & Schedule. 2014. http://www.netmindbody.com/for-practitioners/seminar-information-and-schedule. Last accessed 6th of May 2015.
78. Karpouzis F, Pollard H, Bonello R. A randomized controlled trial of the Neuro Emotional Technique (NET) for childhood Attention Deficit Hyperactivity Disorder (ADHD): a protocol. Trials. 2009;10:6.
79. Karpouzis F. Clinical Investigation of Chiropractic Neuro Emotional Technique (NET) for Attention-Deficit/Hyperactivity Disorder (ADHD) in Children: [Master of Science (Honours)]. Sydney, Australia: Macquarie University; 2011.
80. Brown BT, Bonello R, Pollard H. The biopsychosocial model and hypothyroidism. BMC Chiropr Osteopat. 2005;13:5.
81. Brown BT, Bonello R, Pollard H. The use of traditional Chinese medical principles in chiropractic technique. Chiropr J Aust. 2008;38:18–26.
82. Bablis P, Pollard H, Bonello R. Neuro emotional technique for the treatment of trigger point sensitivity in chronic neck pain sufferers: a controlled clinical trial. Chiropr Osteopat. 2008;16:4.
83. Karpouzis F, Pollard H, Bonello R. Separation anxiety disorder in a 13-year-old boy managed by the Neuro Emotional Technique as a biopsychosocial intervention. J Chiropr Med. 2008;7(3):101–6.
84. Monti DA, Stoner ME, Zivin G, Schlesinger M. Short term correlates of the Neuro Emotional Technique for cancer-related traumatic stress symptoms: A pilot case series. J Cancer Surviv. 2007;1(2):161–6.
85. Brown BT, Bonello R, Pollard H, Graham P. The influence of a biopsychosocial-based treatment approach to primary overt hypothyroidism: A protocol for a pilot study. Trials. 2010;11(106). http://www.trialsjournal.com/content/11/1/106. last accessed accessed 6th of May 2105
86. Lovibond SH, Lovibond PF. Manual for the Depression Anxiety Stress Scales (DASS). 2nd ed. University of New South Wales, NSW 2052, Australia: Psychology Foundation Monograph; 2004.
87. Abbott. Architect System -TSH. Abbott Park, IL, USA: Abbott Ireland Diagnostic Division; 2005c.
88. Abbott. Architect System - Free T3. Abbott Park, IL, USA: Abbott Ireland Diagnostic Division; 2005a.
89. Abbott. Architect System -Free T4. Abbott Park, IL, USA: Abbott Ireland Diagnostic Division; 2005b.
90. Siemens. Immulite 2500 Anti-TG Ab. Los Angeles, CA, USA: Siemens Medical Solutions Diagnostics; 2005.
91. Siemens. Immulite 2500 Anti-TPO Ab. Los Angeles, CA, USA: Siemens Medical Solutions Diagnostics; 2005.
92. Ware JE, Kosinski M, Bjorner JB, Turner-Bowker DM, Gandek B, Maruish ME. User's manual for the SF-36v2 Health Survey. 2nd ed. Lincoln RI: Quality Metric Incorproated; 2007.
93. Brant R. Inference for means: comparing two independent samples 2015. http://www.stat.ubc.ca/~rollin/stats/ssize/n2.html. last accessed 6th of May 2015.
94. Random Sequence Generator. http://www.random.org/sform.html. Last accessed 6th of May 2015.
95. Hornik K. R: A Language and Environment for Statistical Computing. Vienna, Austria 2011.
96. Little D. Statistical Analysis with Missing Data. New York: Wiley; 1987.
97. Tunbridge WM, Evered DC, Hall R, Appleton D, Brewis M, Clark F, et al. The spectrum of thyroid disease in a community: The Whickham survey. Clin Endocrinol. 1977;7(6):481–93.
98. Schulz KF, Chalmers I, Hayes RJ, Altman DG. Empirical evidence of bias. Dimensions of methodological quality associated with estimates of treatment effects in controlled trials. JAMA. 1995;273:408–12.
99. Lewith G, Barlow F, Eyles C, Flower A, Hall S, Hopwood V, et al. The context and meaning of placebos for complementary medicine. Forsch Komplementmed. 2009;16:404–12.
100. Curran-Everett D. Multiple comparisons: philosophies and illustrations. Am J Physiol Regul Integr Comp Physiol. 2000;279(1):R1–8.
101. Walker S. The Amazing Story of NET [webpage]. 2000. https://www.netmindbody.com/about-us/the-amazing-story-of-net. Last accessed 6th of May 2015.
102. Walker S, NET Basic Seminar Manual 2005. Sydney, Australia.
103. Shang A, Huwiler-Müntener K, Nartey L, Jüni P, Dörig S, Sterne JA, et al. Are the clinical effects of homoeopathy placebo effects? Comparative study of placebo-controlled trials of homoeopathy and allopathy. Lancet. 2005;366(9487):726–32.
104. Cucherat M, Haugh MC, Gooch M, Boissel JP. Evidence of clinical efficacy of homeopathy. A meta-analysis of clinical trials. Eur J Clin Pharmacol. 2000;56(1):27–33.
105. Jonas WB, Kaptchuk TJ, Linde K. A critical overview of homeopathy. Ann Intern Med. 2003;138(5):393–9.
106. National Health and Medical Research Council. NHMRC Statement: Statement on Homeopathy. National Health and Medical Research Council. 2015. March 2015. Report No.: CAM02.
107. Burek CL, Talor MV. Environmental triggers of autoimmune thyroiditis. J Autoimmun. 2009;33(3–4):183–9.
108. Lang EV, Hatsiopoulou O, Koch T, Berbaum K, Lutgendorf S, Kettenmann E, et al. Can words hurt? Patient-provider interactions during invasive procedures. Pain. 2005;114(1–2):303–9.

13

Current preventative and health promotional care offered to patients by chiropractors in the United Kingdom: a survey

Patricia E Fikar[1*], Kent A Edlund[2] and Dave Newell[2]

Abstract

Background: With increasing morbidity and mortality attributable to non-communicable disease, primary healthcare providers are urged to increasingly support people in making healthy lifestyle choices. Many chronic physical diseases associated with lifestyle behaviours have been linked to neuromusculoskeletal disorders and pain. Chiropractors, as primary healthcare professionals, are in a position to provide preventative and promotional healthcare to patients, however, it is unknown to what extent such care is provided, particularly in the United Kingdom (UK).

Method: This study was a cross sectional online questionnaire distributed to four UK chiropractic associations. The responses were collected over a period of two months from March 26th 2012 to May 25th 2012. Descriptive analyses were performed to identify the trends in current practice of chiropractors in the UK. Additionally, subgroup analyses of all items were performed using Pearson Chi-Square tests to determine statistically significant differences between respondents based on gender, years in practice, educational institution and association membership.

Results: Of the 2,448 members in the four participating associations, 509 chiropractors (approximately 21%) completed the survey. The great majority of UK chiropractors surveyed report evaluating and monitoring patients in regards to posture (97.1%), inactivity/overactivity (90.8%) and movement patterns (88.6%). Slightly fewer provide this type of care for psychosocial stress (82.3%), nutrition (74.1%) and disturbed sleep (72.9%). Still fewer do so for smoking (60.7%) and over-consumption of alcohol (56.4%). Verbal advice given by the chiropractor was reported as the most successful resource to encourage positive lifestyle changes as reported by 68.8% of respondents. Goal-setting is utilised by 70.7% to 80.4% of respondents concerning physical fitness issues. For all other lifestyle issues, goal-setting is used by approximately two-fifths (41.7%) or less. For smoking and over-consumption of alcohol, a mere one-fifth (20.0% and 20.6% respectively) of the responding chiropractors set goals.

Conclusions: UK chiropractors are participating in promoting positive lifestyle changes in areas common to preventative healthcare and health promotion areas; however, more can be done, particularly in the areas of smoking and over-consumption of alcohol. In addition, goal-setting to support patient-provider relationships should be more widespread, potentially increasing the utility of such valuable advice and resources.

Keywords: Chiropractic, Health promotion, Health prevention, Wellness, Non-communicable disease, Goal-setting

* Correspondence: patricia.fikar@gmail.com
[1]Private Practice, Vienna, Austria
Full list of author information is available at the end of the article

Background

One of the greatest challenges facing global public health is the burden of non-communicable diseases (NCDs). NCDs are non-infectious and non-transmittable which include chronic, slow progressing diseases. Statistics show that in 2008, of the 57 million deaths globally, 36 million where due to NCDs of which 80% were preventable [1]. Top on the list are cardiovascular disease (most especially coronary heart disease and stroke), cancer, chronic respiratory disease and diabetes. Additionally, many countries report mental health issues as contributors to the burden by increasing the instance of the other NCDs [2]. Consequently, the World Health Organization (WHO), in its Global Strategy on Diet, Physical Activity and Health [3], is encouraging individuals to make appropriate lifestyle changes and is looking to healthcare professionals of all disciplines to be facilitators in this task on both an individual patient basis and for society as a whole. It emphasised that primary care providers have an important duty to make routine inquiries regarding these issues, helping individuals where possible to develop sustained behavioural change.

In 2006, the Council on Chiropractic Education (CCE) in the United States of America (USA) suggested a set of standards indicating specific health promotional efforts that every chiropractor should perform and health promotion and prevention methods that ideally should be part of the curriculum at accredited USA chiropractic colleges [4]. According to this standard, accepted principles of health promotion include assessing the patients' health status, screening for risky lifestyle behaviours, and using multiple health outcome instruments. Preventative care includes educating patients regarding the impact of lifestyle on health, providing appropriate recommendations and counselling, and providing the necessary resources to promote health and wellness. For the purpose of this paper, health promotion and preventative care will take these two definitions.

Acknowledging the debate within the chiropractic profession as to whether chiropractors serve as primary care providers or spine specialists, Evans and Rupert [5] argue that health promotion and prevention are important to all chiropractors regardless of their view on their role in healthcare. They state that since many chiropractic patients seek care as part of a health maintenance programme, chiropractors are well-positioned to make routine inquiry and initiate preventative care and health promotion. In a study by Von Korff et al. [6], the authors concluded that chronic spinal pain may be co morbid with another conditions including stroke, hypertension, asthma, COPD, irritable bowel syndrome, ulcers, HIV/AIDS, epilepsy and vision problems, which are by association relevant to chiropractors. In a systematic review by Goldberg et al. [7], it was found that smoking is likely to be associated with the incidence and prevalence of non-specific back pain. Additionally, in a multiphase cross-sectional survey of muscu loskeletal pain in the United Kingdom (UK) general population, Webb et al. [8] reported obesity as an important independent predictor of back pain and its severity. Furthermore, Fishbain et al. [9] found depression to be more common in chronic pain patients than in healthy controls as a consequence of the presence of chronic pain, further highlighting the importance of addressing these issues in all types of chiropractic practices.

Although some patients seek chiropractic care for pain relief and end treatment when they become asymptomatic, Evans and Rupert [5] suggest that if a patient indicates willingness to attempt to change any unhealthy behaviour, chiropractors should not simply stress personal empowerment, but be able to provide specific information and resources. UK chiropractic education not only consists of chiropractic technique and diagnosis, but provides chiropractors with a broad base in health knowledge including nutrition, physical fitness and psychosocial considerations in patient care [10]. Additionally, UK chiropractors can further their knowledge in these areas by completing continuing professional development hours through self-directed study, continuing post-graduate education or by attending national and international seminars [11].

Preventative health care and health promotion are of emerging importance to the chiropractic profession. Previous work in this area has been done by Evans et al. [12] who focused on the patients' perspective of health promotional advice in a chiropractic teaching clinic in the USA, however, the chiropractors' perspective on providing this type of care to their patients is unknown. Therefore, the purpose of this UK-based study is two-fold. Firstly, to determine if care is being provided by UK chiropractors in regards to preventative healthcare and health promotion, particularly in the areas of nutrition, physical fitness and exercise, psychosocial well-being, smoking and alcohol consumption. Secondly, to identify to what extent such care is provided.

Methods

The survey questionnaire was generated from November, 2011 to March, 2012. The items were organised into categories, namely, nutrition, physical activity, psychosocial well-being, smoking and alcohol consumption. Additionally, every item on the questionnaire had a comment box where the participants could leave additional issues that did not appear on the item lists. The information submitted in these comment boxes were not included in the data analysis, but rather used for interpretation and to direct future research.

To reach a large number of chiropractors throughout the UK, the survey was distributed electronically through four UK chiropractic associations. The four participating

UK associations were the British Chiropractic Association (BCA) [13], the McTimoney Chiropractic Association (MCA) [14], the Scottish Chiropractic Association (SCA) [15], and the United Chiropractic Association (UCA) [16]. The survey items were entered into the open source online survey application Limesurvey® [17]. An email bulletin with a link to the survey requesting members to participate was sent to the chiropractors by the associations' secretaries. The survey ran once for a two-month period from the 26th of March, 2012 to the 25th of May, 2012. A reminder bulletin was sent at the end of April 2012 to all members regardless if they had already completed the survey or not, however, the bulletin indicated that they should only complete the survey once. Descriptive analyses were performed to identify the trends in current practice of chiropractors in the UK. Additionally, with the use of Statistical Package for the Social Sciences (SPSS 21.0), subgroup analyses of all items were performed using Pearson Chi-Square tests to determine statistically significant differences between respondents based on gender, years in practice, educational institution and association membership.

Ethics

This research was ethically approved by the Anglo-European College of Chiropractic undergraduate ethics panel in March 2012.

Results

Cohort characteristics

Five hundred and nine participants returned fully completed surveys. The total number of members of the four participating associations, which was provided through email request by the associations' secretaries, sums up to 2,448 member chiropractors. The 509 respondents represent approximately 21% of chiropractic membership in these four associations; however, as individual chiropractors can be members of multiple associations, the response rate is potentially higher than 21%. Furthermore, the associations' secretaries where unable to determine the number of members on their mailing lists, so the exact number of bulletin recipients as well as the actual response rate is unknown. Of the total respondents, 63% were BCA members, with another 25% representing the UCA, 11% representing the MCA, 3% representing the SCA and 4% representing other associations. Table 1 shows the total number of members of each association at the time the study was conducted and the proportion of chiropractors in those associations who completed the survey.

Just under half of all respondents (44.6%) were female. Most (52.1%) had practiced for 10 years or less and the majority (54.2%) were trained at the AECC. Table 2 illustrates the demographic and professional characteristics of the entire cohort.

Of all respondents, 89.0% consider themselves to be evidence informed practitioners. Depending on the issue, 61.7 to 97.1% of the respondents agreed that the items associated with lifestyle issues were their responsibility to discuss. These issues included decreasing alcohol consumption, decreasing psychosocial stress, regular exercise, improving eating habits, improving posture, improving movement patterns, normalising sleep patterns and smoking cessation. The specific values for each issue are shown in Table 3. Similar proportions of chiropractors indicated they would evaluate/monitor (56.4-97.1%) or give advice/resources (53.8-96.3%), again depending on the specific issues listed. However, respondents' perceived responsibility to discuss lifestyle issues with patients and the actual proportion that evaluate/monitor, give advice/resources or set goals in practice differed across all categories. These differences are visually highlighted in Figure 1. In this survey, the highest number (70.7-80.4%) of chiropractors who incorporate goal-setting and re-evaluation of goals did so in regards to physical activity. However, in all of the other areas, up to approximately two-fifths (20.0-41.7%) of the chiropractors set goals and re-evaluate. For over-consumption of alcohol and smoking, merely one-fifth (20.0% and 20.6% respectively) provide this service. Additionally, fewer chiropractors indicated they "set goals" or "re-

Table 1 Association membership and survey response rate

Association	Members[1]	Respondents	Survey respondents[2] (%)	Membership (%)
BCA	1352	319	63	24
MCA	544	55	11	10
SCA	145	15	3	10
UCA	407	127	25	31
Other*	unknown	19	4	N/A
Total	2448	516	106	21

[1]The number of members in each association was obtained through email request and the figures shown were given directly by each association.
[2]Multiplicity of membership included.
*Other associations indicated: American Chiropractic Association, Associazione Italiana Chiropratici, China Hong Kong Macao Chiropractic' Association, Chiropractic Association of South Africa, Chiropractors' Association of Australia, College of Chiropractors, Danish Chiropractors Association, European Chiropractors' Union, International Chiropractic Pediatric Association, International Chiropractors Association, SOTO Europe, Swedish Chiropractic Association.

Table 2 Demographic and professional characteristics of whole cohort (N= 509)

Variable	Proportion (%)	N
Gender (F)	44.6	227
Years in practice		
0-5	27.1	138
6-10	25.0	127
11-15	14.5	74
16-20	11.6	59
>20	21.8	111
Chiropractic education		
AECC	54.2	276
McTimoney	12.2	62
WIOC	19.4	99
Other*	14.2	72

*Other countries indicated for chiropractic education: Australia, Canada, New Zealand, South Africa, Sweden, UK, USA.

evaluated goals", with less than half (41.6%) setting/re-evaluating goals at the majority of visits. When asked which resource the respondents think is the most successful to prevent illness and promote their patients' health, the majority (68.8%) indicated verbal advice, followed in descending order by written advice (10.6%), referral to another health professional (internal or external) (6.3%), brochures and pamphlets (3.3%), internet website address (1.4%) and a place address or contact number (0.2%). Table 3 summarises the respondents' practice characteristics and behaviours.

Subgroup analysis

In order to determine any differences between subgroups, analyses were carried out using Pearson Chi-Square tests. This revealed that there was a statistically significant greater proportion of males with >20 years in practice, χ^2 (4, N =489) =13.85, p = .008) reflecting an increasing female representation in the profession over the most recent decades. Additionally, in regards to years in practice and association membership, the UCA had a statistically significant over-representation of respondents with fewer years in practice, χ^2 (4, N =489) =17.18, p = .002), while the BCA was over-represented by respondents with greater years in practice, χ^2 (4, N =489) =16.66, p = .002). This was not seen in the MCA or SCA.

In relation to patient behaviours, a significantly greater number of female respondents reported disturbed sleep, χ^2 (1, N =489) =9.74, p = .002), and psychosocial stress, χ^2 (1, N =489) =6.99, p = .008), as being behaviours they evaluate and/or monitor. Conversely, males reported poor posture, χ^2 (1, N =489) =5.98, p = .014), with higher frequency than females. In regards to the lifestyle changes for which the respondents set and/or re-evaluate goals with their patients, respondents in practice for ≤20 years reported doing so more frequently in regards to poor posture, χ^2 (4, N =489) =12.97, p = .011). On the other hand, respondents in practice for >20 years reported with higher frequency goal setting/re-evaluation for smoking, χ^2 (4, N =489) =11.35, p = .023).

Discussion

This study indicates that the surveyed UK chiropractors are participating in preventative healthcare and health promotion activities, encouraging patients to make positive lifestyle changes especially in regards to physical activity and fitness. Although less in comparison to physical activity, our findings indicate that a fair degree of nutritional and psychosocial care is provided. These are potentially important components not only to individual patients, but to public health initiatives as highlighted by O'Connor et al. [18]. The authors suggest that chiropractors, given the practicalities of their work, have the opportunity to be opportunistic screeners and referrers for a variety of conditions that can potentially decrease mortality and morbidity at minimal cost, an important consideration emerging across the global health care sector.

The results also show that just over half of the chiropractors reported smoking and over-consumption of alcohol as their responsibility to discuss. However, less of these same clinicians evaluate and monitor their patients for these behaviours. This is surprising as over-consumption of alcohol and smoking are not only known to lead directly to the development of NCDs, but additionally have quite severe consequences on skeletal and nervous system health [19-21]. Nevertheless, the proportion of UK chiropractors reporting that they provide advice for smoking cessation is similar to the amount of advice being offered by other healthcare professionals to patients in the USA [22,23]. In the UK, Coleman et al. [24] states that many opportunities to discuss smoking with patients are not being utilised by general practitioners in order to avoid negative responses from patients and many practitioners do not raise the topic unless the patients present with smoking-related problems. It appears to be an area of care that needs more attention from healthcare professionals as a whole and chiropractors could have a positive role to play.

As preventative care and health promotion focus on the daily choices an individual makes regarding their long-term health objectives, goal-setting should be a core component. In a study by Holliday et al. [25], neurological rehabilitation patients in the UK who were encouraged to participate in goal-setting found such goals to be more relevant than those set primarily by the providers as they felt a greater sense of autonomy and satisfaction when they were part of the process. Goal-setting where patients and providers co-create health by focusing on a specific problem, setting realistic objectives, and developing action

Table 3 Practice characteristics and behaviours of whole cohort (N= 509)

Question	Proportion (%)	N
Evidence informed?		
Yes	89.0	453
No	2.4	12
No answer	8.6	44
Lifestyle issues considered responsible to discuss		
Decrease alcohol consumption	61.7	314
Decrease psychosocial stress	80.4	409
Regular exercise	95.9	488
Improve eating	81.1	413
Improve posture	97.1	494
Improve movement patterns	90.2	459
Normalise sleep patterns	71.9	366
Smoking cessation	65.8	335
Other	11.8	60
Behaviours Evaluated/monitored		
Over-consumption alcohol	56.4	787
Psychosocial stress	82.3	419
Inactivity/Over activity	90.8	462
Poor diet	74.1	377
Poor posture	97.1	494
Faulty movement patterns	88.6	451
Disturbed sleep	72.9	371
Smoking	60.7	309
Other	7.7	39
Advice/resources given		
Over-consumption alcohol	53.8	274
Psychosocial stress	82.3	419
Inactivity/Over activity	91.6	466
Poor diet	78.6	400
Poor posture	96.3	490
Faulty movement patterns	88.0	448
Disturbed sleep	75.4	384
Smoking	56.6	288
Other	8.8	45
Set goals/re-evaluate progress		
Over-consumption alcohol	20.6	105
Psychosocial stress	40.5	206
Inactivity/Over activity	72.7	370
Poor diet	41.7	212
Poor posture	80.4	409
Faulty movement patterns	70.7	360
Disturbed sleep	34.8	177
Smoking	20.0	102
Other	6.7	34
Frequency of setting/review goals		
Up to 50% of visits	48.5	247
51-100% of visits	41.6	212
Never	4.7	24
Only per patient request	5.1	26
Successful resources to prevent disease/promote health		
Verbal advice from chiropractor	68.8	350
Written advice from chiropractor	10.6	54
Brochures/Pamphlets	3.3	17
Internal/External referral	6.3	32
Internet website address	1.4	7
Place address/contact number	0.2	1
No answer	9.4	48

plans should be viewed as a core service according to Von Korff et al. [26]. In our study, other than for physical fitness issues, goal-setting appears to be under-utilised with only up to two-fifths (41.7%) of the chiropractors setting and re-evaluating goals depending on the specific lifestyle issue and only one-fifth doing so for issues of over-consumption of alcohol (20.0%) and smoking (20.6%). A case therefore could be made to encourage more chiropractors to adopt goal-setting in key areas of preventative healthcare and health promotion.

Study limitations

A significant limitation of this study is the estimated 79% non-response rate from the UK chiropractors in this survey. Although the approximate 21% response rate allows us to draw conclusions regarding the practices of those who responded, the UK chiropractic profession is not represented in its entirety. This leads to less than robust confidence in the generalisability of these attitudes and practices to the wider profession.

Additionally, the chiropractors were asked to report general tendencies, not specific patient encounters, and interpretation between chiropractors may differ. This is particularly important where clinicians were asked to report the number of patient visits where goal-setting and re-evaluation of goals took place. Additionally, false reports, conscious or subconscious, might have occurred; however, this is an unavoidable limitation of the study design.

Lastly, some issues were not included in the survey, but may have an impact on decreasing NCDs as suggested by the respondents in the comment boxes. These included

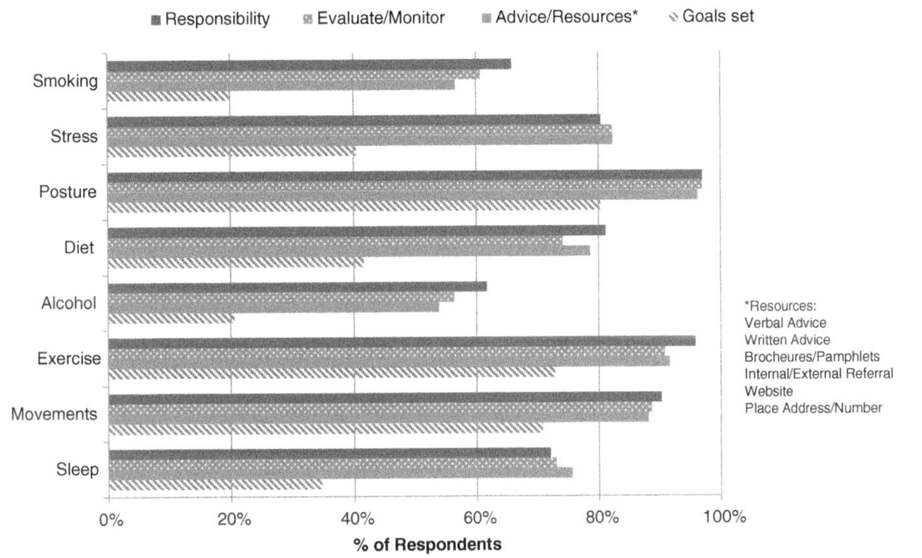

Figure 1 Proportion of respondents who perceived responsibility to discuss lifestyle issues and proportion who evaluate/monitor, give advice/resources or set goals for lifestyle issues in practice.

pregnancy and birth plans, regular weight checks, work-life balance, supplements, prescription drugs, vaccinations, ergonomics, exposing oneself to adequate sunlight and spiritual pursuits.

Future research

This survey explored the degree with which UK chiropractors engage with patients concerning efforts to support the potential reduction in the burden of NCDs. While being only a snapshot of the current situation for the chiropractors who responded, this study could serve as a starting point for further work in this area in the UK. Future studies in this field will not only be of interest to patients and chiropractors, but potentially to other health care professionals as well as policy makers. Further exploration of the patients' perspective and the reasons why chiropractors do or do not consider it their responsibility to incorporate such care into their practices as well as seeking insight into successful methods being utilised in chiropractic practices should be explored.

Conclusion

Links have been shown between chronic disease, smoking, obesity and depression with pain, particularly spinal pain. With the WHO calling on primary healthcare professionals to assist patients in developing sustained lifestyle changes, the goal of this study was to explore the chiropractic professions' engagement with preventative healthcare and health promotion. This survey of a subset of UK chiropractors shows that a good degree of preventative healthcare and health promotion is already provided, especially in regards to physical activity, nutrition and psychosocial stress. However, goal-setting and re-evaluation of goals could be incorporated more routinely by UK chiropractors into their practices. The chiropractic profession has a valuable role in preventative healthcare and health promotion and many of those surveyed are already participating in decreasing the burden of NCDs in various aspects of patient care. However, as in most things, there is considerable room for improvement if desired.

Abbreviations

BCA: British Chiropractic Association; CAM: Complementary and alternative medicine; MCA: McTimoney Chiropractic Association; NCD: Non-communicable disease; SCA: Scottish Chiropractic Association; SPSS: Statistical Package for the Social Sciences; UCA: United Chiropractic Association; UK: United Kingdom; USA: United States of America; WHO: World Health Organization.

Competing interests

The authors declare that this paper is original and has not been published nor is being considered elsewhere for publication. The authors, individually and collectively, declare no conflicts of interests.

Authors' contributions

The corresponding author, PEF, planned the design, was responsible for the concept development, communication with the chiropractic associations, data collection/processing, analysis/interpretation, literature search, and writing of this manuscript. KAE was integral for concept development, survey supervision, and critical review of this manuscript. DN also helped with concept development, data analysis/interpretation and critical review of this manuscript. All authors read and approved the final manuscript.

Authors' information

Patricia E Fikar, MChiro, BA, CNA, Chiropractor, Private Practice, Vienna, Austria. Kent A Edlund, DC, BSc, ICSSD, Senior Clinical Tutor, Anglo-European College of Chiropractic, 13–15 Parkwood Road, Bournemouth, Dorset, BH5 2DF, UK. Dave Newell, BSc MSc PhD FRCC (Hon) FEAC, Director of Research, Anglo-European College of Chiropractic, 13–15 Parkwood Road, Bournemouth, Dorset, BH5 2DF, UK.

Acknowledgements
The authors would like to acknowledge the members of the AECC faculty and staff who participated in the pilot survey and gave feedback. Additionally, the authors would like to acknowledge the secretaries of the four participating chiropractic associations (BCA, MCA, SCA and UCA) who were most helpful in distributing the survey to their members and sending reminder bulletins.

Author details
[1]Private Practice, Vienna, Austria. [2]AECC-Anglo-European College of Chiropractic, 13-15 Parkwood Road, Bournemouth, Dorset BH5 2DF, UK.

References

1. WHO. Global Status Report on Noncommunicable Diseases 2010. Geneva, Switzerland: World Health Organization; 2011.
2. Beaglehole R, Yach D. Globalisation and the prevention and control of non-communicable disease: the neglected chronic diseases of adults. Lancet. 2003;362(9387):903–8.
3. WHO. Global strategy on diet, physical activity and health. Geneva, Switzerland: World Health Organization; 2004.
4. The Council on Chiropractic Education. Standards for Doctor of Chiropractic Programs and Requirements for Institutional Status Scottsdale, AZ. 2007; 45–47.
5. Evans MW, Rupert R. The council on chiropractic education's new wellness standard: a call to action for the chiropractic profession. Chiropr Osteopat. 2006;14:23.
6. Von Korff M, Crance P, Lane M, Miglioretti, Simon G, Saunders K, et al. Chronic spinal pain and physical-mental comorbidity in the United States: results from the national comorbidity survey replication. Pain. 2005;113:331–9.
7. Goldberg MS, Scott SC, Mayo NE. A review of the association between cigarette smoking and the development of nonspecific back pain and related outcomes. Spine. 2000;25(8):995–1014.
8. Webb R, Brammah T, Lunt M, Urwin M, Allison T, Symmons D. Prevalence and predictors of intense, chronic, and disabling neck and back pain in the UK general population. Spine. 2003;28(11):1195–202.
9. Fishbain DA, Cutler R, Rosomoff HL, Rosomoff RS. Chronic pain-associated depression: antecedent or consequence of chronic pain? A review. Clin J Pain. 1997;13(2):116–37.
10. CCE. Standards for doctor of chiropractic programs and requirements for institutional status. Scottsdale: Council on Chiropractic Education; 2007.
11. Stuber KJ, Grod JP, Smith DL, Powers P. An online survey of chiropractors' opinions of continuing education. Chiropr Osteopat. 2005;13:22.
12. Evans MW, Page G, Ndetan H, Martinez D, Brandon P, Daniel D, et al. Are patients receiving health promotional advice in the chiropractic teaching clinic setting? An impact assessment of a brief intervention to increase advising rates and goal setting. J Chiropract Educ. 2011;25(2):132–41.
13. British Chiropractic Association [http://www.chiropractic-uk.co.uk/]
14. McTimoney Chiropractic Association [http://www.mctimoneychiropractic.org/]
15. Scottish Chiropractic Association [http://www.sca-chiropractic.org/]
16. United Chiropractic Association [http://www.united-chiropractic.org/]
17. Limesurvey® [www.limesurvey.org]
18. O'Connor L, Walker BF, Watts C. The early detection and prevention of skin cancer by complementary health professionals. COMSIG Rev. 1994;3(2):54–60.
19. Hollenbach KA, Barrett-Connor E, Edelstein SL, Holbrook T. Cigarette smoking and bone mineral density in older men and women. Am J Public Health. 1993;83(9):1265–70.
20. Laitinen K, Välimäki M. Factors affecting bone metabolism and osteoporosis: alcohol and bone. Calcif Tissue Int. 1991;49(1):70–3.
21. Thomas VS, Rockwood KJ. Alcohol abuse, cognitive impairment, and mortality among older people. J Am Geriatr Soc. 2001;49(4):415–20.
22. Kruger J, Shaw L, Kahende J, Frank E. Health care providers' advice to quit smoking, National health interview survey, 2000, 2005, and 2010 CME. Prev Chronic Dis. 2012;9:110340.
23. Fiore MC, Bailey WC, Cohen SJ. Treating Tobacco Use and Dependence: Quick Reference Guide for Clinicians. Rockville, MD: US Department of Health and Human Services. The Public Health Service; 2000.
24. Coleman T, Murphy E, Cheater F. Factors influencing discussion of smoking between general practitioners and patients who smoke: a qualitative study. Br J Gen Pract. 2000;50(452):207–10.
25. Holliday RC, Cano S, Freeman JA, Playford ED. Should patients participate in clinical decision making? An optimised balance block design controlled study of goal setting in a rehabilitation unit. J Neurol Neurosurg Psychiatry. 2007;78(6):576–80.
26. Von Korff M, Gruman J, Schaefer J, Curry SJ, Wagner EH. Collaborative management of chronic illness. Ann Intern Med. 1997;127(12):1097–102.

Patients' experiences and expectations of chiropractic care: a national cross-sectional survey

Hugh MacPherson[1*], Elizabeth Newbronner[2], Ruth Chamberlain[3] and Ann Hopton[1]

Abstract

Background: Not enough is understood about patients' views of chiropractic care. The aims of this research were to explore patients' experiences and expectations, their perceptions of benefits and risks, and the implications for chiropractors' continuing fitness to practise.

Methods: Survey questions were formulated from existing literature, published guidance on good practice from the General Chiropractic Council, and from 28 telephone interviews and a small focus group with chiropractic patients using a semi-structured topic guide. In its final form, the survey elicited patients' ratings on expectations regarding 33 aspects of care. In a national cross-sectional survey, a number of sampling methods were required as a consequence of the low practitioner response rate.

Results: In total, 544 completed questionnaires were received from chiropractic patients, a lower response rate than expected (8%). The two main benefits that patients reported regarding their chiropractic care were reduced pain (92%) and increased mobility (80%). Of respondents, 20% reported unexpected or unpleasant reactions to their treatment, most commonly tiredness or fatigue (32%), and extra pain (36%). In most cases they expressed low levels of concern about these reactions. Patients' expectations were met for most aspects of care. The four aspects of practice where expectations were least well met comprised: having more information on the cost of the treatment plan at the first consultation (80%); the chiropractor contacting the patient's general practitioner if necessary (62%); having a discussion about a referral to another healthcare practitioner (62%); and providing a method for confidential feedback (66%).

Conclusions: Overall, patients reported a high level of satisfaction with the benefits of their chiropractic care, although there is a likelihood of bias towards patients with a positive experience of chiropractic. There were no serious adverse reactions; however, patients reported concern about pain, tingling and numbness in the limbs after chiropractic. In general, patients' expectations were being well met.

Keywords: Chiropractic, Patients' expectations, Patients' experiences, Risk, Benefit, Fitness to practice

Background

There is a growing body of research into patients' expectations and experiences (including adverse reactions) of complementary therapies. The OPEn Study [1] funded by the UK's General Osteopathic Council explored patients' expectations and experiences in relation to the benefits, risks and side effects of osteopathic treatment. It prioritised five areas of practice for the profession and the regulator to consider: the clinic environment; professionalism; treatment; relationship; and outcomes. It found a high level of satisfaction amongst patients consulting osteopaths working in private practice and most of the more widely held expectations were being met. Many of these related to the overall 'customer experience' but others were concerned with the therapeutic process and included the importance of "informing patients about what to expect in relation to treatment and outcomes including side effects" [1]. The study identified some gaps between expectations and delivery of care which could have a negative effect on the outcomes of care, and suggested that these gaps could be reduced by improving care and/or managing expectations better.

* Correspondence: hugh.macpherson@york.ac.uk
[1]Department of Health Sciences, University of York, York, UK
Full list of author information is available at the end of the article

There has been relatively little work on the expectations of patients of chiropractic. One study conducted in Sweden [2] found that whilst patients and chiropractors had similar expectations in relation to key areas such as the chiropractor diagnosing and explaining the nature of the problems to the patients, there were other important areas where expectations differed. In particular, patients were more likely than their chiropractor to expect a rapid (i.e. within one to two treatments) improvement in their condition. They were also more likely to expect to be given advice about how to manage their problem and exercises to do between treatments. Interestingly, the OPEn Study highlighted this as an area where the level of unmet positive expectation was relatively high.

In a Dutch study [3] on the benefits and risks of chiropractic care for neck pain, 529 patients provided data that showed that adverse reactions are rarely severe in nature and for most patients the benefits outweighed the risks. Two studies [4] commissioned by the UK's General Chiropractic Council (GCC) in 2009/10 brought together information from clinical research about the risks of chiropractic, and examined the possible costs of adverse reactions and sub-optimal outcomes. They concluded that 'suboptimal outcomes', such as delayed or missed diagnosis, missed recognition of contra-indications, inadequate care-management and poor record keeping, were of more concern (and had greater cost implications) than significant adverse reactions.

Whilst much can be learned from these and other studies, both from their direct work with patients and the wider literature reviews, the GCC identified an evidence gap in relation to UK chiropractic patients' views and expectations. Moreover the GCC was also reviewing its approach to the revalidation of registrants, and as part of this process wanted to gain a fuller understanding of patients' views of chiropractic care, in particular people's assessment of the risks and benefits of chiropractic treatment, their expectations of chiropractors, and their experience of them. In this context, the GCC commissioned independent researchers from Firefly Research & Evaluation, in partnership with the Department of Health Sciences at the University of York, to carry-out research with a focus on the experiences and expectations of patients and the extent to which these expectations were met. The results of the research outlined in this report were designed to inform the GCC's work on revalidation. This paper presents an overview of the survey results.

Methods

Design and setting of the qualitative interviews and focus group

We used qualitative methods as a preparation for designing and conducting a national survey. Three areas (Cardiff, the Scottish Borders, and Mansfield/Chesterfield) were chosen for the interviews and focus group to reflect city, town and rural communities. The chiropractors in each area were asked to assist with the study by inviting up to 10 of their current and former patients (including as far as possible a mix of age, gender, ethnicity and condition or disability) to take part in either a focus group, a telephone interview or face-to-face interview. In total, 12 chiropractors agreed to be involved and through them 30 patients gave written consent to take part in the study: 56% of these patients were female and 73% were aged under 65. Twenty-eight patients chose to take part in individual telephone interviews and two attended a focus group (in Mansfield/Chesterfield). The interviews and focus group were conducted by two experienced female health services researchers (LN, RC), using a semi-structured topic guide covering four main topics: 'choosing your chiropractor'; 'expectations'; 'risks and benefits'; and 'fitness to practice'. The topic guide used in the interviews provided an initial framework which was then expanded. The interviews were digitally recorded and typically lasted around 40 minutes. The interviews and focus group recordings were transcribed in full and the data were then analysed thematically [5] by two researchers (LN, RC). Ethical approval was obtained from the Research Governance Committee of the University of York's Department of Health Sciences (Ref no. HSRGC/2012/06)

Development of the questionnaire

The questionnaire used in the national cross-sectional survey was developed from reviewing the existing literature about patients' experiences and expectations of manual therapies, the General Chiropractic Code of Practice and Standard of Proficiency [6] and the telephone interviews and the focus group, as described above. The sections of the questionnaire were informed by five questions that were set out by the GCC to inform the research:

- What do patients of chiropractors see as the benefits of receiving chiropractic care?
- What do patients see as the potential risks of receiving chiropractic care?
- Has their perception of benefits and risks changed over time? If so, how?
- What has influenced their perceptions of the benefits and risks?
- Once a chiropractor is on the GCC register, what do patients expect will happen to assure an Individual chiropractor's continuing fitness to practise?

The core of the questionnaire focused on patients' experiences and expectations of chiropractic care and treatment at different stages in their contact with the chiropractor. We also asked patients directly about benefits, adverse reactions and what systems would reassure them that their chiropractor was keeping their knowledge and skills up to date. We tested the first draft of the questionnaire with a small number of patients who had taken part in the interviews and volunteered to assist us at this stage. Building on their comments and following discussions with colleagues at the GCC and within the research team, we developed a second draft of the questionnaire with was then tested with a sample of patients from a single chiropractic practice. Following this second pilot, the final version of the questionnaire was developed and agreed with colleagues at the GCC. A copy of the final questionnaire is attached in Additional file 1.

Survey participants

During November 2012 a random sample of 600 chiropractors (drawn from the GCC's database of registrants; n =960) were invited to participate in a national cross-sectional survey by distributing a questionnaire (available in paper-based form or electronically) to at least 10 of their current and former patients: four to current patients who were receiving regular chiropractic care over the past three months or more; two to new patients (i.e. at their first consultation); two to former patients who ceased treatment within the past 6 months by mutual agreement with the chiropractor and/or because the presenting problem was resolved; two to former patients who ceased treatment within the past 6 months but who ended their treatment unilaterally (i.e. before, in the chiropractor's view, the presenting problem was resolved). Practitioners were also asked to try to include a mix of age, gender, ethnicity and disability. In the first approach involving 600 practitioners, 47 chiropractors agreed to take part (8%). We subsequently contacted an additional sample of 360 chiropractors and of these 21 agreed to take part (6%). A further two chiropractors volunteered to be involved when the British Chiropractic Association (BCA) sent an email to its members. This resulted in a total of 70 chiropractors who agreed to help recruit patients for the survey. Information about the survey was also circulated by email to chiropractic patients registered with Care Response, an organisation that supports the collection of routine patient-related data (http://www.careresponse.co.uk/)

Data analysis

Data was entered onto an Excel spreadsheet and two researchers (Martin Baxter, Liz Newbronner) conducted a random audit of 10% of questionnaires to check for accuracy. Analysis of the survey data was conducted to characterise the survey respondents to assess the distribution of age within the sample, and the analysis included calculation of the mean, median and interquartile range values and the calculation of Z scores to assess the distribution of ages. Demographic data, comprising sex, ethnicity, educational attainment, living environment and nationality, were analysed using frequencies and proportions. Other survey data regarding the experiences and expectations of chiropractic treatment were also analysed using frequencies and proportions. Associations between adverse reactions were analysed using Chi-squared statistics. Questions that were not answered (i.e. missing data) were also reported as frequencies and proportions.

Results

Patient participation rates and patient profile

We sent 1075 information sheets and questionnaires to the 70 recruited chiropractors and asked them to distribute these to their patients. This generated 401 usable questionnaires, a 37% response rate. A total of 5167 patients registered with 36 Care Response member chiropractors were emailed and 112 (2%) patients completed the survey through this route. In addition, the Chiropractic Patients Association also informed its members of the survey (N = 350) and 27 (9%) members and four of their friends and family responded as a result of this. Together all these recruitment methods generated a total of 544 respondents. Excluding the four family and friends, for whom we have no denominator, this represents an overall response rate of 8% (540/6592). The majority of questions (82%) had been answered; however, five questions (questions 40–44) contained between 16% and 20% of missing data. These questions with the greater proportion of missing data corresponded with the less well met expectations.

Of the 544 respondents, 360 (66%) were women; 4 (0.7%) did not give their gender (Table 1). The age distribution showed a significant negative skew ($z = -2.12$). The median age of respondents was 54.5 years (interquartile range = 43–71); yet when examined more closely, the age profile for women followed a normal distribution whilst the age profile for men showed a significant negative skew ($z = -2.810$) whereby 70% of the male participants were aged 50 and over. The majority of respondents lived in England (89%), classified their ethnic origin as white (96%), and lived within a city or town environment (58%). With regard to their highest level of educational qualification, 50% of the respondents had either first degrees or second degrees. This compares with 30% of the UK working age population having a first degree or higher [7].

Experiences of chiropractic care

Before receiving chiropractic treatment, 58% of patients had limited knowledge of what the treatment involved, 41% were unsure of the likely benefits and 71% had little knowledge of the possible reactions to treatment (Table 2). Over half (53%) attended every other month, 25% were no longer receiving treatment and 59% no

Table 1 Demographic of chiropractic patients surveyed (Total n = 544)

Questions asked		
What is your age? (n = 544)	**Years**	
Range =	16-87	
Median=	54.50	
Interquartile range 1; Interquartile range 3 =	43 ; 71	
Missing	0	
Are you? (n = 540)	**n =**	**(%)**
Male	180	33%
Female	360	66%
Missing	4	0.7%
What is your ethnicity? (n = 543)		
White	519	96%
Black or Black British	6	1%
Asian or Asian British	6	1%
Chinese or Chinese British	2	0.4%
Mixed heritage	0	0
Other ethnic group	8	1.4%
Missing	1	0.2%
Do you consider yourself to have a disability? (n =536)		
Yes	44	8%
No	492	91%
Missing	8	1.4%
What is your highest level of academic education/attainment? (n = 527)		
No academic qualifications	38	7%
GCSE or equivalent (e.g. O level, CSE, NVQ1)	96	18%
A levels or equivalent (e.g. NVQ2-3, BTec certificate, City and Guilds crafts)	117	22%
BA or BSC degree or equivalent (e.g. NVQ4, BTEC diploma, City and Guilds level 3+, nursing or teaching qualifications)	193	36%
Master's Degree, PhD, Post graduate certificate or NVQ level 5	79	15%
Other	4	0.7%
Missing	18	3%
How would you describe the area that you live in? (n = 534)		
City/Urban area	50	9%
Town or suburb	267	49%
Village or rural area	217	41%
Missing	10	1.8%
Which of the four UK nations do you live in? (n = 535)		
England	484	90%
Scotland	13	2%
Wales	28	5%
Northern Ireland	8	1.4%
Missing	9	1.6%

Table 2 Experiences of chiropractic treatment (n = 544)

Statements		
Before you first had chiropractic treatment, how much did you know about:		
a. What the treatment involved	n =	%
I knew very little	318	58%
Some knowledge	148	27%
I knew a lot	75	14%
Missing	2	0.4%
b. The likely benefits of the treatment		
I knew very little	224	41%
Some knowledge	182	33%
I knew a lot	134	25%
Missing	2	0.4%
c. Possible reactions to the treatment		
I knew very little	387	71%
Some knowledge	112	21%
I knew a lot	41	7%
Missing	2	0.4%
Approximately how many chiropractic treatments have you had in the last 12 months?	n = treatments	
Range =	0-55	
Median =	6	
Interquartile range 1; Interquartile range 3 =	4 ; 10	
Are you currently receiving treatment?	n =	%
YES	409	75%
NO	135	25%
Reasons given in answer to the question, "If 'NO', why did you stop chiropractic treatment?" (n = 135)		
	n =	%
The problem being treated improved/got better, I no longer needed treatment	79	59%
The problem being treated has improved and I am currently able to manage it myself	47	35%
I did not feel the treatment was benefitting me	6	4%
I was unhappy with the chiropractor's approach/manner	2	1.5%
I had an unpleasant reaction to treatment	0	0%
I was unhappy with the cost of treatment	3	2%
I am currently unable to afford treatment	7	5%
Other health problems have prevented me from having chiropractic treatment	1	0.7%
NB. 10 people (7%) gave more than one reason for stopping chiropractic treatment	145	107%

longer needed treatment. One third of the patients had changed their chiropractor at some point in the past with the main reasons being: linked to the patient moving to a new area; finding a chiropractor at a more convenient location; or the chiropractor moving away. Eight people (5%) said that the approach or manner of the chiropractor did not suit them or the treatment was not benefiting them.

Experiences of benefits and adverse reactions

The majority of patients surveyed reported benefits associated with chiropractic. These benefits included a reduction in the pain (92%) and an improvement in mobility (80%) (Table 3). More than half reported that chiropractic treatment had an ongoing effect of reducing future problems (55%) and provided a better understanding of their health problem (53%).

Approximately 20% (n = 110) of respondents reported one or more reactions to treatment that they found unexpected or unpleasant. Of a total of 153 reactions, among respondents 45% (n = 49) had one reaction, 34% (n = 37) had two reactions and the remainder had 3 or more (n = 15) (Table 4). Where patients reported on more than one type of reaction, they reported a single level of concern associated with their reactions. Extra pain and/or radiating pain was the symptom associated with the greatest level of concern (n = 19). Where patients had more than one reaction, extra pain was more commonly combined with tingling and stiffness.

Expectations of chiropractic care

Patients reported their expectations prior to the first consultation and what they experienced in practice (Table 5). Where patients responded 'Yes' to the question 'Did it happen' their expectation was met, but a response of 'No' signified their expectation was not met. For these questions, more than 80% of patients expected these aspects of care to happen and they did happen, which suggests there was a high level of satisfaction with this stage of the 'patient journey'.

Similar results were obtained for the patients' first consultation (Table 6). An area where there was a noticeable gap between expectations (86%) and experience (80%) was in regard to an explanation of the cost of the treatment plan at the first consultation. Though there was a small difference of 3% between the expectation the chiropractor would talk about the possibility of adverse reactions and what happened, 13% of patients reported that this did not happen.

Questions were asked of respondents about on-going treatment processes (Table 7). In most cases, more than 90% of patients' expectations and experiences corresponded well. In some areas, chiropractors exceeded their patients' expectations, for example by displaying information about their length of time in practice and about their special interests or additional skills. In the survey, 99% of the respondents expected that their chiropractor would allow sufficient time for their consultation and this expectation was largely met, with 97% saying that it had happened. People responding to the survey had slightly lower expectations (85%) relating to when treatment should be reviewed.

When considering referral to other agencies, 86% of survey respondents expected that the chiropractor would refer them to other healthcare practitioners if appropriate and 87% expected them to contact their general practitioner, should this be needed (Table 8). In both cases, nearly two-thirds (62%) said this happened although 20% and 18% respectively did not answer the questions (q40, q41). It is not clear whether this relates to the expectation not being delivered or whether a referral was not required. Another area where there appeared to be a gap between expectations (76%) and experiences (66%) was with regard to a system for patients to provide confidential feedback; between 16% and 20% of patients did not answer these questions. A high percentage (97%) of survey respondents expected the chiropractor to provide advice on how to manage symptoms between treatments and this expectation was largely met, with 96% of respondents saying they had been given this type of support.

Expectations with regard to fitness to practice

With regards to the chiropractors' fitness to practice, almost half of the patients responding to the survey (49%) would feel reassured if patients were provided with information about the chiropractors' on-going training and development, whereas 19% disagreed and 30% were undecided. Between half and two-thirds of patients (61%) agreed that chiropractors should review their practice regularly (61%), be assessed by an independent assessor (66%) and have a practice-level system for gathering and showing patient feedback (59%). Half (50%) agreed that there should be a national system for gathering patient feedback and that patients could access.

Table 3 Experiences of chiropractic treatment: main benefits of treatment (n = 544)

	n =	%
It has reduced or removed the pain I was experiencing.	503	92%
It has increased my mobility/flexibility.	434	80%
It has helped me maintain my general health and wellbeing.	344	63%
It is helping to prevent or reduce future problems.	297	55%
It has given me a better understanding of my health problem.	286	53%
It has increased my ability/confidence to manage my health problem.	239	44%
It has enabled me to return to work, sport or other activities.	204	38%

Discussion

In a survey comprising 544 patients, the positive experiences reported were the benefits of reduced pain and increased mobility and an understanding of how to

Table 4 Experiences of chiropractic treatment: frequency of adverse reactions and reported level of concern (n = 110 of 544 patients)

Reaction	Level of concern (n =)		
	Of lower concern (1,2)	Of greater concern (3,4,5)	Total number of reactions
Tiredness or fatigue	33	2	35
Headache	19	4	23
Extra Pain and/or Radiating Pain	21	19	40
Tingling/numbness in legs or arms	3	9	12
Stiffness	13	7	20
Dizziness or light headedness	13	6	19
Nausea	1	3	4
Total	103	50	153

NB. Where patients reported on more than one type of reaction, they reported a single level of concern associated with their reactions.

maintain the improvements gained. There were no serious adverse reactions. Regarding minor reactions to treatment, some people reported greater concern about extra pain, tingling and numbness, whereas tiredness, fatigue and headache were of low concern. The survey showed that the patients' expectations of advice on how to manage symptoms between treatments were largely met. There were four areas where patients had relatively high expectations (i.e. >75% expected an aspect of care to happen) but these were not met for a significant proportion of patients (between 10 to 25%). These were: if necessary and with consent, the chiropractor would contact the patient's general practitioner; if the problem is not improving or the patient has other health needs the chiropractor will discuss referral to another healthcare practitioner; having the cost of the treatment plan explained at the first consultation; and the chiropractic practice having a system for patients to provide confidential feedback.

Strengths and limitations of the study

In terms of strengths, the study was conducted by a research group that was independent of associations or regulatory bodies associated with chiropractic. This independence meant that the study was not biased by prior agendas or partiality towards particular styles of chiropractic. The use of interviews with patients receiving chiropractic care prior to the national survey helped shape a more appropriate and targeted questionnaire. The piloting of the survey questions helped clarify the focus of the survey and reduced ambiguity. Nevertheless, the survey did require patients to recall their first consultation and so there is a risk of recall bias.

For many questions the level of expectation is high and the estimation of expectations being met may be reflected accurately. However, where the level of expectation is below 80% there may be a possibility of a substantial over-estimation of expectations being met. Furthermore, the missing data on questions relating to

Table 5 Expectations of chiropractic care: responses to questions related to 'before seeing the chiropractor' (n = 544); n/a = not answered

Statements	Expected			Did it happen?		
	Yes	No	n/a	Yes	No	n/a
Q11. Before seeing the Chiropractor I expect to be given general information about chiropractic treatment and what it involves.	91%	8%	1%	92%	7%	1%
Q12. Before seeing the Chiropractor I expect to be given general information about possible reactions (both positive and negative) to chiropractic treatment.	82%	15%	3%	82%	15%	3%
Q13. Before seeing the Chiropractor I expect to be given information about what will happen at my first consultation.	91%	7%	2%	91%	7%	2%
Q14. Before seeing the Chiropractor I expect to be told about the cost of treatments.	97%	2%	1%	95%	4%	1%
Q15. Before seeing the Chiropractor I expect to be told how long the first consultation is likely to last.	90%	8%	1%	91%	7%	2%
Q16. Before seeing the Chiropractor I expect to fill-in and sign a consent form for the first consultation.	83%	13%	3%	90%	6%	4%
Q17. Before seeing the Chiropractor I expect to provide my General Practitioner's name and contact details.	83%	15%	2%	91%	6%	3%

Table 6 Expectations of chiropractic care: responses to questions about the first consultation (n = 544); n/a = not answered

Statements	Expected			Did it happen?		
	Yes	No	n/a	Yes	No	n/a
Q18. At the First Consultation I expect to be given time to tell the chiropractor about my problem and how it was affecting me.	99%	0%	1%	99%	0%	1%
Q19. At the First Consultation I expect the chiropractor to take a detailed account of my personal case history.	96%	3%	1%	96%	1%	2%
Q20. At the First Consultation I expect to be given a gown and/or towels to cover up if I had to undress.	83%	12%	4%	84%	9%	7%
Q21. At the First Consultation I expect to be able to undress and dress in privacy.	90%	6%	5%	88%	5%	7%
Q22. At the First Consultation I expect the chiropractor to explain why any further investigations (e.g. X-Rays) were necessary and any risks associated with them.	72%	18%	10%	67%	20%	14%
Q23. At the First Consultation I expect the chiropractor to give me a diagnosis or rationale for my care.	93%	5%	2%	95%	3%	3%
Q24. At the First Consultation I expect the chiropractor to explain what treatment I will need (e.g. the type, frequency and duration of treatment).	97%	2%	1%	94%	4%	2%
Q25. At the First Consultation I expect the chiropractor to talk to me about any possible adverse reactions to the treatment.	87%	9%	3%	83%	13%	3%
Q26. At the First Consultation I expect the chiropractor to talk to me about the likely success of the treatment.	93%	6%	2%	91%	7%	2%
Q27. At the First Consultation I expect the chiropractor to explain what the cost of the agreed treatment plan would be.	86%	12%	3%	80%	17%	3%
Q28. At the First Consultation I expect the chiropractor to give me time to ask questions about the proposed treatment plan.	96%	3%	1%	94%	4%	2%

referral and the patients' complaint procedure may also reflect that the question was not applicable to them, because they had not previously considered the questions and therefore found it difficult to answer whether or not they expected to be told of either referral or complaints procedures.

A limitation of the survey was related to the difficulty we had in engaging chiropractors in the study, though we did eventually recruit 70, two of whom were not contacted directly. We only achieved a response rate of 7% (n = 68) from the 960 chiropractors that we contacted directly. Moreover the response rate from their patients was also poor, with 37% of the questionnaires sent to chiropractors returned in paper form or on-line by their patients. It is possible that, despite the guidance provided by the research team, the chiropractors could have selected patients who they felt would provide a positive response, thereby biasing the sample. Therefore it could be argued that among respondents, largely consisting of patients selected by their own chiropractor or those who have joined a Chiropractic Patient's Association, attitudes towards chiropractic were biased towards being more favourable.

Table 7 Expectations of chiropractic care: responses to questions related to on-going treatment (n = 544); n/a = not answered

Statements	Expected			Did it happen?		
	Yes	No	n/a	Yes	No	n/a
Q29. I expect to be given time to tell the chiropractor about how I felt after my last treatment, and discuss any problems or concerns.	98%	1%	0%	97%	1%	1%
Q30. I expect the chiropractor to ask me if there has been any change in my condition, general health or medication.	97%	2%	1%	97%	2%	1%
Q31. I expect the chiropractor to allow sufficient time for the consultation.	99%	0%	1%	97%	2%	1%
Q32. I expect the chiropractor to talk to me about further treatment options.	91%	6%	2%	87%	9%	4%
Q33. I expect the chiropractor to allow me time to decide what I wish to do about future treatment.	92%	5%	3%	91%	5%	4%
Q34. I expect the chiropractor to agree with me when my treatment should be reviewed.	85%	11%	4%	84%	10%	6%
Q35. I expect the chiropractor to give me advice about how I manage my problems/symptoms between treatments.	97%	2%	1%	96	3%	1%

Table 8 Expectations of chiropractic care: assuring chiropractors are 'Fit to practice' responses to questions related to the chiropractor's knowledge and experience; (n=544); n/a = not answered

Statements	Expected			Did it happen?		
	Yes	No	n/a	Yes	No	n/a
Q36. I expect that information about the chiropractor's qualifications and registration will be displayed in the clinic/available in leaflets/included on the practice website.	90%	8%	2%	95%	4%	2%
Q37. I expect that information about the chiropractor's experience (e.g. length of time in practice) will be displayed in the clinic/available in leaflets/included on the practice website.	76%	22%	3%	82%	13%	6%
Q38. I expect that information about the chiropractor's special interests or additional skills (e.g. soft tissue massage) will be displayed in the clinic/available in leaflets/included on the practice website.	69%	26%	5%	75%	17%	9%
Q39. I expect that information about how the chiropractor is maintaining/improving their professional knowledge (e.g. further training) will be displayed in the clinic/included on the practice website.	56%	38%	6%	59%	28%	13%
Q40. I expect that if my problem is not improving with chiropractic treatment and/or I have other health needs, the chiropractor will discuss referral to another healthcare practitioner.	86%	8%	6%	62%	18%	20%
Q41. I expect that, if necessary, and with my consent, the chiropractor will contact my GP.	87%	10%	4%	62%	20%	18%
Responses to statements related to patient feedback and complaints						
Q42. I expect the chiropractic practice to have a clear system to enable me to provide confidential feedback (whether positive or negative).	76%	20%	4%	66%	18%	16%
Q43. I expect to be given information about the practice's complaints procedure.	54%	39%	7%	44%	38%	18%
Q44. I expect to be told about my right to refer a complaint to the General Chiropractic Council and be given the GCC's contact details.	51%	41%	9%	40%	40%	20%

There is some research evidence [8] that the overall population of chiropractic patients is fairly evenly split between women and men. We also noted the relatively high proportion of participants with either first degrees or second degrees compared to the UK working age population and speculate that this may reflect an affordability issue, in that chiropractic is more likely to be used by professional classes. In terms of how representative the patients involved in this study are of all patients who seek chiropractic care, it is important to sound a note of caution. The nature of this study means that most of the patients who contributed were either currently receiving treatment or had had on-going chiropractic care in the recent past. Those patients who ceased chiropractic care after a small number of treatments, perhaps because they were unhappy with their care may well be under-represented. Nevertheless, our study data also suggests that where patients are unhappy with their treatment, this does not necessarily deter them from seeking further treatment from another chiropractor.

Comparison to previous literature

The positive experiences related to expectations of chiropractic care reported in this study are consistent with a previous quantitative study of expectations related to osteopathic treatment,[9] in which the majority of people were satisfied with the treatment they received and their expectations of care were largely met. Also consistent with qualitative evidence within the osteopathic literature is that the most important expectations relate to the themes of individual agency, professional expertise, customer experience, therapeutic process and interpersonal relationships [10]. In a survey of chiropractic patients in Sweden, patients were found to have lower expectations of the chiropractic treatment than the chiropractors had, but higher expectations of being given advice and exercises than the chiropractors had [2]. Moreover, patients expected to get better faster than the chiropractors expected them to. We found that patients' expectations about being given advice about managing symptoms were largely met. In another study involving chiropractic patients, the researcher found that patients had an inaccurate or rudimentary understanding of the mechanisms that underpin chiropractic treatment, were not particularly interested in how it worked and despite the explanations of the chiropractor, patients showed only a limited understanding of the mechanisms [11]. In our study more than 90% expected to be given information about chiropractic and what it involved and to be given a diagnosis and rationale for their treatment. However, our survey did not ask whether the patients understood any of the information provided. There remains a gap in the literature, as previously identified [2], on whether unmet expectations contribute to lower levels of effectiveness.

Implications for practice

With regard to clinical practice, the less well met expectations can provide guidance on how chiropractic care could be improved from the perspective of patients. These areas where there could be some improvement include: allowing sufficient time for the consultation; being told about the cost of treatments; having the treatment needed explained; being given time to ask questions about the treatment plan; being told about the likely success of the treatment and adverse reactions; being told about further treatment options; and being able to undress and dress in privacy. A more substantial expectation/experience gap that could be addressed by changes in practice include: if necessary and with consent, the chiropractor would contact the patient's general practitioner; if the problem is not improving or the patient has other health needs the chiropractor will discuss referral to another healthcare practitioner; having the cost of the treatment plan explained at the first consultation; and the chiropractic practice having a system for patients to provide confidential feedback. These gaps between expectations and delivery of care are mostly a consequence of poor communication and may lead to negative effects on outcomes of care and/or patient dissatisfaction. By closing the gaps, chiropractors individually and as a profession can improve their clinical practice. In terms of future research, this paper provides a platform from which a more comprehensive survey can be conducted, with better methods of recruiting chiropractic patients to improve the response rate and to limit selection bias.

Conclusion

In general, patients reported a high level of satisfaction with the benefits of their chiropractic care, most commonly related to reduced pain and increased mobility. There were no serious adverse reactions. Among the minor reactions reported, there was greater concern about extra pain, tingling and numbness attributed to chiropractic and a lower level of concern about reactions of tiredness or fatigue. As reported by patients, expectations were largely met for most of the 33 aspects of practice. The areas where expectations were less well met were mostly due to inadequate or limited communication. By addressing these areas, chiropractors can improve the quality of their clinical practice and delivery of patient care.

Additional files

Additional file 1: Questionnaire for national survey -final.pdf, 339 K http://www.chiromt.com/imedia/1336971084126552/supp1.pdf.

Competing interests

The authors declare that they have no competing interests.

Authors' contributions

HM is a senior research fellow specialising in the effectiveness, cost-effectiveness, mechanisms and safety in the evaluation of complementary medicine. He provided academic supervision for the study, drafted the article and gave final approval for publication. LN is an independent health and social care researcher whose research focuses on long term conditions, disability and self-management. She conducted the interviews and analysis, managed the survey, interpreted the data and helped revise the article. RC is an independent health and social care researcher who specialises in qualitative research. She conducted the interviews and analysis. AH is a research fellow from a nursing background whose research focuses on the non-pharmacological management of chronic pain and depression. She contributed to the design of the survey and revised the article. All authors read and approved the final manuscript.

Acknowledgements

We would like to thank all the patients who kindly agreed to be interviewed for this study and those who took the time to complete the survey. We are also very grateful to the chiropractors who agreed to assist us with the research as without their help in recruiting patients for the interviews and distributing the survey the study would not have been possible. We would also like to thank those professional associations who assisted us by publicising the study. Lastly we are indebted to Carol Latto from Chiropractic Plus for all her help and advice throughout the study, to Jonathan Field who distributed information about the survey to the Care Response patients from consenting practices, to Martin Baxter who provided technical support in managing the data from the survey and to Janet Eldred for her copy-editing.

Funding statement

The General Chiropractic Council, 44 Wicklow Street, London WC1X 9HL, UK commissioned and funded the independent research organisation, Firefly Research & Evaluation, North Yorkshire, to conduct this study. The GCC provided practical assistance in sampling from their database of registered chiropractors but had no involvement in the sampling decisions. The data collection, analysis and interpretation of the data of the project and the preparation, review and final approval of the manuscript were undertaken independently of the GCC by Firefly Research and by the Complementary Medicine Evaluation Group at the University of York.

Author details

[1]Department of Health Sciences, University of York, York, UK. [2]Firefly Research & Evaluation and Visiting Fellow, Department of Health Sciences, University of York, York, UK. [3]Firefly Research & Evaluation, North Yorkshire, UK.

References

1. Leach J, Cross V, Fawkes C, Mandy A, Hankins M, Fiske A, et al. Investigating osteopathic patients' expectations of osteopathic care: the OPEn project. Brighton: University of Brighton; 2011 [http://www.osteopathy.org.uk/resources/Research-and-surveys/GOsC-research/Osteopathic-patient-expectations-study/]
2. Sigrell H. Expectations of chiropractic treatment: what are the expectations of new patients consulting a chiropractor, and do chiropractors and patients have similar expectations? J Manip Physiol Ther. 2002;25(5):300–5.
3. Rubinstein SM, Leboeuf-Yde C, Knol DL, De Koekkoek TE, Pfeifle CE, Van Tulder MW. The benefits outweigh the risks for patients undergoing chiropractic care for neck pain: a prospective, multicenter, cohort study. J Manip Physiol Ther. 2007;30(6):408–18.
4. European Economics for the GCC: Report to the General Chiropractic Council and Counterfactual for Revalidation – Report to the General Chiropractic Council. General Chiropractic Council; 2010.
5. Braun V, Clarke V. Using thematic analysis in psychology. Qual Res Psychol. 2006;3:77–101.
6. General Chiropractic Code of Practice and Standard of Proficiency. General Chiropractic Council; 2010 [cited 2014 Apr 7]. [http://www.gccuk.org/UserFiles/Docs/COPSOP_2010.pdf]
7. Office for National Statistics. Census Population of working age by level of highest qualification, second quarter 2009. 2012, [http://www.ons.gov.uk/ons/publications/re-reference-tables.html?edition=tcm%3A77-363799]

8. Pedersen P, Breen AC. An overview of European chiropractic practice. J Manip Physiol Ther. 1994;17(4):228–37.
9. Leach C, Mandy A, Hankins M, Bottomley LM, Cross V, Fawkes CA, et al. Patients' expectations of private osteopathic care in the UK: a national survey of patients. BMC Comp Altern Med. 2013;13(1):122.
10. Cross V, Leach CMJ, Fawkes CA, Moore AP. Patients' expectations of osteopathic care: a qualitative study. Health Expect; 2013 May. doi:10.1111/hex.12084
11. Hennius BJ. Contemporary chiropractic practice in the UK: a field study of a chiropractor and his patients in a suburban chiropractic clinic. Chiropr Man Ther. 2013;21(1):25.

Helping address the national research and research capacity needs of Australian chiropractic: introducing the Australian Chiropractic Research Network (ACORN) project

Jon Adams[1*], Amie Steel[1,2], Sungwon Chang[1] and David Sibbritt[1]

Abstract

Chiropractic is a popular health care choice in Australia and yet major gaps in our empirical understanding of this area of practice remain. Furthermore, while some research excellence exists, a largely uncoordinated approach to research activity and development has in effect led to silos of interest and a lack of strategic 'big-picture' planning essential to producing a sustainable research culture and capacity for the profession. This commentary identifies the significance of a number of key features - including a national, coordinated focus, and a rich engagement with the practitioner and patient base amongst others – arguably important to the future development of research and research capacity within Australian chiropractic. The design features and phases of the Australian Chiropractic Research Network (ACORN) project are also outlined. ACORN is one contemporary initiative specifically developed to address chiropractic's research and research capacity building needs and help grow a broad evidence-base to inform safe, effective patient care.

Keywords: Chiropractic, Research, Practice based research networks, Research capacity building

Background

Chiropractic is a popular health care choice in Australia as elsewhere constituting a major component of health care utilisation (estimated to be worth over $3 M in out-of-pocket expenses in 2005 [1]) and attracting reports of good patient satisfaction [2-10]. Despite emerging research activity and developments within chiropractic in Australia and overseas [11-13], major gaps in our empirical understanding of this area of health care practice remain. There is much room for the further development of a broad range of methods and disciplinary perspectives to help assess and advance the evidence-base for chiropractic care. Given the prevalence of chiropractic use in Australia, further research development - providing insights of benefit for practitioners, patients and policymakers - is essential to ensuring effective, safe, coordinated chiropractic care and provision [14].

* Correspondence: jon.adams@uts.edu.au
[1]Australian Research Centre in Complementary and Integrative Medicine, Faculty of Health, University of Technology Sydney, Australia
Full list of author information is available at the end of the article

A key challenge that has faced research of chiropractic in Australia to date has been the piecemeal and often largely uncoordinated nature of research activity. While some research excellence and emerging evidence exists, a largely uncoordinated approach has in effect led to silos of interest and a lack of strategic 'big-picture' planning essential to producing a sustainable research culture for the profession [15]. Following the lead of other health professional groups it is vital that Australian chiropractic invest substantial effort and resources to facilitate a coordinated approach to producing a sustainable culture of research [11,12,15-19]. A failure to significantly invest in research capacity building runs the very real risk of substantially limiting the prospects of the profession and its research base for the foreseeable future [16-20].

Discussion

Key features essential to future development of chiropractic research and research capacity building

In order to directly and successfully address the contemporary research and research capacity building needs of

Australian chiropractic and to ensure necessary credibility and strength in design, there is an arguably urgent need for initiatives to build upon a number of interrelated, distinct features. In particular, we would argue, it is essential such initiatives wherever possible: be based upon a critical, non-partisan research approach; adopt and build upon rigorous health and medical research methods and designs; be coordinated, broad and multidisciplinary in research focus; be national in design and scope; be longitudinal and sustainable providing short term, mid-term and long term outcomes as well as helping build a wider incremental program of research; incorporate practitioner engagement and research capacity building wherever possible; reflect and connect with the clinical and practice realities of contemporary chiropractic and wider health care in order to ensure translation and impact of results for practitioners and patient care; and be inclusive and research network building (housing an ability to facilitate, promote and advance research networks where already established and help encourage and grow networks and research activity elsewhere as necessary).

One new strategy of response: introducing the ACORN project

The Australian Chiropractic Research Network (ACORN) project is one contemporary initiative which has been designed and launched in direct response to these research and research capacity building needs. In the following sections of this paper, the overarching design and phases of the ACORN project will be explained along with a discussion of the specific ways in which the project will address the essential research and research capacity building issues facing Australian chiropractic.

ACORN is the first long-term, national project built upon a Practice-Based Research Network (PBRN) design to examine chiropractic care in Australia. A PBRN design has been previously utilised in a range of health care fields including general practice [21-23], pharmacy [24] and dentistry [25]. Chiropractic PBRN work has developed outside Australia [26] and, while not constituting a PBRN, practice-based research has also previously been undertaken in Australian chiropractic on a regional level [4,27]. PBRN studies act as 'research laboratories' for health and medical care [22] drawing upon groups of practitioners/practices (small or large in number) in order to systematically answer questions that arise from clinical practice [28] as well as undertake research of relevance to both grass-roots practitioners and patient care [29]. The notion of a PBRN being sustainable and capacity building has also been highlighted [30,31]. Examples of the type of issues that have previously been investigated via PBRN designs include an examination of a range of information sources practitioners draw upon to inform their clinical decision-making [32] and the comparative effectiveness of different models of health care [33]. A PBRN is extremely well positioned to help address research questions around professional standards of practice and clinical characteristics and behaviours and can provide an opportunity for more rigorous sub-studies to examine the efficacy of particular protocols within particular patient sub-groups of *direct relevance* to frontline practice settings [30].

The ACORN project, funded by the Chiropractors' Association of Australia, has been independently designed and is independently led and conducted by the Australian Research Centre in Complementary and Integrative Medicine (ARCCIM), Faculty of Health, University of Technology Sydney (UTS). The project will provide extensive data collection and analysis as well as develop essential national infrastructure for future research on chiropractic. The ACORN project draws upon and promotes critical multidisciplinary, longitudinal investigation based upon rigorous scientific design and methods, strongly encourages (and relies upon) collaborative involvement from across the chiropractic profession – both in terms of practitioners and researchers/research groups – and introduces a national coordinated agenda for chiropractic research that is translational in output and reflective of practice realities. While the project is capable of facilitating a diverse range of research sub-studies and addressing a very broad range of distinct but interrelated research questions, the platform focus of the ACORN project is upon examining issues around chiropractic best practice, safety and cost-effectiveness. The ACORN project will employ a diverse dissemination strategy to ensure empirical findings reach practitioner, patient, researcher and policymaker audiences. Dissemination of the empirical findings from the ACORN project will include publication in relevant national and international peer-reviewed journals as well as practitioner-friendly webpage dissemination.

The ACORN project has three initial core phases - all covered by the initial period of funding - that will be implemented over the first three years of the project (with a view to establishing a longer-term, programmatic initiative to be maintained over a much longer period). *Phase One* is focused upon the design, preparation and promotion activities. *Phase Two* involves distribution of a brief (2 page) baseline practitioner questionnaire, practitioner recruitment for the wider project (establishing a national chiropractor database), the launch of an Expression of Interest (EOI) round and initial approval for nested sub-studies and PhD proposals. Finally, *Phase Three* will facilitate additional and ongoing nested sub-study activity available to senior researchers and their teams and PhD development opportunities alongside maintaining the national chiropractor database. The ACORN project is available to those already developing and conducting chiropractic research to take advantage of a national chiropractic network to address a broad spectrum of related research questions.

In the remaining sections of this paper we outline the three phases of the ACORN project providing a general overview of the project's approach and methods and highlighting how the project incorporates key design features which ensure short term and long term critical investigation and evaluation as well as the capacity building necessary to enable the profession and field to develop and prosper.

Phase one: ethics, design, preparation and promotion

In this initial phase of ACORN, the project Steering Committee is focused upon a number of platform-building tasks. It is imperative for a national-scale PBRN project such as ACORN to attract as high a response rate as possible [30] from the target population (*all* practising chiropractors across Australia) and critical to this is a well-developed promotion campaign. In response, Phase One of the project includes an extensive promotions strategy to be administered via regional and national events in order to reach and engage as many of the registered practising chiropractors across Australia as possible. To this end, ACORN senior Chief Investigators will present introductory ACORN project talks at relevant venues and events (including regional and national Executive and Membership Meetings, AGMs and research-focused events) and provide regular updates and information briefings via relevant newsletters (e.g. via Chiropractor's Association of Australia and Chiropractic and Osteopathic College of Australasia) throughout 2014 and early 2015. Further information regarding the ACORN project will also be available via the project webpage [34].

Drawing upon previous relevant research in Australia and overseas [26,27] the ACORN project team will design, pilot and finalise a brief 2 page questionnaire which will be administered in Phase Two to collect baseline practitioner and practice data regarding chiropractor characteristics, practice characteristics, patient management and case-load mix amongst other topics. All the initial phase design features of the ACORN project will also be subject to ethical review and approval by relevant University Ethics Committees.

Phase two: administering a baseline chiropractor survey, establishing a national chiropractor research database and launching an expression of interest (EOI) call

An initial focus of Phase Two of the project will be to administer the questionnaire instrument designed and finalised in Phase One. The questionnaire will be as short as possible (maximum of 2 pages) to encourage and maximise a good response rate. Initial pilot-testing shows the questionnaire will take approximately 6–8 minutes to complete. The questionnaire will include examination of practitioner's demographics, their practice characteristics including the frequency of patient types and presentations as well as the techniques and methods of care employed. The survey will be administered to *all* registered chiropractors across Australia (via both electronic and hard copy mail out) and will constitute the first national-scale mapping of chiropractors' clinical management and patient care undertaken in Australia. In addition, the national mapping of chiropractic provided from the brief questionnaire will also be critical to establishing a broad data resource with which others can build, value-add, examine specific lines of investigation and address additional research questions.

Alongside the 2 page questionnaire, chiropractors will also receive an additional invitation to participate in the longer-term ACORN project. The contact details of each consenting chiropractor will be added to a secure database (to be securely housed at ARCCIM, UTS) which will be an ongoing resource for further research investigation via approved EOI applications (see below). The ACORN project has been assessed for formal learning hours and the allocation of Continuing Professional Development hours is subject to an individual's level and amount of engagement.

Phase Two will also include an initial call for EOIs to be conducted by other interested researchers, practitioners and research teams/groups who may wish to access the ACORN chiropractor database for the purpose of developing and conducting nested sub-studies. Such EOIs regarding sub-study proposals will follow a formal application process and will be peer-reviewed by the ACORN Steering Committee headed by Senior ARCCIM academics with a view to ensuring appropriate standards of scientific validity, feasibility and design/methodological expertise are maintained.

Alongside accommodating more senior researchers, sub-study applications which primarily build upon or contain PhD studentships/study are also strongly encouraged. Indeed, all established chiropractic departments and research groups are encouraged to seek additional funding to facilitate separate PhD studentships/stipends which can be nested in the ACORN project and thereby take advantage of the infrastructure established by the project. Sub-studies suitable for EOI submission can include a vast array of possible designs and features including (but not restricted to): qualitative, quantitative and mixed-method research design; data collected via both chiropractors and/or their patients; and cross-sectional as well as longitudinal studies.

Phase three: facilitating chiropractor and patient Sub-studies, PhD development and further funding opportunities

In Phase Three the EOI call will remain open to encourage ongoing sub-study development and applications. The

ACORN project database provides an ideal platform for nesting future PhD projects and can therefore be harnessed and utilised as a rich and valuable resource for doctoral level studies that will ultimately build chiropractic research capacity. In addition, the core ACORN project research team at ARCCIM will prepare further funding applications and seek input from relevant and interested partners to support applications for Federal Government research funding where possible. With this in mind, the ARCCIM will also explore opportunities to maintain and regularly update the ACORN practitioner database providing a valuable and ongoing resource for research and research capacity building in chiropractic over the three initial years of funding and beyond.

Addressing key needs for research and research capacity building via the ACORN project

The ACORN project has been designed to directly address the key features essential to growing the broad evidence base and research capacity of Australian chiropractic (outlined earlier). These features are now outlined in more detail below.

Adopting a critical, non-partisan research approach built upon rigorous health and medical research methods and designs

Chiropractic, like other areas of health care practice located beyond conventional medicine, has generated emotive debate and commentary over recent years [35,36]. Such debate has tended to be a barrier to the scientific, rigorous examination and assessment of chiropractic within the Australian health care system. Indeed, there is an urgent need for chiropractic to be subject to critical investigation utilising rigorous designs and methods in order to promote a balanced, non-partisan approach to empirical study and appraisal – a situation no different to that demanded of all health care professions regardless of origins or orientation [37]. Such a balanced, non-partisan approach is at the very core of the ACORN project which has been designed and is independently led and conducted by a team of senior multi-disciplinary health care researchers (research methodologists) and yet inclusive of field-practitioner participation and input to assist in making the project more relevant to frontline practice. The ARCCIM team have extensive training and experience in successfully applying robust designs and methods to the critical study of health care topics (across complementary medicine, conventional health care and beyond) as well as established track records in attracting a significant portfolio of National Health and Medical Research Council (NHMRC) and Australian Research Council (ARC) grant and Fellowship funding.

Accommodating a coordinated, broad, multidisciplinary research focus

It is important that chiropractic research, at this significant juncture in its development, be co-ordinated and sufficiently broad (both disciplinarily and methodologically) in its focus as to ensure a suitable platform to accommodate as many sub-studies as possible. While increasing expertise and detailed engagement with specific areas of chiropractic care is wanting, the immediate task facing this research field is guaranteeing the research activity of today provides the most efficient use of resources and energy for future endeavours [38]. A PBRN design such as that adopted in the ACORN project is an excellent vehicle to ensure this is achieved within the real-life setting of frontline practice [39].

At the heart of the ACORN project is a multi-disciplinary approach incorporating a wide spectrum of clinical, public health and health services research methods, designs and disciplinary-based perspectives. The ACORN project (especially Phases Two and Three via the EOI process) encourages the conduct of a multitude of nested-study designs which can include observational studies and experimental studies.

First national scale, longitudinal project of its type in Australia

It is vital that any serious attempt to build a significant chiropractic research agenda and culture that will have substantial influence and impact within and beyond the profession be designed around a study of national scale. ACORN has been designed to provide the first national research project of its type in Australian chiropractic. Through recruitment from registered chiropractors across Australia, ACORN will be able to provide the first national-scale mapping of chiropractors' clinical management and patient care undertaken in Australia. This scope of study also provides excellent opportunity for analyses to be large scale (national) as well as regionally and locally significant – the national data collected can also be analysed in terms of States/Territories, regional areas (i.e. a major urban area) or based upon urban/rural/remote settings amongst other criteria.

Similarly, PBRN designs such as that adopted by the ACORN project allow excellent infrastructure to conduct longitudinal analyses whereby patients and treatment outcomes are tracked over specific time periods. Such work is particularly important in addressing questions around the effectiveness of different treatments and will be strongly encouraged in terms of partnering and/or outside teams of investigators looking to submit sub-study proposals.

Sustainable and research capacity building

Essential to harnessing and promoting a well-developed research culture within chiropractic is a commitment to ensuring research activity is more than short-term and involves developing the research training and careers of those within chiropractic. Chiropractic, not dissimilar to other professions outside of conventional health care, is in much need of research growth starting with expanding the pool of people with PhDs in the field [38]. In response, the ACORN project actively encourages and comfortably accommodates PhD candidates and other early career researchers via the EOI process. Crucially, the ACORN project also facilitates not only immediate but also mid to long-term research activity around chiropractic in much needed areas - the ACORN project effectively establishes the necessary infrastructure upon which others can build and value-add.

The EOI and nested sub-study design also provide excellent opportunity for chiropractors to engage in conducting empirical research study. As previous PBRN studies have illustrated, so long as time and effort is taken to promote closer researcher-practitioner relations and develop research collaborations where practitioners are mentored by senior researchers, a PBRN such as the ACORN project can comfortably accommodate those chiropractors looking to develop their research experience and skills [30].

Incorporating practitioner engagement and reflective of practice realities

A PBRN design such as that adopted within the ACORN project necessitates that the research perspective be directly linked to and contextualised within everyday practice activity and behaviours. The ACORN project design – drawing upon data from both grass-roots practitioners and their patients – will ensure that the research focus is of direct relevance to (and thereby impact upon) practice realities. As with other quality health research, the ACORN project will accommodate an ability to approach the practitioner and/or patient as *a partner/partners* in investigations and the project acknowledges the essential engagement and involvement of both chiropractors and their patients in ensuring the project and project findings are translational and impactful for patient care. The ACORN project provides a national platform for chiropractors in the field to directly participate within significant research projects, which can influence the future of the profession in Australia.

Encouraging inclusivity and research network building

In order to maximise and help support the pockets of research excellence and activity already established around chiropractic, the ACORN project houses a fundamentally *inclusive* research design. The success of the project is significantly dependent upon the engagement and commitment of interested researchers and research teams (which can, and in many cases should, include key practitioner collaborators) beyond the core ARCCIM investigators. Indeed, the EOI process has been developed to encourage partnership and input beyond the immediate ARCCIM team and the ACORN project actively encourages the submission of nested sub-studies led by qualified and interested groups/parties across Australia and/or on the international stage.

Conclusion

It is imperative that chiropractors and chiropractic profession, like all health care practitioners and practices currently available and utilised by Australians, be subject to sufficient critical, rigorous examination and assessment. While addressing the many research gaps on this topic via a coordinated effort has obvious and far-reaching benefits for chiropractors and the wider profession in Australia, the ACORN project also constitutes a significant initiative for others beyond the profession. To examine and assess fundamental aspects and features of contemporary chiropractic will produce insights of benefit to all interested and engaged in researching, practicing and managing evidence-based, safe and effective patient care.

Addressing the research and research capacity building needs of Australian chiropractic will certainly require long-term commitment and engagement from a number of stakeholders across the profession (especially practitioners and researchers). However, the establishment of the ACORN project constitutes a solid national platform for helping address these needs in an inclusive manner which ensures investigations can accommodate an appropriate wealth of interests, designs and expertise as well as provide an evidence-base assessment and reflect the grass-roots features of chiropractic patient care.

Competing interests

The authors declared that they have no competing interests.

Authors' contributions

JA designed and produced first draft of the paper. JA, AS, SC and DS all contributed substantial revisions to the manuscript, read and approved final manuscript prior to submission.

Funding

The ACORN project is funded by the Chiropractor's Association of Australia (CAA).

Author details

[1]Australian Research Centre in Complementary and Integrative Medicine, Faculty of Health, University of Technology Sydney, Australia. [2]Office of Research, Endeavour College of Natural Health, Brisbane, Australia.

References

1. Xue CC, Zhang AL, Vin C, Myers R, Polus B, Story DF. Acupuncture, chiropractic and osteopathy use in Australia: a national population survey. BMC Public Health. 2008;8:105.
2. Adams J, Sibbritt D, Broom A, Loxton D, Pirotta M, Humphreys J, et al. A comparison of complementary and alternative medicine users and use across geographical areas: a national survey of 1,427 women. BMC Complement Altern Med. 2011;11(1):85.

3. Adams J, Sibbritt D, Lui C. The urban–rural divide in complementary and alternative medicine use: a longitudinal study of 10,638 women. BMC Complement Altern Med. 2011;11(1):2.
4. French SD, Densley K, Charity MJ, Gunn JM. Who uses chiropractic services? Chiropr Man Therap. 2013;21:31.
5. Sibbritt D, Adams J. Back pain amongst 8,910 young Australian women: a longitudinal analysis of the use of conventional providers, complementary and alternative medicine (CAM) practitioners and self-prescribed CAM. Clin Rheumtol. 2010;29:25–32.
6. Steel A, Adams J, Sibbritt D, Broom A, Gallois C, Frawley J. Utilisation of complementary and alternative medicine (CAM) practitioners within maternity care provision: results from a nationally representative cohort study of 1,835 pregnant women. BMC Pregnancy Childbirth. 2012;12:146.
7. Wardle J, Sibbritt D, Adams J. Referrals to chiropractors and osteopaths: a survey of general practitioners in rural and regional New South Wales, Australia. Chiropr Man Therap. 2013;21:5.
8. Xue C, Zhang AL, Lin V, Da Costa C, Story DF. Complementary and alternative medicine use in Australia: a national population-based survey. J Altern Complement Med. 2007;13:643–50.
9. Zodet M, Stevans J. The 2008 prevalence of chiropractic use in the US adult population. J Manipulative Physiol Ther. 2012;35(8):580–8.
10. Brown BT, Bonello R, Fernandez-Caamano R, Eaton S, Graham PL, Green H. Consumer characteristics and perceptions of chiropractic and chiropractic services in Australia: results from a cross-sectional survey. J Manipulative Physiol Ther. 2014;37(4):219–29.
11. Rubenstein SM, Bolton J, Webb AC, Hartvigsen J. The first research agenda for the chiropractic profession in Europe. Chiropr Man Therap. 2014;22:9.
12. Mootz RD, Coulter ID, Hansen DT. Health services research related to chiropractic: review and recommendations for research prioritization by the chiropractic profession. J Manipulative Physiol Ther. 1996;20(3):201–17.
13. Triano JJ, Goertz C, Weeks J, Murphy DR, Kranz KC, McClelland GC, et al. Chiropractic in North America: toward a strategic plan for professional renewal-outcomes from the 2006 chiropractic strategic planning conference. J Manipulative Physiol Ther. 2006;2010(33):395–405.
14. Adams J, Broom A, Jennaway M. Qualitative methods in chiropractic research: one framework for future enquiry. J Manipulative Physiol Ther. 2008;31(6):455–60.
15. Stuber K, Bussieres A, Gotlib A. Chiropractic research capacity in Canada in 2008. J Can Chiropr Assoc. 2009;53(2):78–86.
16. Adams J, Sibbritt D, Broom A, Wardle J, Steel A, Murthy V, et al. Research capacity building in traditional, complementary and integrative medicine: grass-roots action towards a broader vision. In: Adams J, Andrews G, Barnes J, Broom A, Magin P, editors. Traditional, complementary and integrative medicine: an international reader 2012. Buckinghamshire: Palgrave MacMillan; 2012.
17. Farmer E, Weston K. A conceptual model for capacity building in Australian primary health care research. Aust Fam Physician. 2002;31(12):1139–42.
18. Hay AD, Rortviet G, Purdy S, Adams J, Sanci LA, Schermer TR, et al. Primary care research – an international responsibility. Fam Pract. 2012;29:499–500.
19. Van Weel C, Rosser WW. Improving health care globally: a critical review of the necessity of family medicine research and recommendations to build research capacity. Ann Fam Med. 2004;2(2):S5–15.
20. Adams J, Smith A. Qualitative methods in radiography research: a proposed framework. Radiography. 2003;9(3):193–9.
21. Britt HC, Miller GC. The BEACH study of general practice. Med J Aust. 2000;173(2):63–4.
22. Green LA, Dovey SM. Practice based primary care research networks: they work and are ready for full development and support. Br Med J. 2001;322(7286):567–8.
23. Green LA, Hickner J. A short history of primary care practice-based research networks: from concept to essential research laboratories. J Am Board Fam Med. 2006;19(1):1–10.
24. MacLaughlin EJ, Ardery G, Jackson E, Ives T, Young R, Fike D, et al. Institutional review board barriers and solutions encountered in the collaboration among pharmacists and physicians to improve outcomes now study: a national multicentre practice-based implementation trial. Pharmacother. 2013;33(9):902–11.
25. Gilbert GH, Williams OD, Rindal DB, Pihlstrom DJ, Benjamin PL, Wallace MC, et al. The creation and development of the dental practice-based research network. J Am Dent Assoc. 2008;139(1):74–81.
26. Hawk C, Long CR, Boulanger KT. Prevalence of nonmusculoskeletal complaints in chiropractic practice: report from a practice-based research program. J Manipulative Physiol Ther. 2001;24(3):157–69.
27. French SD, Charity ML, Forsdike K, Gunn JM, Polus BI, Walker BF, et al. Chiropractic observation and analysis study (COAST): providing an understanding of current chiropractic practice. Med J Aust. 2013;199(10):687–91.
28. Jones C. Laboratories of primary care practice-based networks in Canada. Can Fam Physician. 2006;52:1045–6.
29. Dwan KM, Magin PJ. The desire for research in general practice. Aust Fam Physician. 2008;37(10):871–3.
30. Gilbert GH, Richman JS, Gordan W, Rindal DB, Fellows JL, Benjamin PL, et al. Lessons learned during the conduct of clinical studies in the dental PBRN. J Dent Educ. 2011;75(4):453–65.
31. Pearce KA, Love MM, Barron MA, Matheny SC, Mahfoud ZM. How and why to study the practice content of a practice-based research network. Ann Fam Med. 2004;2(5):425–8.
32. Andrews J, Pearce K, Love M. Information-seeking behaviours of practitioners in a primary care practice-based research network (PBRN). J Med Libr Assoc. 2005;93(2):206–12.
33. Curro F, Vena D, Naftolin F, Terracio L, Thompson V. The PBRN initiative: transforming new technologies to improve patient care. J Dent Res. 2012;91(7):12–20.
34. ACORN Project webpage. Available at http://www.acorn-arccim.com/. 2015. Accessed 30 January 2015.
35. Dwyer J. There's no place for pseudo-scientific chiropractic in Australian universities. The Conversation 6 Dec 2011. Available at http://theconversation.com/theres-no-place-for-pseudo-scientific-chiropractic-in-australian-universities-4576. 2011. Accessed 30 January 2015.
36. O'Neill A, Willis E. Chiropractic and the politics of health care. Aust N Z J Public Health. 1994;18(3):325–31.
37. Adams J. Utilising and promoting public health and health services research in complementary and alternative medicine: the founding of NORPHCAM. Complement Ther Med. 2008;16(5):245–6.
38. Swain M, Downie A, Brown B, Lystad RP. A commentary to address the state of chiropractic research in Australia. Chiropr J Aust. 2013;43(2):73–4.
39. Peterson KA, Lipman PD, Lange CJ, Cohen RA, Durako S. Supporting better science in primary care: a description of practice-based research networks (PBRNs) in 2011. J Am Board Fam Med. 2012;25(5):565–71.

Altered postural sway in patients suffering from non-specific neck pain and whiplash associated disorder - A systematic review of the literature

Alexander Ruhe[1*], René Fejer[2] and Bruce Walker[3]

Abstract

Study design: Systematic literature review.

Objectives: To assess differences in center of pressure (COP) measures in patients suffering from non-specific neck pain (NSNP) or whiplash-associated disorder (WAD) compared to healthy controls and any relationship between changes in postural sway and the presence of pain, its intensity, previous pain duration and the perceived level of disability.

Summary of Background data: Over the past 20 years, the center of pressure (COP) has been commonly used as an index of postural stability in standing. While several studies investigated COP excursions in neck pain and WAD patients and compared these to healthy individuals, no comprehensive analysis of the reported differences in postural sway pattern exists.

Search methods: Six online databases were systematically searched followed by a manual search of the retrieved papers.

Selection Criteria: Papers comparing COP measures derived from bipedal static task conditions on a force plate of people with NSNP and WAD to those of healthy controls.

Data collection and analysis: Two reviewers independently screened titles and abstracts for relevance. Screening for final inclusion, data extraction and quality assessment were carried out with a third reviewer to reconcile differences.

Results: Ten papers met the inclusion criteria. Heterogeneity in study designs prevented pooling of the data and no direct comparison of data across the studies was possible. Instead, a qualitative data analysis was conducted. There was broad consensus that patients with either type of neck pain have increased COP excursions compared to healthy individuals, a difference that was more pronounced in people with WAD. An increased sway in antero-posterior direction was observed in both groups.

Conclusions: Patients with neck pain (due to either NSNP or WAD) exhibit greater postural instability than healthy controls, signified by greater COP excursions irrespective of the COP parameter chosen. Further, the decreased postural stability in people with neck pain appears to be associated with the presence of pain and correlates with the extent of proprioceptive impairment, but appears unrelated to pain duration.

Keywords: Balance, center of pressure, force-plate, neck pain, whiplash, systematic review

* Correspondence: alexander_ruhe@hotmail.com
[1]Murdoch University. Praxis fuer Chiropraktik Wolfsburg, Porschestrasse 1, 38440 Wolfsburg, Germany
Full list of author information is available at the end of the article

Background

Rationale

Ideally, the body should be able to generate quick center of pressure (COP) transitions that just exceed the current position of the center of mass (COM) [1] and accelerate it into the opposite direction in order to maintain balance. Any condition effecting the afferent sensory pathways may interfere with this process. The neck is particularly prone to this due to the abundant cervical sensory receptors in joints and muscles [2,3] as well as their central and reflex connections to visual, vestibular and postural control systems [4].

The debate continues however, as to whether the cause of abnormal cervical afferent input is primarily proprioceptive or nocioceptive in nature. Deterioration of this proprioceptive information from the neck may be the determining factor in reducing the accuracy in the sensory integration process. The resulting imprecise estimation of the COM position may then lead to an increase in the safety margin of the adaptive COP shifts with regard to the predicted COM oscillations [5].

The excitation of chemosensitive nociceptors in cervical facet joints and muscles may alter the sensitivity of the muscle spindles by reflex activation of fusimotor neurones [6], leading to a decreased proprioceptive acuity. This effect may be triggered by marked activation of mechanosensitive nociceptors as occurs in whiplash injuries [7]. Acute "pain inhibition" [8] may be another mechanism where discharge from high-threshold nociceptive afferents interferes with spinal motor-pathways as well as the motor cortex. Pain may also cause an increased pre-synaptic inhibition of muscle afferents [9] as well as affect the central modulation of proprioceptive spindles of muscles [10], causing prolonged latencies. Such alterations may lead to decreased muscle control and result in increased postural sway.

In the case of whiplash associated disorder (WAD), facet joint components may be at risk of injury due to compression during rear-impact accelerations while capsular ligaments are at risk of injury at higher accelerations [11]. Depending on the magnitude of trauma, the resulting impairment of the sensory system is therefore likely to be more pronounced compared to cases of non-specific neck pain (NSNP).

Several attempts have been made to investigate differences in COP sway pattern between people with NSNP and healthy controls by means of forceplate tilting [12], body leaning [13] or vibratory stimulation to structures of the neck [14]. Although these approaches contribute important knowledge to the field, an experimental setup without additional equipment for stimulation or external perturbation that can be applied comprehensively for a broad spectrum of complaints may be of additional use. We previously described that such a simple static setup is not only highly discriminative for non-specific low back pain [15] but also allowed the observation of a linear relationship between the perceived pain intensity and COP sway velocity [16]. If people with NSNP can also be identified by COP measurements during such basic postural tasks, similar relationships are likely and may allow for comparison of postural sway between painful regions.

This literature review will attempt to identify possible differences in COP pattern between people with WAD, people with NSNP and healthy controls that may relate to the mechanisms described above. As COP measures are commonly used in a clinical setting, this will allow the researcher or clinician to put their results into context. To our knowledge no comprehensive systematic review has been conducted to investigate the possible impact of neck pain on COP pattern during bipedal static tasks and the possible association of this effect with pain intensity or disability.

Objective

The objective of this systematic literature review is to 1) determine if there are significant differences in postural sway between people with NSNP and WAD patients and healthy controls, 2) investigate whether the magnitude of these COP excursions are related to the level of pain perception, previous pain duration or perceived level of disability.

Methods

Search

A comprehensive search strategy was developed by identifying all potentially relevant search terms, categorizing these terms into specific search phases and subsequently combining them by using Boolean terms. This search strategy was applied to six different electronic databases: PubMed, MEDLINE, EMBASE, Web of Science, ScienceDirect and the Cochrane library. The date range of publications searched was from January 1980 to January 2011.

The following key words were used in the search strategy: "neck pain", "cervical pain", "whiplash", "WAD", "center of pressure", "COP", "balance", "posture", "postural stability", postural control". The detailed search strategy is available upon contacting the corresponding author.

The hand search included analyzing references cited in studies selected from the original online search. Citation searches of relevant studies were conducted using the PubMed, MEDLINE and ScienceDirect databases.

Eligibility criteria

Papers were limited to those published in peer-reviewed journals without language restrictions.

The inclusion criteria were: the study investigated force changes over time (postural sway) exhibited by participants with NSNP or WAD derived from bipedal static task conditions on a forceplate, ideally compared to measures of healthy controls. For the purpose of this review, NSNP was broadly defined as pain in the cervical area of musculoskeletal origin in the absence of any neurological symptomatology or serious pathology such as cancer or infection. Induced neck pain in otherwise healthy participants is considered as non-specific neck pain.

The selection criteria for this review does not concern study type as the focus is comparing COP sway data irrespective of the original research purpose of the study. Further, the quality of the various postural sway measures depends on technical aspects of the experimental setup. Therefore all study designs were considered.

We excluded studies with insufficient documentation of patient demographics or experimental setup where this rendered data extraction impossible. In addition, papers that were anecdotal, speculative or editorial in nature or studies that employed dynamic task conditions such as one-leg hopping, walking or some form of translation of the force platform were excluded.

Information sources

Study selection

For the purpose of this review AR acted as the principal reviewer. A colleague (TB) was involved independently in the process of identifying relevant studies but did not participate in further analysis of the finally included papers. Where discrepancies between AR and TB were not reconciled by discussion, a third reviewer was used for a majority decision.

Data collection process

To standardize the procedure between the reviewers, the main author developed a detailed data extraction sheet to acquire general information on objectives, design, participant's demographics and outcomes. If any title and abstract did not provide enough information to decide whether or not the inclusion criteria were met, the article was included for the full text selection.

With regard to the research question, data extraction was concerned with four main areas regarding the association between neck pain and postural sway: 1) perceived pain intensity, 2) previous pain duration, 3) reported disability levels and 4) the experimental setup applied.

For the latter, we extracted data on 1) sampling duration, 2) number of trials, 3) sampling and cut-off frequency, 4) foot position, 5) visual condition (eyes open/closed), 6) surface condition (firm/compliant) as well as 7) the COP parameters used. These points were based on recommendations for obtaining reliable COP measures [17].

Summary measures

The principle summary measure in the included studies was differences in means.

Synthesis of results

We planned to combine the results of the included studies to conduct inter-study comparisons of means and statistical differences. We also planned to do this for NSNP and WAD separately and combined to investigate differences between the two.

Results

Study selection

Initially, the database search strategy identified 203 studies of which titles and abstracts were screened individually by the reviewers. The application of inclusion/exclusion criteria and consensus by the reviewers on the titles and abstracts eliminated 182 papers. From the titles and abstracts of papers selected (n = 23), full papers were reviewed by the same two reviewers (AR and TB) who applied the inclusion criteria to the full text. Of these, 10 studies met the inclusion criteria and were included in this review (Figure 1). There was full consensus between the reviewers during the selection process of included papers.

Study characteristics

Combining results was not possible due to the heterogeneous study designs and patient characteristics across the included studies. Therefore only a general trend is noted.

Both subject demographics and health status for all studies are shown in Table 1. The number of symptomatic participants and the matching number of controls was generally small and ranged between seven [18] and fifty [19]. All but two of the included studies (8/10,

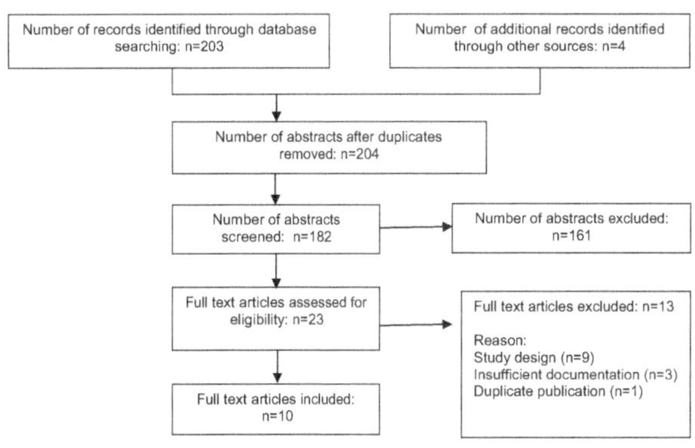

Figure 1 Flowchart of considered studies.

Table 1 Participant demographics and health status

Study	Participant status	Gender (n) Female	Male	Age in years Mean (SD)	Weight in kg Mean (SD)	Height in cm Mean (SD)
McPartland et al. [18]	NSNP *	6	1	39.1	-	-
	healthy *	4	3	39.4	-	-
Michaelson et al. [21]	chronic NSNP	9	0	40 (9)	73 (18)	165 (7)
	chronic WAD	6	3	44 (10)	79 (14)	171 (10)
	healthy	13	3	41 (9)	70 (14)	168 (8)
Madeleine et al. [23]	chronic WAD *	7	4	33.3 (6.7)	73.4 (11.4)	173.3 (7.2)
	healthy/induced NP	7	4	33.1 (6.8)	68.0 (12.5)	171.5 (6.3)
Treleaven et al. [19]	WAD (dizziness)	38	12	35.6	-	-
	WAD (no dizziness)	38	12	35.8	-	-
	healthy	28	22	29.9	-	-
Storaci et al. [26]	WAD	24	16	28.4 (8.8)	-	-
	healthy	23	17	33.9 (12.7)	-	-
Endo et al. [25]	WAD	19	13	39.0 (10.1)	-	-
	healthy	4	16	37.9 (9.3)	-	-
Treleaven et al. [27]	WAD	15	5	46.5	-	-
	healthy	14	6	49.5	-	-
Field et al. [22]	WAD	24	6	30.3 (1.3)	-	-
	NSNP	23	7	27.9 (1.3)	-	-
	healthy	23	7	26.8 (1.3)	-	-
Poole et al. [24]	NSNP	20	0	65-82	-	-
	healthy	20	0	65-82	-	-
Vuillerme et al. [20]	healthy/induced NP	0	16	22.2 (1.8)	73.0 (11.8)	181.4 (6.4)

NP: neck pain, NSNP: non-specific neck pain, SD: standard deviation, WAD: whiplash-associated disorder.
* one patient and one control participants did not participate in COP measurement.
- : not described.

80%) enrolled mixed gender groups of healthy and symptomatic participants. The studies employed different age ranges of participants, with 20-40 years being most commonly enrolled (7/10, 70%).

General shortfalls in the documentation of technical aspects of COP acquirement were apparent. In addition, few authors described the baseline demographics of the participants in appropriate detail, including weight, height, age and gender (3/10, 30%).

There was a marked variation present in the included studies in terms of sampling duration, number of trials or the selection of the COP parameters. The studies often employed a combination of different positional and visual setups in order to investigate postural sway in various challenging positions. The resulting variation in results can be observed irrespective of the COP parameter chosen.

Table 2 shows the study characteristics for sway assessment in people with NSNP. The majority of trials were performed under both eyes open (EO) and eyes closed (EC) condition (4/6, 67%) with only a single repetition (5/6, 83%). Sway area and root mean square (RMS) amplitude were the most commonly used COP parameters.

The study characteristics for trials enrolling WAD patients are presented in Table 3. Only a single recording was used in most cases (6/7, 86%), but in contrast to the NSNP studies, all study designs employed both visual conditions.

Reliability of COP data

Table 4 gives an overview of how the studies included meet the ideal experimental setup for reliable data.

With the exception of one paper that only measured postural sway under visual deprivation [20], all of the studies included assessed COP with both eyes open and eyes closed. No study applied best practice experimental setup throughout.

Pain assessment

All symptomatic participants experienced pain at the time of recording. About 75% of studies described the total neck pain duration prior to the COP measurements whereby the pain history ranged from acute, induced pain to 97 (SD 68) months. Of these studies, half (5/8, 63%) assessed both the duration and the perceived pain intensity by using either the visual analogue scale (VAS) [19-22] or the 11-box numeric rating scale (NRS-11) [23].

The perceived pain levels varied between the studies (Table 5). The pain intensity of WAD patients ranged between VAS 2.2 (SD 0.9) [22] and 4.9 (SD 2.3) [21],

Table 2 Study characteristics and selected COP parameters measured in people with NSNP

Study	Condition	Duration (sec)	Number of trials	Parameter	Neck pain Result (SD)	Healthy controls Result (SD)	p value
McPartland et al. [18]	normal stance EO/EC/F	30	6	absolute	EO/F: 4.2	EO/F: 3.3	p < 0.05
				sway Vel †	EC/F: 4.3	EC/F: 3.4	ns
	narrow stance EO/EC/F	30	6	absolute	EO/F: 4.4	EO/F: 3.7	ns
				sway Vel †	EC/F: 5.3	EC/F: 4.4	ns
Michaelson et al. [21]	narrow stance, EO/EC/F	20	1	sway area (mm^2)	EO: 105 (73)	EO: 66 (47)	-
					EC: 166 (117)	EC: 109 (65)	-
Madeleine et al. [23]∞	narrow stance, EO/F	45	1	displacement ampl. AP (mm)	EO: ~2.7 *	EO: ~2.1	-
				displacement ampl. ML (mm)	EO: ~1.7 *	EO: ~1.0	-
Field et al. [22]∞	normal stance EO/EC/F/C	30	1	AP RMS amplitude (mm)	EO/F: ~1.3	EO/F: ~1.2	ns
					EC/F: ~1.4	EC/F: ~1.1	p < 0.05
					EO/C: ~2.2	EO/C: ~2.3	ns
					EC/C: ~2.5	EC/C: ~2.4	ns
				ML RMS amplitude (mm)	EO/F: ~2.6	EO/F: ~2.4	ns
					EC/F: ~3.4	EC/F: ~2.8	ns
					EO/C: ~4.1	EO/C: ~4.1	ns
					EC/C: ~6.2	EC/C: ~5.6	ns
	narrow stance, EO/EC/F/C	30	1	AP RMS amplitude (mm)	EO/F: ~3.3	EO/F: ~3.1	ns
					EC/F: ~4.5	EC/F: ~4.0	ns
					EO/C: ~4.5	EO/C: ~4.4	ns
					EC/C: ~7.6	EC/C: ~6.9	ns
				ML RMS amplitude (mm)	EO/F: ~5.2	EO/F: ~5.1	ns
					EC/F: ~6.5	EC/F: ~5.6	p < 0.05
					EO/C: ~6.1	EO/C: ~6.0	ns
					EC/C: ~9.0	EC/C: ~8.2	ns
Poole et al. [24] ∞	normal stance, EC/EO/F/C	30	1	AP RMS amplitude (mm)	EO/F: ~2.3	EO/F: ~3.1	ns
					EC/F: ~5.0	EC/F: ~3.0	p = 0.02
					EO/C: ~5.8	EO/C: ~4.2	p = 0.01
					EC/C: ~7.5	EC/C: ~6.2	ns
		30	1	ML RMS amplitude (mm)	EO/F: ~1.7	EO/F: ~1.8	ns
					EC/F: ~1.9	EC/F: ~1.6	ns
					EO/C: ~3.8	EO/C: ~2.8	ns
					EC/C: ~3.8	EC/C: ~3.5	ns
	narrow stance, EC/EO/F/C	30	1	AP RMS amplitude (mm)	EO/F: ~4.2	EO/F: ~3.6	ns
					EC/F: ~4.4	EC/F: ~4.2	ns
					EO/C: ~5.9	EO/C: ~5.1	p = 0.01
					EC/C: ~8.2	EC/C: ~8.3	ns
		30	1	ML RMS amplitude (mm)	EO/F: ~6.6	EO/F: ~5.0	p = 0.02
					EC/F: ~7.3	EC/F: ~6.0	ns
					EO/C: ~8.3	EO/C: ~7.5	ns
					EC/C: ~10.6	EC/C: ~10.7	ns
Vuillerme et al. [20] ∞	normal stance, EC/F	10	1	Variance (mm^2)	~19.5 *	~13.5	p < 0.05

Table 2 Study characteristics and selected COP parameters measured in people with NSNP *(Continued)*

				range (mm)	~ 20.3*	~15.5	p < 0.01
				mVel (mm/s)	~17.0 *	~11.3	p < 0.001

∞ The results presented have been extracted from bar-charts.

* Induced neck pain cases and healthy participants are identical.

- : not described

†: unit not described

AP: antero-posterior, BP: bipedal, displ. ampl: displacement amplitude, C: compliant (foam) surface, COP: center of pressure, EC: eyes closed, EO: eyes open, F: firm surface, ML: medial-lateral, mPos: mean position, mVel: mean velocity, ns: not significant (p > 0.05), NSNP: non-specific neck pain, RMS: root mean square, vel: velocity

Table 3 Study characteristics and selected COP parameters measured in people with WAD

Study	Condition	Duration (sec)	Number of trials	Parameter	WAD Result (SD)	Healthy controls Result (SD)	p value
Michaelson et al. [21]	narrow stance, EO/EC/F	20	1	sway area (mm^2)	EO: 96 (57)	EO: 66 (47)	ns
					EC: 269 (147)	EC: 109 (65)	p < 0.01
Madeleine et al. [23]	narrow stance, EO/EC/F	45	1	displacement ampl. AP (mm)	EO: ~4.6	EO: ~2.1	-
					EC: ~6.0	EC: ~2.5	-
				displacement ampl. ML (mm)	EO: ~2.2	EO: ~1.0	-
					EC: ~3.2	EC: ~1.2	-
Treleaven et al. [19] ∞	normal stance, EO/EC/F/C	30	1	total energy	EO/F: ~0.80	EO/F: ~0.66	ns
					EC/F: ~0.93	EC/F: ~0.70	p < 0.05
					EO/C: ~1.30	EO/C: ~1.15	ns
					EC/C: ~1.52	EC/C: ~1.38	ns
Storaci et al. [26]	unclear stance, EO/EC/F	-	2	sway area (mm^2)	EO: 136.6 (76.3)	EO: 84.1 (44.8)	-
					EC: 246.3 (127)	EC: 180.1 (102)	-
				path length (mm)	EO: 407.5 (103)	EO: 338 (85.6)	-
					EC: 565.8 (151)	EC: 494.5 (145)	-
Endo et al. [25]	unclear stance, EO/EC/F	60	1	sway area (mm^2)	EO: 102.8 (109)	EO: 35.0 (14.7)	p < 0.01
					EC: 218.6 (207)	EC: 41.9 (25.2)	p < 0.05
				mVel (mm/s)	EO: 18.6 (12.5)	EO: 13.8 (4.3)	p < 0.001
					EC: 32.8 (22.2)	EC: 17.9 (6.0)	p < 0.001
Treleaven et al. [27] ∞	Normal stance, EO/EC/F/C	-	1	total energy AP	EO/F: ~ 1.2	EO/F: ~0.7	p < 0.01
					EO/C: ~1.6	EO/C: ~1.2	p < 0.01
					EC/F: ~1.4	EC/F: ~0.9	p < 0.01
					EC/C: ~1.9	EC/C: ~1.6	p < 0.01
		-	1	total energy ML	EO/F: ~0.6	EO/F: ~0.2	p < 0.01
					EO/C: ~1.3	EO/C: ~0.7	p < 0.01
					EC/F: ~0.7	EC/F: ~0.2	p < 0.01
					EC/C: ~1.5	EC/C: ~0.9	p < 0.01
	narrow stance, EO/EC/F/C	-	1	total energy AP	EO/F: ~1.2	EO/F: ~1.1	ns
					EO/C: ~1.6	EO/C: ~1.3	p < 0.03
					EC/F: ~1.6	EC/F: ~1.3	p < 0.02
					EC/C: ~1.9	EC/C: ~1.6	p < 0.03
		-	1	total energy ML	EO/F: ~1.5	EO/F: ~1.3	ns

Table 3 Study characteristics and selected COP parameters measured in people with WAD *(Continued)*

					EO/C:~1.7	EO/C: ~1.6	ns
					EC/F: ~1.7	EC/F: ~1.5	p < 0.02
					EC/C: ~1.9	EC/C: ~1.9	ns
Field et al. [22] ∞	normal stance EO/EC/F/C	30	1	AP RMS amplitude (mm)	EO/F: ~1.4	EO/F: ~1.2	p < 0.05
					EC/F: ~1.5	EC/F: ~1.1	p < 0.05
					EO/C: ~3.1	EO/C: ~2.3	ns
					EC/C: ~3.9	EC/C: ~2.4	p < 0.05
				ML RMS amplitude (mm)	EO/F: ~2.9	EO/F: ~2.4	ns
					EC/F: ~3.5	EC/F: ~2.8	ns
					EO/C: ~5.0	EO/C: ~4.1	p < 0.05
					EC/C: ~7.0	EC/C: ~5.6	p < 0.05
	narrow stance, EO/EC/F/C	30	1	AP RMS amplitude (mm)	EO/F: ~4.2	EO/F: ~3.1	p < 0.05
					EC/F: ~4.8	EC/F: ~4.0	p < 0.05
					EO/C: ~5.3	EO/C: ~4.4	p < 0.05
					EC/C: ~7.9	EC/C: ~6.9	ns
				ML RMS amplitude (mm)	EO/F: ~5.5	EO/F: ~5.1	ns
					EC/F: ~6.3	EC/F: ~5.6	ns
					EO/C: ~6.3	EO/C: ~6.0	ns
					EC/C: ~9.2	EC/C: ~8.2	ns

- : not described.

∞ The results presented have been extracted from bar-charts.

ampl: amplitude, AP: antero-posterior, BP: Bipedal, C: compliant surface, COP: center of pressure, EC: eyes closed, EO: eyes open, F: firm surface, ML: medial-lateral, mPos: mean position, mVel: mean velocity, RMS: root mean square, WAD: whiplash associated disorder.

indicating mild to moderate pain. Individuals with NSNP perceived pain within a similar range and rated their intensity from VAS 3.2 (SD 0.4) [22] to 5.2 (SD 1.6) [21].

Neck pain and postural sway

Generally there was a great variability in the reported COP measures. The results of the included studies indicated that patients with any form of neck pain exhibited a greater postural instability than healthy controls, a difference that was more pronounced in WAD patients.

In people with NSNP, a significant difference compared to healthy individuals was only observed in a minority of recordings (9/38, 24%) across all positional and visual conditions. Statistical significance was reached only in normal stance under visual deprivation on a firm surface [20,22,24] as well as with open eyes on both firm [18] and compliant surface [24]. In narrow stance the differences reached $p \leq 0.05$ with eyes open [24] and closed [22] on a firm surface as well as on a foam pad with eyes open [24]. One study failed to report levels of significance [21].

Table 4 Reliability criteria

Study	Sampling frequency	Cut-off frequency	Duration	Number of repetitions	Visual condition	Surface	Total
Recommended	~100 Hz	10 Hz	≥ 90 sec	3-5	eyes closed	firm	
McPartland et al. [18]	+	0	0	+	+	+	++++
Michaelson et al. [21]	0	0	0	0	+	+	++
Madeleine et al. [23]	+	+	0	0	+	+	++++
Treleaven et al. [19]	0	0	0	0	+	+	++
Storaci et al. [26]	0	0	0	0	+	+	++
Endo et al. [25]	0	0	0	0	+	+	++
Treleaven et al. [27]	0	0	0	0	+	+	++
Field et al. [22]	0	0	0	0	+	+	++
Poole et al. [24]	0	0	0	0	+	+	++
Vuillerme et al. [20]	0	0	0	0	+	+	++

Table 5 Pain definition, intensity and characteristics of included studies

Study	WAD	NSNP	Pain presence in months (SD)	Pain present at time of trial	Pain intensity evaluation (pre-trial)	Score mean (SD)
McPartland et al. [18]		X	-	yes	-	-
Michaelson et al. [21]	X		87 (77)	yes	VAS	4.9 (2.3)
		X	97 (68)	yes	VAS	5.2 (1.6)
Madeleine et al. [23]	X		≥ 6	yes	NRS-11	6.0 (0.7)
		X	induced	yes	NRS-11	2.6-4.5 (0.5)
Treleaven et al. [19]	X		-	yes	VAS	2.8
	X		-	yes	VAS	4.1
Storaci et al. [26]	X		-	-	-	-
Endo et al. [25]	X		6	yes	-	-
Treleaven et al. [27]	X		17	yes	-	-
Field et al. [22]	X		≥ 3	yes	VAS	2.2 (0.9)
		X	≥ 3	yes	VAS	3.2 (0.4)
Poole et al. [24]		X	> 5	yes	VAS	-
Vuillerme et al. [20]		X	induced	yes	VAS	7.1 (1.7)

- : not reported, NDI: Neck Disability Index, NSNP: non-specific neck pain, SD: standard deviation, WAD: whiplash associated disorder.
∞ : induced pain.
Visual Analogue Scale (VAS) ranging from 0-10: 0-2: light pain, 3-5: light to moderate pain, 6-7: moderate to intense pain, 8-10: unbearable pain.

In cases of acutely induced neck pain, a marked immediate increase in postural sway could be observed. While Vuillerme et al. [20] found a significantly increased mean sway velocity and area, no *p*-values were calculated for the study by Madeleine et al. [23] (Table 2).

People with WAD also showed an increased postural sway, indicated by a greater COP sway area [21,25,26], total energy [19,27], root mean square (RMS) amplitude and mean sway velocity [22,25]. In contrast to NSNP patients, the variance in COP excursion compared to healthy controls was significant in the majority of experimental setups, although two studies did not report levels of significance [23,26]. The increase in postural sway in antero-posterior (AP) direction was more significant than in the medio-lateral (ML) plane [22,23] (Table 3).

Disability assessment

Only three studies [19,22,24] assessed the level of disability in neck pain patients using the neck disability index (NDI) [28]. The NSNP patients scored NDI disability percentages between 21.5% (SD 1.4) [22] and 23.95% (SD 2.3) [24] while people with WAD had higher levels of impairment at 36.9% (SD 2.8) [22]. Scores from 21-40% indicate moderate disability.

Discussion

Summary of evidence

The heterogeneous study designs and experimental setups did not allow pooling of data or any direct comparison of results across the studies. In addition, the poor overall documentation of the experimental setups, particularly with regards to participant demographics and technical aspects such as sampling frequency and cut-off frequency, impaired full interpretation. However, despite the great variability there was enough consistency in results to show that patients suffering from NSNP and WAD exhibit an increased COP sway compared to healthy individuals, especially in AP direction. Unfortunately, the magnitude of these differences in postural sway cannot be summarily expressed in terms of specific percentages or values. As a result, only a general trend is noted.

As we outlined in a previous systematic review [17], the reliability of COP measurements is primarily determined by the six main factors (Table 4). Although only two of the included studies fulfilled more than half of the recommended reliability criteria [18,23], it is worth bearing in mind that studies considering less than all six criteria may still present fairly reliable results.

While a general trend towards decreased postural stability can be observed irrespective of the origin of the pain, the altered sway pattern appears to correlate with the associated degree of proprioceptive impairment. This is signified by the generally greater COP excursions in WAD cases [21-23] where damage to proprioceptive structures and neck musculature due to the sustained trauma may be expected. In addition, higher pain intensities or the underlying neurological or vestibular impairments observed in several studies [21,25] may be the determining factor in the reported highly significant differences in sway pattern compared to healthy controls. The lack of comparable data does not allow the interpretation of previous pain duration or associated perceived disability in this context. While some WAD patients may have also been included in NSNP studies, it appears unlikely that this affected the overall results.

We have decided to include studies using induced pain in our review. While this cannot be considered similar to (chronic) NSNP, it may nevertheless mimic many alterations in sensorimotor functions documented in acute clinical pain conditions, although it should be noted that it does not replicate any potential long term neurological adaptation. Both experiments resulted in significantly altered sway pattern which may underline the role of acute "pain inhibition" [8] in the observed postural response. However, the COP sway area measured was nevertheless smaller than reported in people with WAD [23] which may underline the likely role of proprioceptive impairment associated with the pain in the development of COP excursions of larger magnitude.

Visual deprivation caused an increase in postural sway in numerous studies of healthy participants [29-32] and has shown to be a major challenge to the balance systems in studies investigating the effect of non-specific low back pain on postural stability [29,33,34]. Nevertheless, statistically significant differences were not found in a number of NSNP studies (Table 2). In addition to issues arising from the experimental setups and the generally small sample sizes of seven [18] to thirty [22] symptomatic participants, the variations in the perceived pain intensities may offer an explanation.

Pain severity has shown to be a determining factor in non-specific low back pain cases [16] where a significant, linear increase in postural sway was observed beginning at a NRS-11 score of 5. If this can be applied to NSNP patients as well, low pain intensities at the time of recording such as those reported by Field et al. [22] may well explain the fact that no significant differences could be identified, while patients suffering from more severe pain exhibited significantly increased postural sway compared to healthy controls [20].

If rather small differences in COP measures between the groups can be anticipated, the choice of appropriate sway parameters is important. However, only Vuillerme et al. [20] and Endo et al. [25] used mean velocity (mVel), a parameter that has shown both consistently high reliability [17] and discriminative value in pain conditions [15]. Despite a small sample size and low scores for the reliability of the experimental setup, they found highly significant differences with eyes open [25] and under both visual conditions [20].

The effect of ageing can be observed when comparing the studies by Field et al. [22] and Poole et al. [24]. Although the methodologies are very similar, varying results were reported. This may be explained by the fact that the latter enrolled elderly patients (65-82 years compared to 27-30 years). Older individuals exhibit increased COP excursions [35] and any pre-existing deficits in proprioception associated with ageing may add to the alterations caused by the neck pain.

Overall, the lack of data available, no conclusions can be drawn regarding a possible relationship between postural stability and perceived pain or disability levels. For the same reason, no conclusion about the effect of impairments in cervical ROM is possible.

Clinical considerations

At this point, there are several important limitations to the application of COP measures in the assessment of postural sway in a clinical setting:

Although the results tempt us to hypothesize a correlation between the magnitude of COP excursions and the extent of damage to proprioceptive structures, the causative factor for the altered postural sway pattern remains largely unclear in people with WAD and NSNP. The question still remains whether the increased COP excursions are predominantly related to the previously described physiological changes due to chronic pain perception, acute or chronic damage to proprioceptive structures in the neck or acute "pain inhibition" [8]. If the latter mechanism is mainly responsible or if the proprioceptive impairment is of acute and reversible nature, monitoring neck pain patients during their treatment and rehabilitation process may aid as an objective tool in assessing the patient's progress. If long-term neuro physiological changes are primarily involved, individually varying recovery time frames may render such measurements less useful.

Finally, the data available is insufficient to determine whether some form of correlation between the neck pain intensity, its duration or the perceived disability and the magnitude of postural sway exists. As a linear relationship between pain intensity and COP sway velocity has been demonstrated in patients with non-specific low back pain [16], further research is necessary to investigate whether this also applies to people with neck pain. If this can be established COP may have a clinical role as an instrument of measurement for neck pain patients.

Limitations

Although employing two reviewers to individually search the literature constitutes a major strength of this review, there are limitations. For example, the search strategy was limited to six key databases which might not have identified all relevant papers. To overcome this, a dynamic search strategy was employed with selected hand searches of reference lists. Due to the aim of this review, only COP measures derived from bipedal static tasks were included.

Conclusions

Patients with neck pain of both whiplash associated disorder and non specific neck pain exhibit greater postural instability than healthy controls. This difference is more pronounced under visual obstruction and may be attributed to either acute pain inhibition or diminished proprioceptive input from the cervical spine and neck muscles due to long-term neurological adaptations although additional cognitive and behavioral factors cannot be ruled out. People with WAD show greater COP excursions than NSNP patients and this may be due to the potentially increased damage to cervical proprioceptive structures associated with the sustained neck trauma,

While the presence of pain itself appears associated with increased postural sway, there is insufficient data to suggest a relationship between pain intensity, previous pain duration or the level of perceived disability and the magnitude of COP excursions.

Author details

[1]Murdoch University. Praxis fuer Chiropraktik Wolfsburg, Porschestrasse 1, 38440 Wolfsburg, Germany. [2]Research Department, Spine Centre of Southern Denmark, Hospital Lillebaelt and University of Southern Denmark, Middelfart, Denmark. [3]School of Chiropractic and Sports Science, Murdoch University, Murdoch, 6150, Western Australia, Australia.

Authors' contributions

AR and Tino Bos (TB) carried out the literature search and both participated in the selection of the included papers. AR drafted the manuscript and performed the statistical analysis. RF and BW helped with the design of the study and drafting the manuscript. All authors read and approved the final manuscript.

Competing interests

The authors declare that they have no competing interests.

References

1. L Baratto, PG Morasso, C Re, G Spada, A new look at posturographic analysis in the clinical context: sway-density versus other parameterization techniques. Motor control. **6**, 246–270 (2002)
2. JM Cavanaugh, Y Lu, C Chen, S Kallakuri, Pain generation in lumbar and cervical facet joints. The Journal of Bone and Joint Surgery. **88**, 63–67 (2006). doi:10.2106/JBJS.E.01411
3. BA Winkelstein, RW Nightingale, WJ Richardson, BS Myers, The cervical facet capsule and its role in whiplash injury: a biomechanical investigation. Spine. **25**, 1238–1246 (2000). doi:10.1097/00007632-200005150-00007
4. W Yin, N Bogduk, The nature of neck pain in a private pain clinic in the United States. Pain Med. **9**, 196–203 (2008). doi:10.1111/j.1526-4637.2007.00369.x
5. M Casadio, PG Morasso, V Sanguineti, Direct measurement of ankle stiffness during quiet standing: implications for control modelling and clinical application. Gait & posture. **21**, 410–424 (2005). doi:10.1016/j.gaitpost.2004.05.005
6. J Thunberg, F Hellstrom, P Sjolander, M Bergenheim, B Wenngren, H Johansson, Influences on the fusimotor-muscle spindle system from chemosensitive nerve endings in cervical facet joints in the cat: possible implications for whiplash induced disorders. Pain. **91**, 15–22 (2001). doi:10.1016/S0304-3959(00)00415-2
7. P Sjolander, P Michaelson, S Jaric, M Djupsjobacka, Sensorimotor disturbances in chronic neck pain–range of motion, peak velocity, smoothness of movement, and repositioning acuity. Man Ther. **13**, 122–131 (2008). doi:10.1016/j.math.2006.10.002
8. GL Moseley, PW Hodges, Are the changes in postural control associated with low back pain caused by pain interference? The Clinical journal of pain. **21**, 323–329 (2005). doi:10.1097/01.ajp.0000131414.84596.99
9. KM Sibley, MG Carpenter, JC Perry, JS Frank, Effects of postural anxiety on the soleus H-reflex. Human movement science. **26**, 103–112 (2007). doi:10.1016/j.humov.2006.09.004
10. NF Capra, JY Ro, Experimental muscle pain produces central modulation of proprioceptive signals arising from jaw muscle spindles. Pain. **86**, 151–162 (2000). doi:10.1016/S0304-3959(00)00231-1
11. AM Pearson, PC Ivancic, S Ito, MM Panjabi, Facet joint kinematics and injury mechanisms during simulated whiplash. Spine. **29**, 390–397 (2004). doi:10.1097/01.BRS.0000090836.50508.F7
12. A Conte, G Caruso, R Mora, Static and dynamic posturography in prevalent laterally directed whiplash injuries. Eur Arch Otorhinolaryngol. **254**, 186–192 (1997). doi:10.1007/BF00879271
13. H Sjostrom, JH Allum, MG Carpenter, AL Adkin, F Honegger, T Ettlin, Trunk sway measures of postural stability during clinical balance tests in patients with chronic whiplash injury symptoms. Spine. **28**, 1725–1734 (2003)
14. M Karlberg, L Persson, M Magnusson, Impaired postural control in patients with cervico-brachial pain. Acta Otolaryngol Suppl. **520**(Pt 2):440–442 (1995)
15. A Ruhe, R Fejer, B Walker, Center of pressure excursion as a measure of balance performance in patients with non-specific low back pain compared to healthy controls: a systematic review of the literature. European spine journal : official publication of the European Spine Society, the European Spinal Deformity Society, and the European Section of the Cervical Spine Research Society. **20**, 358–368 (2011)
16. A Ruhe, R Fejer, B Walker, Is there a relationship between pain intensity and postural sway in patients with non-specific low back pain? European Spine Journal (under review). (2010)
17. A Ruhe, R Fejer, BF Walker, The test-retest reliability of centre of pressure measures in bipedal static task conditions - A systematic review of the literature. Gait Posture. **32**, 436–445 (2010). doi:10.1016/j.gaitpost.2010.09.012
18. JM McPartland, RR Brodeur, RC Hallgren, Chronic neck pain, standing balance, and suboccipital muscle atrophy–a pilot study. Journal of manipulative and physiological therapeutics. **20**, 24–29 (1997)
19. J Treleaven, G Jull, N Lowchoy, Standing balance in persistent whiplash: a comparison between subjects with and without dizziness. Journal of rehabilitation medicine : official journal of the UEMS European Board of Physical and Rehabilitation Medicine. **37**, 224–229 (2005)
20. N Vuillerme, N Pinsault, Experimental neck muscle pain impairs standing balance in humans. Exp Brain Res. **192**, 723–729 (2009). doi:10.1007/s00221-008-1639-7
21. P Michaelson, M Michaelson, S Jaric, ML Latash, P Sjolander, M Djupsjobacka, Vertical posture and head stability in patients with chronic neck pain. Journal of rehabilitation medicine : official journal of the UEMS European Board of Physical and Rehabilitation Medicine. **35**, 229–235 (2003)
22. S Field, J Treleaven, G Jull, Standing balance: a comparison between idiopathic and whiplash-induced neck pain. Man Ther. **13**, 183–191 (2008). doi:10.1016/j.math.2006.12.005
23. P Madeleine, H Prietzel, H Svarrer, L Arendt-Nielsen, Quantitative posturography in altered sensory conditions: a way to assess balance instability in patients with chronic whiplash injury. Arch Phys Med Rehabil. **85**, 432–438 (2004). doi:10.1016/j.apmr.2003.03.003
24. E Poole, J Treleaven, G Jull, The influence of neck pain on balance and gait parameters in community-dwelling elders. Man Ther. **13**, 317–324 (2008). doi:10.1016/j.math.2007.02.002
25. K Endo, H Suzuki, K Yamamoto, Consciously postural sway and cervical vertigo after whiplash injury. Spine. **33**, E539–542 (2008). doi:10.1097/BRS.0b013e31817c55fe
26. R Storaci, A Manelli, N Schiavone, L Mangia, G Prigione, S Sangiorgi, Whiplash injury and oculomotor dysfunctions: clinical-posturographic correlations. European spine journal : official publication of the European Spine Society, the European Spinal Deformity Society, and the European Section of the Cervical Spine Research Society. **15**, 1811–1816 (2006)
27. J Treleaven, N LowChoy, R Darnell, B Panizza, D Brown-Rothwell, G Jull, Comparison of sensorimotor disturbance between subjects with persistent whiplash-associated disorder and subjects with vestibular pathology

associated with acoustic neuroma. Arch Phys Med Rehabil. **89**, 522–530 (2008). doi:10.1016/j.apmr.2007.11.002

28. H Vernon, S Mior, The Neck Disability Index: a study of reliability and validity. Journal of manipulative and physiological therapeutics. **14**, 409–415 (1991)
29. T Popa, M Bonifazi, R Della Volpe, A Rossi, R Mazzocchio, Adaptive changes in postural strategy selection in chronic low back pain. Experimental brain research Experimentelle Hirnforschung Experimentation cerebrale. **177**, 411–418 (2007)
30. L Mann, JF Kleinpaul, ARP Moro, CB Mota, FP Carpes, Effect of low back pain on postural stability in younger women: Influence of visual deprivation. Journal of Bodywork & Movement Therapies. **14**(4):361–6 (2009)
31. V Leinonen, M Kankaanpaa, M Luukkonen, M Kansanen, O Hanninen, O Airaksinen, S Taimela, Lumbar paraspinal muscle function, perception of lumbar position, and postural control in disc herniation-related back pain. Spine. **28**, 842–848 (2003)
32. TM Kuukkanen, EA Malkia, An experimental controlled study on postural sway and therapeutic exercise in subjects with low back pain. Clinical rehabilitation. **14**, 192–202 (2000). doi:10.1191/026921500667300454
33. A Hamaoui, Mc Do, L Poupard, S Bouisset, Does respiration perturb body balance more in chronic low back pain subjects than in healthy subjects? Clinical biomechanics (Bristol, Avon). **17**, 548–550 (2002). doi:10.1016/S0268-0033(02)00042-6
34. A Hamaoui, MC Do, S Bouisset, Postural sway increase in low back pain subjects is not related to reduced spine range of motion. Neuroscience letters. **357**, 135–138 (2004). doi:10.1016/j.neulet.2003.12.047
35. P Era, P Sainio, S Koskinen, P Haavisto, M Vaara, A Aromaa, Postural balance in a random sample of 7,979 subjects aged 30 years and over. Gerontology. **52**, 204–213 (2006). doi:10.1159/000093652

Passive standing as an adjunct rehabilitation intervention after stroke: a randomized controlled trial

Francesco Ferrarello[1*], Gabriella Deluca[2], Assunta Pizzi[2], Carlo Baldini[2], Francesca Iori[2], Niccolò Marchionni[3] and Mauro Di Bari[3]

Abstract

Background: Early physical rehabilitation enhances functional recovery in stroke survivors. Supported standing is a common adjunctive therapeutic practice in subjects with several central nervous diseases who are unable to stand actively. Data on the effect of supported positioning on standing frames in individuals with recent stroke are scarce and contradictory.

Objectives: To verify if the addition of supported standing practice (SSP), delivered by means of a standing frame in two durations, to conventional physical therapy (CPT), may improve motor function, autonomy, and mobility in individuals with disability due to recent stroke.

Methods: After baseline assessment, 75 participants with severe disability due to stroke, all receiving CPT, were randomly assigned to adjunctive 20 or 40 min of SSP, or CPT only (control). Motor function, autonomy, and mobility were assessed before and after training, and three months later.

Results: All participants assessed received the planned dose of intervention. No adverse events of SSP were detected. Most outcome measures improved from baseline through the end of treatment and in the follow-up in all groups; the extent of change was comparable across the three randomization groups.

Conclusions: In this randomized trial, SSP was unable to provide any sizeable adjunctive benefit, above and beyond CPT, in subjects with recent stroke.

Keywords: Stroke, Supported standing, Randomized controlled trial

Background

Stroke is a major cause of disability and death worldwide [1], with only a small proportion of survivors achieving full functional recovery after acute event. Indeed, at 40 % of survivors have difficulties in performing basic self-care tasks after 6 months [2], and more than 30 % report participation restrictions as long as 4 years after stroke [3]. Systematic reviews show that organized multidisciplinary care and rehabilitation are effective in the early phase of a stroke, improving survival and independence, and reducing length of hospital stay and need for institutionalization [4].

Physical rehabilitation enhances substantially the functional recovery in stroke survivors, and improvements are greater with earlier beginning and higher intensity of rehabilitation [5]. Early mobilization lessens the likelihood of acute phase complications (e.g., pneumonia, pressure sores, deep vein thrombosis) and usually begins when clinical conditions are stable [6]. Beyond sitting, the standing position brings additional benefits such as prevention of hip and knee flexors contractures, circulatory training, autonomic nervous system stimulation, and sensory activation [7]. Moreover, recovery of the ability to stand up and sustain load on the affected limb is crucial to gait training and recovery of upper limb functionality [8, 9]. Supported standing on tilt table or standing frame is an adjunctive therapeutic practice commonly adopted in subjects with several central nervous

* Correspondence: francescoferrarello@tiscali.it
[1]Functional Rehabilitation Unit, Azienda USL 4, Via Cavour 118/120, 59100 Prato, Italy
Full list of author information is available at the end of the article

diseases who are unable to stand actively. Its aim is to improve antigravity muscles strength and head and trunk postural control, maintain standing ability, and prepare for gait training [10].

Data on the effect of supported positioning on standing frames in patients with recent stroke are scarce and contradictory. In a randomized controlled trial (RCT), 14 sessions of supported standing, added with flexible duration and schedules to conventional rehabilitation within nine weeks after stroke onset, did not significantly improve functional status [11]. However, potential weaknesses should be recognized in this study: the intervention was administered late in the course of the disease, its intensity was low, its duration was left to the therapists' discretion [11], and the first post-treatment assessment often did not coincide with the end of the intervention [10]. In another pilot RCT, an intervention combining passive standing on a variety of stabilizers and task training, achieved some improvement in balance [12]. Thus, we deemed as necessary a study conducted with more stringent selection criteria and a rigorously controlled intensity of the intervention, in order to ascertain the merit of passive standing in post-stroke rehabilitation.

We conducted the present RCT to verify whether the addition to early conventional physical therapy (CPT) of supported standing practice (SSP) delivered by means of a standing frame in two durations, improves motor function, autonomy, and mobility in individuals with disability due to recent stroke.

Methods

The reporting of this study conforms to the CONSORT (Consolidated Standards of Reporting Trials) Statement for non-pharmacologic trials [13]. The study was approved by the IRCCS Fondazione Don Gnocchi ethics committee.

Subjects

Persons with recent stroke, admitted for early rehabilitation to the inpatient Neurology Unit of the IRCCS Fondazione Don Gnocchi in Florence, Italy, from April 2011 to February 2012, were screened for enrollment. Inclusion criteria were: (1) first ever ischemic or hemorrhagic stroke, (2) age ≥18 years, (3) admission within 4 weeks from stroke onset, (4) severe functional limitation in walking (score 0 or 1 in the Functional Ambulation Classification, FAC) [14], (5) tolerance to the standing frame of at least 10 min (assessed two days after admission), (6) stable clinical conditions, (7) adequate participation and cognitive capacity, and (8) ability to provide informed consent.

Exclusion criteria were: (1) clinical contraindications to prolonged upright position (e.g. postural hypotension), (2) previous stroke, (3) severe limitations of the range of motion, particularly the lack of hip and knee extension, and ankle dorsiflexion, (4) the presence of recent fractures of the pelvis or lower limb (if full weight- bearing was not allowed) and (5) any other co-morbidity or disability that would preclude participation in the training program. Eligible subjects signed an informed consent conforming to the Helsinki Declaration, which contained detailed information on study design and data management.

Study design and procedures

After inclusion and baseline assessment, participants were stratified according to the FAC score (0 and 1). They were then randomly assigned to either adjunctive 20 or 40 min of SSP (experimental interventions), or standard (see below) CPT only (control). The random sequence was generated by an investigator not involved in participants' assessment (MDB) using a web-based application (http://www.randomizer.org). Allocation assignment was kept concealed using serially numbered, opaque, sealed envelopes.

Baseline and follow-up evaluations were performed by an independent physical therapist (GD), blinded to group allocation and otherwise uninvolved in the study. Treatments were administered by physical therapists five days a week for three weeks, in an inpatient setting. Assessments were done at enrollment (T0), at the end of the 3-week treatment (T1), and three months later (T2).

A formal sample size calculation was not performed because of lack of adequate preliminary data on the expected effect size. In particular, the present RCT differed from previous studies in the outcome measures chosen, in the overall duration of the treatment period and in the double dosing (20 and 40 min/day) of the intervention.

Experimental treatment

Participants randomized to the 40-min daily SSP treatment received 2 20-min sessions (morning and afternoon). The standing frame STANDY (Ormesa®, www.ormesa.com) was utilized for the experiment. Equipped with heel rests, knee pads and back rest (both adjustable in width, depth, and height) it allows a flexible and safe static regimen.

Patients' positioning on the standing and monitoring were conducted by the treating physical therapists. Exercise duration was timed and inconveniences or discomforts were recorded. The standing session was not performed, or could be interrupted, if participants showed intolerance or hypotension.

Conventional physical therapy treatment

All participants underwent individual CPT sessions, which included 60 min of neuromuscular and musculoskeletal interventions, and practice of functional activities [15]. Moreover, 20 min of passive cycling (upper- and/or lower- limbs), hydrokinetic and occupational therapy were administered, as well as cognitive and speech therapy when needed.

Data

Demographic and main clinical characteristics (stroke type, days from event, and affected side) were recorded. Stroke severity was assessed with the National Institute of Health Stroke Scale (NIHSS). The clinical history of participants was investigated for any contraindications to upright position. Goniometric measurement of the range of movement of the lower limbs was performed to exclude limitations that might affect the ability to stand. Moreover, the ability to control the trunk in an upright position (sitting and standing) was recorded. Tolerance to the standing frame was assessed by measuring blood pressure, heart and respiratory rate first in the supine and seated positions, and then after 5 min of standing. Signs and symptoms of hypotension were monitored. As a safety measure, blood pressure and heart rate were recorded also during the interventions.

Primary outcome measures

The Fugl-Meyer Assessment of Motor Recovery after Stroke - motor domain (FM) scale, the Functional Independence Measure (FIM), and the FAC were chosen as primary outcome measures.

The FM, used in both clinical and research settings, is one of the most widely used quantitative measures of motor impairment, with excellent intra- and inter- rater reliability and construct validity, particularly of the motor

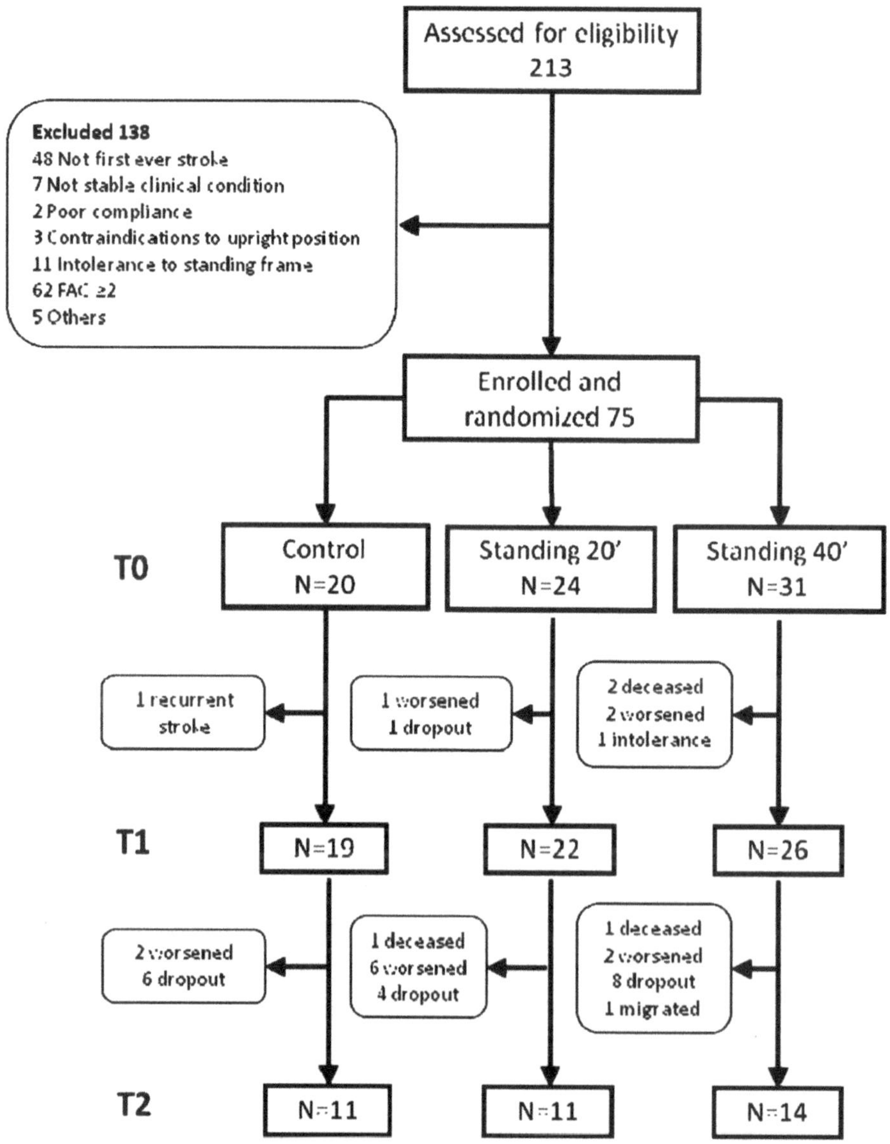

Fig. 1 Study flow chart. Abbreviations: FAC = Functional Ambulation Categories; T0 = baseline; T1 = end of treatment; T2 = follow-up (3 months)

domain, as shown by numerous studies [16]. The motor domain includes items measuring movement, coordination, and reflex action about upper- and lower- limb; motor score ranges from 0 (hemiplegia) to 100 points (normal motor performance), divided into 66 points for the upper extremity and 34 points for the lower extremity. The FIM measures the level of disability and indicates how much assistance is required to perform activities of daily living [17]. The FAC categorizes subjects according to basic motor skills necessary for functional ambulation [14].

Secondary outcome measures

The Modified Ashworth scale (MAS), the Timed-Up-and-Go test (TUG) at three months (T2), the drop in systolic blood pressure from supine to standing position, and the ability to control the trunk while sitting or standing were taken as secondary outcome measures.

The MAS [18] evaluates spasticity in patients with lesions of the central nervous system; knee flexors and extensors, ankle dorsal and plantar flexors, and hip adductors of the affected side were assessed. The TUG is a widely used mobility test, which requires that a person rises from a chair, walks three meters, turns around, walks back to the chair, and sits down again on the chair, while being timed [19].

Moreover, the Trunk Control Test (TCT) [20], which examines four simple aspects of trunk movement, was added to the protocol after the study began, and was therefore administered in a subsample.

Statistical analysis

Data were analyzed by an independent investigator, blind to group allocation. Sample characteristics were analyzed by descriptive statistics. Differences between groups in baseline demographic and pre-training characteristics were examined using one-way ANOVA for continuous and the chi-square test for ordinal and categorical variables respectively, taking into account trends as appropriate. To perform the between-group comparisons, a two-way ANOVA for repeated measures with group x time interaction was used. The Kruskal-Wallis test was utilized to highlight the between-group differences in the TUG test three months after the end of treatment.

Analyses were performed according to the intention-to- treat (ITT) and the per- protocol (PP) principles [21]. For ITT analysis missing data were dealt with by using the last- observation- carried- forward method [21]. The IBM SPSS Statistics for Windows, (version 20.0; IBM Corp, Armonk, NY) was utilized for calculations. The significance level was set at a p value of <0.05.

Table 1 Baseline characteristics of the study groups

	Control (*n* = 20)	20′ SSP (*n* = 24)	40′ SSP (*n* = 31)	P
Variable				
Age	75.15 (±3.64)	76.65 (±1.78)	72 (±2.62)	0.430
Days from event	13.5 (±0.92)	12.13 (±0.86)	11.87 (±0.69)	0.562
Gender F/M	8/12	14/10	16/15	0.476
Type of stroke I/E	10/10	17/7	21/10	0.305
Lesion side DX/SX	6/14	10/14	11/20	0.722
FAC 0/1	14/6	20/4	20/11	0.297
Trunk control upright No/Yes	7/13	12/11	17/14	0.353
NIHSS	7.70 (±1.02)	8.71 (±0.97)	8.68 (±0.82)	0.716
FM	10.55 (±1.11)	8.89 (±1.19)	8.33 (±0.91)	0.600
FIM	53.65 (±3.83)	51.17 (±2.85)	49.45 (±2.89)	0.708
SBP supine	127.75 (±3.44)	129.17 (±3.06)	123.28 (±4.51)	0.752
DBP supine	72.25 (±2)	72.08 (±1.7)	76.61 (±2.09)	0.673
SBP standing	123.75 (±3.44)	124.17 (±3.06)	123.28 (±4.51)	0.916
DBP standing	72.50 (±2.16)	69.79 (±1.69)	74.31 (±1.99)	0.674
MAS	3.5 (±0.43)	4.26 (±0.5)	4.14 (±0.48)	0.538
TCT[a]	55.50 (±8.96)	45.79 (±8.52)	46.19 (±7.94)	0.681

Data are mean (standard error) and proportions for continuous- and ordinal- or categorical- variables respectively

20′ SSP 20 min Supported Standing Practice, *40′ SSP* 40 min Supported Standing Practice, *DBP* Diastolic Blood pressure, *FAC* Functional Ambulation Categories, *FIM* Functional Independence Measure, *FM* Fugl-Meyer Assessment of Motor Recovery after Stroke - motor domain, *NIHSS* National Institute of Health Stroke Scale, *MAS* Modified Ashworth Scale, *SBP* Systolic Blood Pressure, *TCT* Trunk Control Test

[a]Sample at T0: Control = 12, 20′ SSP = 14, 40′ SSP = 16

Table 2 Effects of experimental and conventional interventions

	Control Group			20′ SSP Group			40′ SSP Group		
Variable	T0 (n=20)	T1 (n=19)	T2 (n=11)	T0 (n=24)	T1 (n=22)	T2 (n=11)	T0 (n=31)	T1 (n=26)	T2 (n=14)
FM	10.55 (±1.11)	12.16 (±1.14)	14.45 (±1.46)	8.89 (±1.19)	10.9 (±1.23)	13.82 (±1.55)	8.33 (±0.91)	10 (±0.97)	11.93 (±1.46)
FIM	53.65 (±3.83)	64.79 (±5.44)	79.3 (±9.85)	51.17 (±2.85)	62. 15 (±3.18)	75.92 (±6.84)	49.45 (±2.89)	61.08 (±4.2)	74.43 (±7.4)
FAC	0.3 (±0.1)	1 (±0.24)	2.3 (±0.52)	0.17 (±0.08)	0.73 (±0.18)	2 (±0.43)	0.35 (±0.09)	0.8 (±0.22)	1.93 (±0.53)
MAS	3.5 (±0.43)	3.97 (±0.46)	4.2 (±0.36)	4.26 (±0.5)	4.5 (±0.27)	4.95 (±0.54)	4.14 (±0.48)	4.68 (±0.46)	4.89 (±0.42)
TCT*	55.5 (±8.96)	63.83 (±9.15)	92.2 (±5.2)	45.79 (±8.52)	54.57 (±8.33)	60 (±12.64)	46.19 (7.94)	71.17 (±7.7)	97.4 (±2.6)
SBP Diff	4 (±2.04)	5.53 (±1.79)	0.91 (±2.11)	4.35 (±2.4)	8.42 (±1.95)	0.91 (±2.11)	8.79 (±2.75)	12.2 (±2.47)	-2. 43 (±1.03)

Data are mean (standard error)

20′SSP 20/min Supported Standing Practice, *40′SSP* 40/min Supported Standing Practice, *FAC* Functional Ambulation Categories, *FIM* Functional Independence Measure, *FM* Fugl-Meyer Assessment of Motor Recovery after Stroke - motor domain, *MAS* Modified Ashworth Scale, *SBP Diff* difference in Systolic Blood Pressure between the supine and standing position, *T0* baseline, *T1* end of treatment, *T2* follow-up (3 months), *TCT* Trunk Control Test

[a]The TCT was administered in a subsample (Control/20′ SS/40′ SSP: T0 = 12/14/16, T1 = 12/13/12, T2 = 5/7/5)

Results

Characteristics of the sample

Of 213 individuals with recent stroke screened, 138 did not fulfill the enrolment criteria and were therefore excluded (Fig. 1), leaving a final sample of 75 participants (37 females), who were randomly assigned to 40 min SSP ($n = 31$), 20 min SSP ($n = 24$), or control ($n = 20$). Age ranged from 18 to 97 years (mean 74.0); days from event ranged from 5 to 22 days (mean 12.3). Cases of hemorrhagic etiology, as well as of right-sided hemispheric lesion, were 27 (36 %); at baseline 36 (49 %) participants were not able to manage trunk control while standing, and 56 (72 %) could not ambulate or could ambulate only on parallel bars (FAC category 0). Baseline participants' characteristics were comparable across the three randomization groups (Table 1). At the end of the 3-week treatment period (T1) and three months later (T2), 67 and 36 participants were assessed, respectively (Fig. 1). All subjects assessed received the planned dose of intervention and had complete data. No adverse events occurred; one participant withdrew because of intolerance to the standing frame.

The results of the ITT and PP analysis were comparable. The data shown in tables and figures refer to the PP analysis. As a whole, all participants significantly improved their condition. In between-group comparisons, the study groups obtained similar scoring in final assessment in all outcome measures, both at the end of treatment and three months later (Table 2, Figs. 2 and 3).

Discussion

Supported standing programs are routinely used in many settings, different clinical conditions and age groups [22]. Being passively supported in the upright position by adaptive equipment is a common intervention for individuals who have inadequate postural control or lower limb strength [10]. The stroke rehabilitation community showed interest in the topic, in fact in a systematic review exploring the issue in adults with upper motor neuron injury, slightly more than half of the participants in the studies included had stroke [10]. Evidence related to the effectiveness of SSP in neurorehabilitation is controversial and few firm conclusions can be drawn from systematic reviews, limited to some

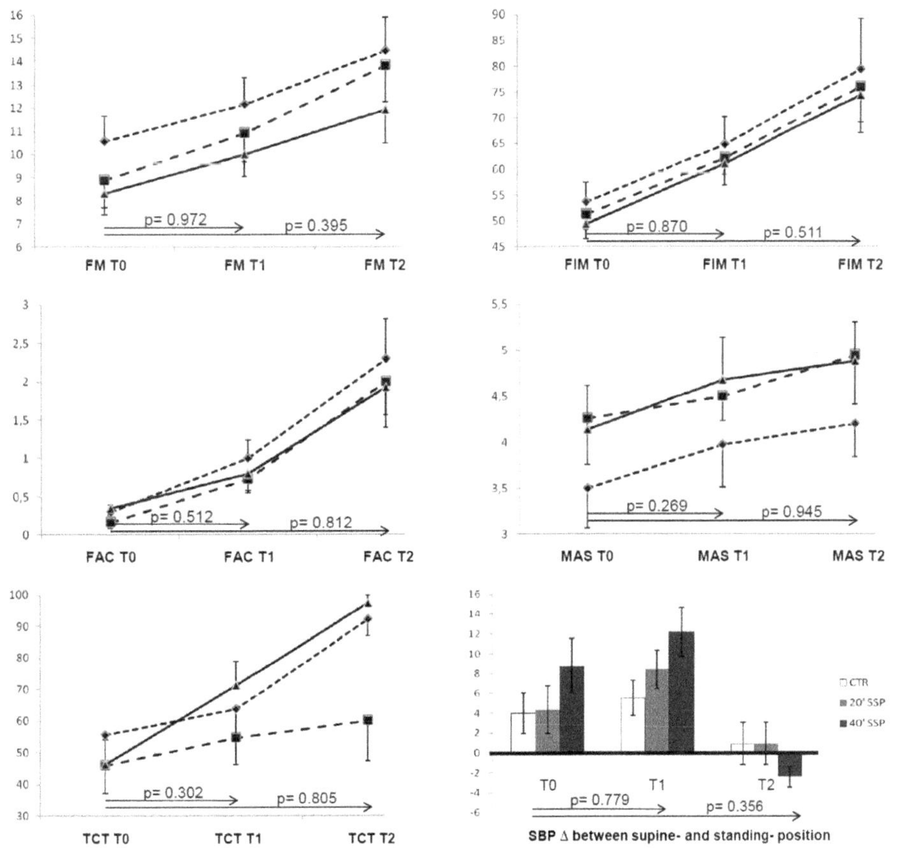

Fig. 2 Mean outcome measures score as a function of time in the three groups. Error bars represent the standard error. The TCT was administered in a subsample. Figure legend. CTR = Control; 20'SSP = 20/min Supported Standing Practice; 40'SSP = 40/min Supported Standing Practice. Abbreviations. As in Table 2

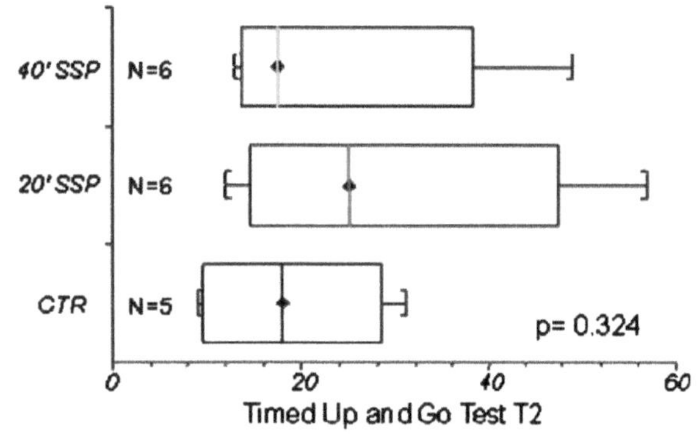

Fig. 3 T2 Timed Up and Go Test, between-groups comparison

positive effects reported in the presence of stabilized symptoms [10, 22, 23].

This study shows that the addition of SSP for 20 or 40 min to CPT, administered in an early phase, does not improve motor function, autonomy, and mobility in individuals with disability due to a stroke. Although outcome measures improved significantly from baseline through the end of treatment and in the follow-up, the extent of change was unrelated to the assignment group. At the same time, the SSP had no adverse effects.

These findings are consistent with those of the largest previous study on this issue [11], which had been considered as inconclusive because of methodological limitations, such as late application and poor standardization of the intervention [10, 11].

In our study, we tried to overcome some of the weaknesses that limited previous experiments [10–12], by narrowing the time gap to enrollment, standardizing and increasing the dose administered, and conducting the first post-treatment assessment soon at the end of the intervention. We administered the adjunctive SSP within 22 days from event and with a precise delivered dose, which might reflect clinical practice for adopted session duration, frequency, and assistive device [10].

As the comparisons with other studies are difficult, because baseline participants' disability level or type of treatment administered were not similar [12, 24, 25], it was not possible to estimate the sample size in our RCT and, therefore, it is possible that our study is underpowered. However, the absence of any trend towards improvement and of a dose-effect relationship (40 min vs. 20 min SSP) in any of our outcome measures discourages the design of further RCTs with larger sample size.

Conclusions

In conclusion, this RCT failed to show any functional benefit of SSP in the rehabilitation of recent stroke. Nevertheless , enough support exists for the use of a standing device as part of a comprehensive 24-h postural management and activity program for individuals chronically ill with severely limited mobility [23]. We cannot exclude that, as shown in other neurological conditions such as multiple sclerosis [26] or cerebral palsy [23], SSP might provide some benefit in the stabilized phase of the disease, to limit the impact of long-term complications on overall well-being and quality of life [27, 28]. However, large, high quality studies are required to definitively verify these potential, late positive effects, which have so far limited support from scientific evidence.

Competing interest

The authors declare that they have no competing interests.

Authors' contributions

GD, AP, and MDB provided concept/idea/research design. FF, GD, and MDB provided writing. GD and AP provided data collection. FF and MDB provided data analysis. GD, AP, CB, and FI provided project management. AP, NM and MDB provided institutional liaisons. AP, CB, FI, and NM provided consultation (including review of manuscript before submission). All authors read and approved the final manuscript.

Author details

[1]Functional Rehabilitation Unit, Azienda USL 4, Via Cavour 118/120, 59100 Prato, Italy. [2]Fondazione Don Carlo Gnocchi ONLUS-IRCCS, Florence, Italy. [3]Research Unit of Medicine of Aging, Department of Experimental and Clinical Medicine, University of Florence, and Azienda Ospedaliero-Universitaria Careggi, Florence, Italy.

References

1. Sacco RL, Kasner SE, Broderick JP, et al. An updated definition of stroke for the 21st century: a statement for healthcare professionals from the American Heart Association/American Stroke Association. Stroke. 2013;44:2064–89.
2. Mayo NE, Wood-Dauphinee S, Cote R, Durcan L, Carlton J. Activity, participation, and quality of life 6 months poststroke. Arch Phys Med Rehabil. 2002;83:1035–42.
3. Gadidi V, Katz-Leurer M, Carmeli E, Bornstein NM. Long-term outcome poststroke: predictors of activity limitation and participation restriction. Arch Phys Med Rehabil. 2011;92:1802–8.
4. Ferrarello F, Baccini M, Rinaldi LA, et al. Efficacy of physiotherapy interventions late after stroke: a meta-analysis. J Neurol Neurosurg Psychiatry. 2011;82:136–43.
5. Pollock A, Baer G, Campbell P, et al. Physical rehabilitation approaches for the recovery of function and mobility following stroke. Cochrane Database Syst Rev. 2014;4:CD001920.
6. Jauch EC, Saver JL, Adams Jr HP, et al. Guidelines for the early management of patients with acute ischemic stroke: a guideline for healthcare professionals from the American Heart Association/American Stroke Association. Stroke. 2013;44:870–947.
7. Knecht S, Hesse S, Oster P. Rehabilitation after stroke. Dtsch Arztebl Int. 2011;108:600–6.
8. Mercer VS, Freburger JK, Chang SH, Purser JL. Measurement of paretic-lower-extremity loading and weight transfer after stroke. Phys Ther. 2009;89:653–64.
9. Higgins J, Mayo NE, Desrosiers J, Salbach NM, Ahmed S. Upper-limb function and recovery in the acute phase poststroke. J Rehabil Res Dev. 2005;42:65–76.
10. Newman M, Barker K. The effect of supported standing in adults with upper motor neurone disorders: a systematic review. Clin Rehabil. 2012;26:1059–77.
11. Bagley P, Hudson M, Forster A, Smith J, Young J. A randomized trial evaluation of the Oswestry Standing Frame for patients after stroke. Clin Rehabil. 2005;19:354–64.
12. Allison R, Dennett R. Pilot randomized controlled trial to assess the impact of additional supported standing practice on functional ability post stroke. Clin Rehabil. 2007;21:614–9.

13. Boutron I, Moher D, Altman DG, Schulz KF. Ravaud P; CONSORT Group. Methods and processes of the CONSORT Group: example of an extension for trials assessing nonpharmacologic treatments. Ann Intern Med. 2008;148:W60–6.
14. Viosca E, Martínez JL, Almagro PL, Gracia A, González C. Proposal and validation of a new functional ambulation classification scale for clinical use. Arch Phys Med Rehabil. 2005;86:1234–8.
15. Dejong G, Horn SD, Gassaway JA, Slavin MD, Dijkers MP. Toward a taxonomy of rehabilitation interventions: Using an inductive approach to examine the "black box" of rehabilitation. Arch Phys Med Rehabil. 2004;85:678–86.
16. Gladstone DJ, Danells CJ, Black SE. The fugl-meyer assessment of motor recovery after stroke: a critical review of its measurement properties. Neurorehabil Neural Repair. 2002;16:232–40.
17. Hamilton BB, Laughlin JA, Fiedler RC, Granger CV. Interrater reliability of the 7-level functional independence measure (FIM). Scand J Rehabil Med. 1994;26:115–9.
18. Bohannon RW, Smith MB. Interrater reliability of a modified Ashworth scale of muscle spasticity. Phys Ther. 1987;67:206–7.
19. Hafsteinsdóttir TB, Rensink M, Schuurmans M. Clinimetric properties of the Timed Up and Go Test for patients with stroke: a systematic review. Top Stroke Rehabil. 2014;21:197–210.
20. Collin C, Wade D. Assessing motor impairment after stroke: a pilot reliability study. J Neurol Neurosurg Psychiatry. 1990;53:576–9.
21. Gupta SK. Intention-to-treat concept: A review. Perspect Clin Res. 2011;2:109–12.
22. Glickman LB, Geigle PR, Paleg GS. A systematic review of supported standing programs. J Pediatr Rehabil Med. 2010;3:197–213.
23. Paleg GS, Smith BA, Glickman LB. Systematic review and evidence-based clinical recommendations for dosing of pediatric supported standing programs. Pediatr Phys Ther. 2013;25:232–47.
24. Lee MY, Wong MK, Tang FT. Clinical evaluation of a new biofeedback standing balance training device. J Med Eng Technol. 1996;20:60–6.
25. Wong AM, Lee MY, Kuo JK, Tang FT. The development and clinical evaluation of a standing biofeedback trainer. J Rehabil Res Dev. 1997;34:322–7.
26. Baker K, Cassidy E, Rone-Adams S. Therapeutic standing for people with multiple sclerosis: efficacy and feasibility. Int J Ther Rehabil. 2007;14:104–9.
27. Nordström B, Näslund A, Eriksson M, Nyberg L, Ekenberg L. The impact of supported standing on well-being and quality of life. Physiother Can. 2013;65:344–52.
28. Nordström B, Nyberg L, Ekenberg L, Näslund A. The psychosocial impact on standing devices. Disabil Rehabil Assist Technol. 2014;9:299–306.

18

Daily functional electrical stimulation during everyday walking activities improves performance and satisfaction in children with unilateral spastic cerebral palsy: a randomized controlled trial

Dayna Pool[1*], Jane Valentine[2], A. Marie Blackmore[3], Jennifer Colegate[4], Natasha Bear[1], Katherine Stannage[5] and Catherine Elliott[6]

Abstract

Background: The aim of this paper is to determine whether daily functional electrical stimulation (FES) is effective in improving self-perceptions of individually identified mobility performance problems in children with unilateral spastic cerebral palsy (USCP). We hypothesized that children receiving 8 weeks of FES treatment would have higher scores for self-perceived performance and satisfaction on the Canadian Occupational Performance Measure (COPM) for individually identified priorities than children not receiving FES.

Methods: Thirty-two children (mean age 10 y 8 mo SD 3y 3mo) with USCP and a Gross Motor Function Classification System I or II were randomly assigned to the FES treatment group (8 weeks of daily FES) and control group (usual treatments). Participants were assessed at baseline (week 0), post treatment (week 8) and 6 weeks follow-up (week 14). The primary outcome measures were self-perceived scores for performance and satisfaction of child- and parent-identified priorities assessed using the COPM post treatment and at follow-up. The secondary outcome measures were the categorization of the performance problems from the COPM and self-report responses according to the International Classification of Functioning Child and Youth version (ICF-CY). This was clinically important because an understanding of mobility performance problems for children with USCP is needed for family-centred service planning.

Results: Performance scores (mean difference 1.6, 95 % CI 0.1 to 3.2, $p = 0.034$) and satisfaction scores post treatment (mean difference 2.4, 95 % CI 0.5 to 4.2, $p = 0.004$) were significantly higher in the treatment group than in the control group. There were no significant differences between the groups for performance scores at follow up, however there was a significant difference between the groups for satisfaction (mean difference 1.9, 95 % CI 0.1 to 3.8, $p = 0.03$) in favour of the treatment group. Priorities were identified across all levels of the ICF-CY but were most commonly identified in the activity and participation domains of the ICF-CY (79.5 %).

Conclusions: Daily FES applied during everyday walking is effective in addressing self-perceptions of individually identified priorities by improving the performance and satisfaction of functional skills after treatment.

Trial registration: Australian New Zealand Clinical Trials Register ACTRN12614000949684. Registered 4 September 2014.

Keywords: Cerebral palsy, Unilateral spastic cerebral palsy, Spastic hemiplegia, Randomized controlled trial, Canadian occupational performance measure, Functional electrical stimulation, Activity, Participation, Satisfaction, Gait

* Correspondence: Dayna.Pool@health.wa.gov.au
[1]Department of Physiotherapy and Paediatric Rehabilitation, Princess Margaret Hospital for Children, Roberts Road, Subiaco, 6008 Perth, Australia
Full list of author information is available at the end of the article

Background

Cerebral palsy describes a group of permanent motor dysfunctions caused by non-progressive damage to the developing brain. It is often accompanied by secondary musculoskeletal impairments that can exacerbate activity limitations [18]. Unilateral spastic cerebral palsy (USCP) is the most common topographical presentation of cerebral palsy [1]. Most children with USCP are classified as having a Gross Motor Function Classification System (GMFCS) level of I or II [13]. This means that though children are independently ambulant, they still have limitations when walking in the community. This is largely attributed to the common lower limb secondary musculoskeletal impairments that are exacerbated with growth in children with USCP. These include a combination of gastrocnemius muscle spasticity, contracture, ankle dorsiflexion weakness and poor ankle selective motor control. The combination of these impairments limits effective foot clearance during the swing phase of gait and can cause tripping or falling when walking [24].

Functional electrical stimulation (FES) applied to the ankle dorsiflexors during the swing phase of gait can be used to address problems with foot clearance. FES refers to the application of neuromuscular electrical stimulation to muscles that may not be able to contract voluntarily within a task-specific functional activity such as walking [12]. An electrical current is used to produce an involuntary muscle contraction by inducing an action potential through the placement of two electrodes over the surface of the skin above the target skeletal muscle [17].

Evidence to support the effectiveness of FES in children with cerebral palsy has been increasing over recent years, particularly because devices suitable for children can now be purchased commercially. They are also more user-friendly, enabling FES to be managed by children and families in the community [11, 14, 15]. Common outcome measurements used to evaluate the effectiveness of FES have been focused mainly on the body structure and function level, which include range of motion, spasticity, strength, muscle volume and gait mechanics [7, 15, 19]. Although these measures have provided useful clinical information, they are not able to indicate how FES impacts the performance of individually specific daily activities in the community and the satisfaction of the user. Given that the application of FES during walking enables the intervention to be applied in the community, there is also a need to determine its effectiveness within these environments.

The Canadian Occupational Performance Measure (COPM) is a valid and reliable client-centred instrument that provides the opportunity to evaluate self-perceived effectiveness of treatment whilst considering the individually specific environment in which it is performed in [2, 5, 22]. Hence the COPM will also be used to evaluate the changes in the self-perception of performance and satisfaction of individually identified priorities following daily FES during everyday walking activities.

The aim of this paper is to determine whether FES in children with USCP is effective in improving self-perceptions of individually identified mobility performance problems when compared to children receiving usual treatments. We hypothesized that children receiving 8 weeks of FES treatment would have higher scores for self-perceived performance and satisfaction on the COPM for individually identified priorities than children not receiving FES. We also hypothesized that children who received FES treatment would continue to have higher scores for self-perceived performance and satisfaction at follow-up than children not receiving FES. The secondary aim of this study was to explore the mobility performance of children with USCP by employing the International Classification of Functioning Child and Youth version (ICF-CY) framework. This is clinically important because an understanding of mobility performance problems for children with USCP is needed for family-centred service planning.

Methods

Study design

The study design was a randomized controlled clinical trial of daily FES during every day walking activities to the ankle dorsiflexors compared with usual treatments (control group).

Participants

Participant inclusion criteria (Table 1) included: USCP, Gross Motor Function Classification System [13] level and Winters Gage and Hicks Classification [24] of I or II, age 5 to 18 years, at least 5 degrees passive ankle dorsiflexion and full knee extension, ability to co-operate with the assessment procedures, and willingness to use FES daily over 8 weeks. The schedule for study commencement was dictated by current clinical care involving botulinum toxin type A injections that is routinely delivered every 6 months. With the exception of 4 children who do not have routine botulinum toxin type A injections (2 children in the treatment group and 2 children in the control group), all remaining children have 6 monthly botulinum toxin type A injections. For these children, baseline measures commenced 3 months after injections which is widely accepted to be after the peak technical response due to motor end plate regeneration [8]. Participants were excluded if they had orthopaedic surgery performed on the affected side less than 12 months before the study commenced, if they had orthopaedic metalware at the site of stimulation, or if they had an uncontrolled seizure disorder.

Table 1 Inclusion and exclusion criteria

Inclusion Criteria	Exclusion Criteria
• Passive dorsiflexion range of affected ankle of at least 5°	• History of uncontrolled seizure disorder
• Full passive knee extension bilaterally	• Orthopaedic lower limb surgery on the affected side in the past 12 months
• Dynamic popliteal angle of no more than 45°	• Orthopaedic metal ware at the site of electrical stimulation
• Able to cooperate with assessment procedures	• Botulinum toxin in lower limb in the past 3 months
• Willing to use the Walk Aide ® at least 4 h a day, 6 days a week for 8 weeks	
• GMFCS I or II, unilateral spastic cerebral palsy (with or without dystonia)	
• Winters Gage and Hicks gait classification of Type I or II	
• Aged between 5 and 18 years	

Participants were referred from Physiotherapists and Paediatric Rehabilitation consultants between June and July 2013 from clinics of the Cerebral Palsy Mobility Service at Princess Margaret Hospital for Children and The Centre for Cerebral Palsy in Perth, Australia. The trial commenced in August 2013 with the final assessments completed by April 2014. Ethics committees at Princess Margaret Hospital for Children and The University of Western Australia approved the trial. The committees' recommendations were adhered to. Written and informed consent for participation and publication was obtained from all participants. This trial was retrospectively registered (ACTRN12614000949684). However no changes were made to the protocol that was approved by the ethics committees.

Procedure

An initial appointment was firstly arranged by the first author (DP): a Physiotherapist, to determine FES tolerance and discuss the study protocol. Randomization to either the FES or control group was achieved through a coin toss, by an individual uninvolved with the study once 2 matched participants were enrolled. Matched participants were of the same GMFCS level, and were within 2 years of age for children aged between 5 and 10, and within 6 years for children aged between 11 and 18. This method was applied to improve the homogeneity of each group in terms of age and gross motor function.

Outcome measures

The primary outcome measures were self-perceptions of performance and satisfaction of individually prioritised mobility performance problems derived from the COPM. The secondary outcomes were the categorization of the priorities identified in the COPM and self-reported parent/participant observations post treatment (FES group only at post treatment) into the domains of the ICF-CY [25].

Canadian occupational performance measure

A single interviewer (JC): an Occupational Therapist performed the COPM at all time points and was blinded to group allocation. At baseline, the interviewer assisted the child and family to identify occupational performance problems in the areas of self-care, productivity or leisure. Once they had identified these problems, they were written positively as goals, which participants and their parents then prioritised by importance on a scale from 1 to 10 (10 indicating greater importance). Scores out of 10 for self-perceived performance and satisfaction were then obtained from each participant (if the child was 12 years or older) or parent (if the child was under 12 years). The scores were summed and averaged over the number of priorities identified to produce two overall scores out of 10 for each participant: one for performance and one for satisfaction. At post-treatment and follow-up, participants were blinded to their previous ratings in order to limit potential bias [23]. A 2 point change in score on the COPM is considered to be clinically meaningful [23].

Participant and parent self-report

At post-treatment, participants and their parents were asked for written comments in answer to the question: "Have you noticed any changes in yourself since using the Walk Aide?" Again, parents answered on behalf of children under 12 years.

FES intervention

Participants in the FES group received the FES device after the baseline assessment. The Walk Aide® (Innovative Neurotronics, Austin, TX, USA) is a small (8.2 cm x 6.1 cm x 2.1 cm, 87.9 g) device that delivers asymmetrical biphasic surface electrical stimulation (ES) in a synchronized manner to stimulate active dorsiflexion of the ankle during the swing phase of gait. The Walk Aide® is attached to the participant's leg by a cuff and sits just below the knee on the affected side. During a gait cycle, the Walk Aide® stimulates the common peroneal nerve, which innervates tibialis anterior and other ankle dorsiflexors (extensor digitorum longus, peroneus tertius and extensor hallucis longus). Ankle dorsiflexion was achieved by the placement of one electrode over the fibular head to stimulate the peroneal nerve and the other electrode on the motor end point of tibialis anterior. Pulse width was set to a maximum of 300 microseconds (μs) and frequency was set at 33 hertz (Hz). Users could adjust intensity (mA) using a dial on the device. The Walk Aide's® tilt sensor was individually synchronized and saved on the device so that the stimulation to the ankle dorsiflexors could occur immediately after toe-off, remaining activated during the swing phase of gait until initial contact.

Weekly to fortnightly community physiotherapy home and school visits were provided for parents and teachers/ education assistants to support FES use in different environments whilst ensuring correct use of the cuff and accurate electrode placement. Participants were asked to change electrodes every two weeks. Any adverse events were to be reported immediately (via text message or email) to the first author (DP) in order to ensure follow-up in a reasonable time frame. Participants were asked to use the FES device for at least 4 h a day, 6 days a week during the 8-week treatment period. This was monitored through the usage log on the device itself. To enable participants an opportunity to accommodate to the device, they were asked to build up gradually to the required dosage over the first week. The 8-week treatment period and 6-week follow-up period was chosen based on the results from our pilot study [14] as well as around current clinical care on the use of botulinum toxin injections (essentially so that the study duration would not be interrupted by botulinum toxin injections in an effort to minimize the confounding effect of the injections to overall outcome).

Participants in the treatment group did not wear their ankle foot orthosis (AFO) either during the FES treatment phase or in the follow-up phase but where appropriate, were provided with customized in-shoe orthosis at the commencement of the study to support foot posture and accommodate for leg length discrepancies. Participants in the control group were asked to continue with their usual orthotic protocol. To maintain consistent contact with the participants, fortnightly home or school visits were also provided for each participant in the control group.

Statistical analysis

Normality was established for the COPM scores through examining distributional plots, Q-plots and the Shapiro-Wilk Test. Means and standard deviations were reported for each group for each phase. Within group differences were assessed for a clinically meaningful change i.e. 2 point score change [23] from baseline. Between group differences were examined using a repeated measures ANOVA to account for the correlation between repeated measures over time. Post-hoc Tukey's test was applied if a main effect for group and time or an interaction of these was found, enabling adjustments for multiple comparisons and calculation of mean differences and 95 % confidence intervals. Assumptions for the repeated ANOVA were examined and met.

Statistical significant was accepted as $p < 0.05$. All statistical analyses were performed using STATA version 12.1 (TestCorp, Texas).

To further explore the performance components of the identified priorities, each priority was analysed using 2 methods. Firstly, each priority was categorized by using the occupational performance model i.e. relating to occupational performance roles, areas or components [9, 10] which secondly, facilitated the translation to the ICF-CY to identify which domain or domains it addressed [16]. Two of the authors (DP and AMB) completed this process with 92 % agreement (differences resolved by discussion).

Self-reported responses concerning overall impressions of the FES device were compiled, thematically analysed and categorized using the ICF-CY by 2 of the authors (DP and AMB). Examples are presented verbatim.

Results

Thirty-two children, mean age 10 y 8 mo (range 5 y 5 mo – 18 y 1 mo) with USCP GMFCS level I or II were recruited for the study. All participants had a Winters Gage and Hicks gait classification of I or II indicating foot clearance problems during walking gait. All participants completed the study in their original group allocation. There were no missing data (Fig. 1).

There were no clinically meaningful differences between the groups at baseline on the COPM (Table 2). Tests for normality showed that COPM scores were approximately normally distributed for performance (Shapiro-Wilk Test $p = 0.133$, Skewness −0.79, Q-plot normal) and satisfaction (Shapiro-Wilk Test $p = 0.49$, Skewness −0.36, Q-plot normal). Participants used the FES daily for a mean of 6.2 (SD 3.2) h over the 8-week intervention period. All participants had a frequency set at 33Hz and pulse width ranging from 25-100 μs. There were no reported unintended effects or adverse events using the FES device.

Primary outcome: COPM

There was a significant main effect for group (performance $p < 0.001$; satisfaction $p < 0.001$), time (performance $p < 0.001$; satisfaction $p < 0.001$) and for interaction of group and time (performance $p = 0.003$; satisfaction $p = 0.002$). Post treatment, performance scores (mean difference 1.6, 95 % CI 0.1 to 3.2, $p = 0.034$) and satisfaction scores (mean difference 2.4, 95 % CI 0.5 to 4.2, $p = 0.004$) were significantly higher in the treatment group than in the control group. At follow-up, there were no significant differences between the groups for performance scores (mean difference 1.2, 95 % CI −0.4 to 2.8, $p = 0.224$). However, there was a significant difference between the groups for satisfaction (mean difference 1.9, 95 % CI 0.1 to 3.8, $p = 0.030$), again in favour of the treatment group.

From the baseline performance score in the treatment group (3.97, SD 1.42), there were clinically meaningful changes (i.e. >2 point change) post treatment (6.97, SD 1.04) and at follow-up (6.66, SD 1.57). From the baseline satisfaction score in the treatment group (4.36, SD 1.69),

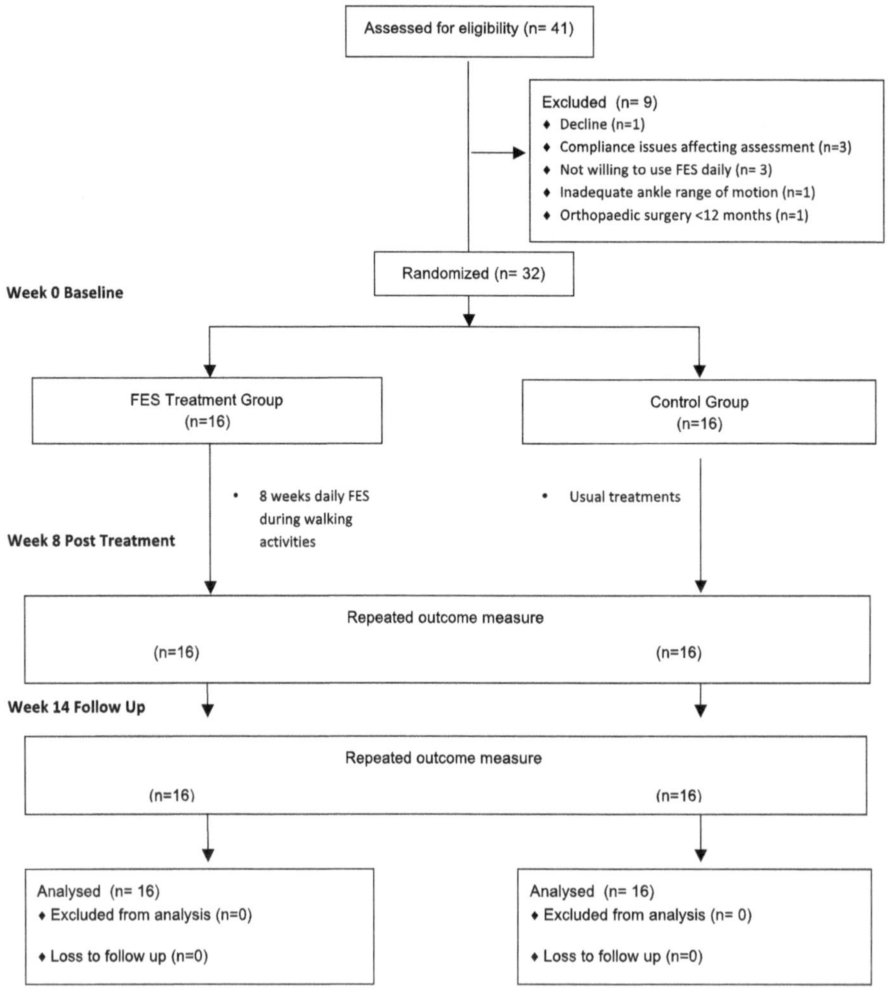

Fig. 1 Flow of participants through the trial. FES, Functional Electrical Stimulation

there were also clinically meaningful changes post treatment (7.45, SD 1.34) and at follow-up (6.99, SD 2.11). There was a trend for the control group having higher scores at post treatment and follow-up than at baseline for performance and satisfaction but these changes were not clinically meaningful. These results are shown graphically in Figs. 2 and 3.

Secondary outcome: ICF-CY classification of priorities

Participants in the study identified 1 to 3 priorities each. There were a total of 80 individual priorities for the 32 participants. Some of the priorities involved more than 1 domain on the ICF-CY. For example, one of the priorities was "to walk consistently with a heel to toe pattern to improve my symmetry (so I don't have to wear an AFO)". This included 2 parts involving (a) improving walking mechanics (activity) (b) not need an AFO (personal). Hence, when the original 80 priorities were divided into their component parts, there were 122 specific priorities. These 122 priorities were categorized into body structure and function, activity and participation domains as well as personal and environmental factors. As shown in Table 3, 17 % of the priorities were directed towards the need to improve impairments in body structure and function, 49 % were directed towards improving functional mobility in the activities domain and 31 % were directed towards improving community mobility and active recreation in the participation domain.

Secondary outcome: ICF-CY classification of self-reported changes in treatment group

ICF-CY analysis identified 5 major themes: (a) improved running and walking (activity, n = 13); (b) improved comfort with more options to wear different shoes (personal factor, n = 6) with comments such as "the walk aide means less blisters on my feet, easier to put on shoes" and "her dad got her 'girlie' shoes and they stay on her feet – really pleased"; (c) reduction in trips and falls (participation, n = 4), (d) improved confidence (personal factor, n = 4) and; (e) increased foot awareness (body structure and

Table 2 Baseline characteristics of participants

	Treatment	Control	*p* value
Weight (kg)	38.5 (15.2)	37.4 (15.9)	0.850[a]
Gender	Male: 9	Male: 8	
	Female: 7	Female: 8	
Side of hemiplegia	Right: 11	Right: 12	0.950[a]
	Left: 5	Left: 4	
GMFCS	I: 10	I: 10	
	II: 6	II: 6	
WGH	I: 1	I: 0	
	II: 15	II: 16	
Age	10y 11mo	10y 5mo	
	(3y 10mo)	(2y 8mo)	
COPM			
Performance	3.97 (1.42)	4.25 (1.42)	0.978[a]
Satisfaction	4.36 (1.69)	4.18 (0.99)	0.719[a]

[a] independent samples t test; GMFCS, Gross Motor Function Classification System, *WGH* Winters Gage and Hicks, *COPM* Canadian Occupational performance Measure

function, n = 2) with comments such as "feel more aware of your foot placement when wearing the walk aide" and "I can feel when it raises my toes when walking".

The comments also yielded some disadvantages of the Walk Aide® (n = 2) which included problems with the size and difficulties in getting clothing to over it, causing the cuff to "fall apart quite often". Three of the participants did not wish to continue wearing Walk Aide® beyond the study period because of difficulties with accurate placement, bulkiness, problems with wearing school uniforms (stockings or leggings), and difficulties in attaining a good fit owing to the cuff sliding down the leg during walking. The remaining 13 participants in the FES group continued to use the Walk Aide® either as an AFO replacement or as an adjunct to their AFO protocol.

Participant 10 wrote a more detailed account of her experiences post treatment:

> "Although compared to many other cases, my CP is quite mild, it has had quite an effect on me over the years; mentally, physically and emotionally.... To be honest I wasn't very keen on it in the beginning; I felt like it added to the things that made me different... but as the study progressed it quickly became the thing that drew me closer to my peers. Emotionally, I struggled with feeling different or out of place; having to wear splints or orthotics, but through the use of the Walk Aide, I began to feel more confident and enthusiastic to do the things I had to do to maintain the physical effects of the Walk Aide. The Walk Aide for me, reduced, in fact eliminated my pain (foot, leg and low back), boosted my confidence, gave me the ability to wear shoes like thongs in summer (one of my goals), increased my energy levels, and gave me the ability to walk long periods of time without growing weak or sore."

Discussion

The FES group achieved significantly higher scores for self-perceived performance and satisfaction on the COPM

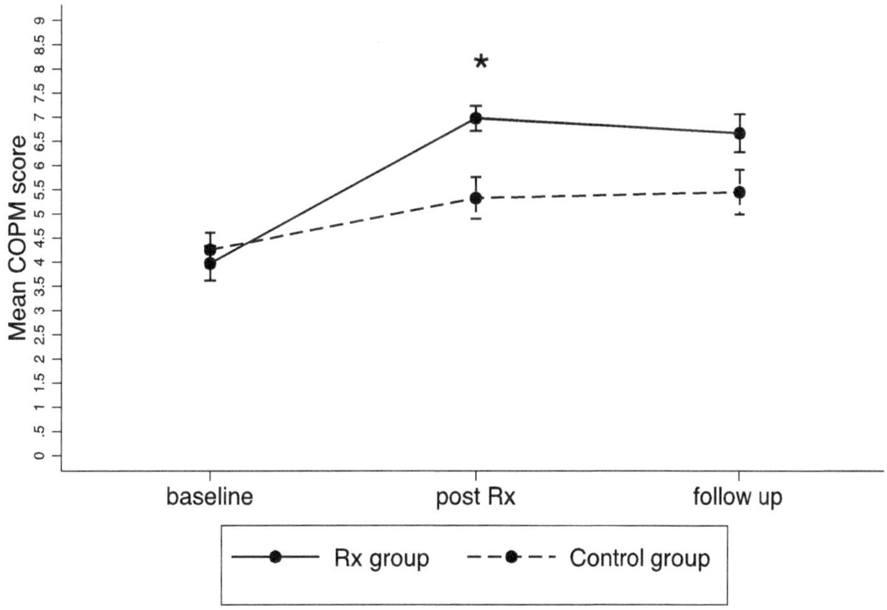

Fig. 2 Mean and standard error of COPM Performance at baseline, post 8 weeks Rx (treatment) and 6 weeks follow-up; *significant difference between groups $p<0.05$

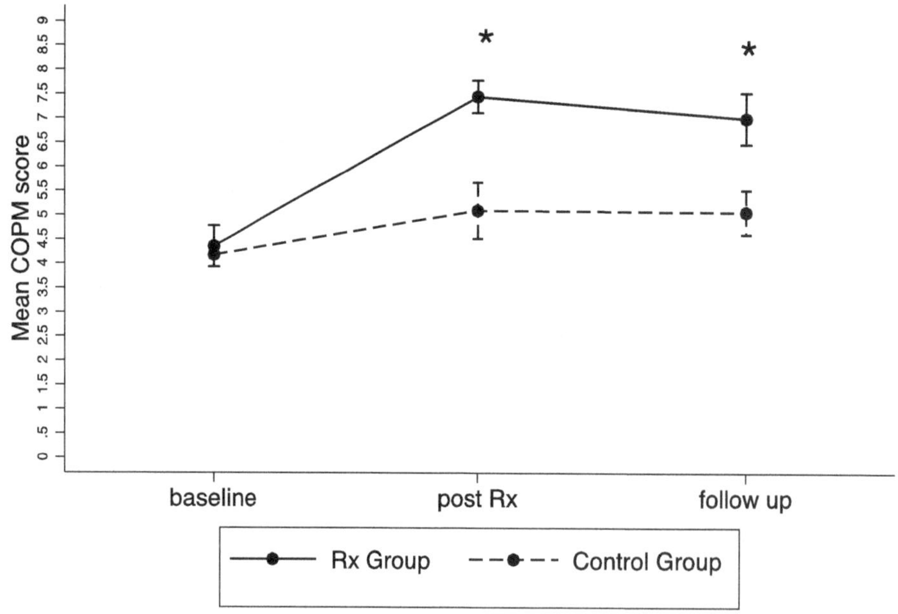

Fig. 3 Mean and standard error of COPM satisfaction at baseline, post 8 weeks Rx (treatment) and 6 weeks follow-up; *significant difference between groups $p<0.05$

at post treatment than the control group. This supports the first hypothesis, that FES is effective in improving self-perceived performance and satisfaction of individually identified mobility performance problems in children with USCP. There has been limited support for the efficacy of FES, particularly in regard to the activity and participation domains of the ICF-CY. This has in part, been attributed to the limited inclusion of valid and reliable activity and participation outcome measures [3, 4]. Therefore, these results not only provide unique evidence supporting the effectiveness of FES on activity and participation but also, that the results are consistent with current knowledge on the effectiveness of FES on the main lower limb impairments observed in children with USCP. Currently, the literature supports that FES can improve selective motor control, range of movement, spasticity, strength and ankle kinematics during gait [11, 14, 15]. Therefore, it appears that by implementing FES during daily walking activities, the main impairments affecting gait in children with USCP are addressed alongside quantifiable functional benefits reflected in the activity and participation domains.

Children who received FES treatment continued to have higher scores for self-perceived satisfaction, but not for performance when compared to children not receiving FES at follow-up. This partially supports the second hypothesis. This is consistent with current findings documenting that the effects of FES on muscular adaptations are use-dependent [7]. This provides a plausible explanation for why the self-perceived performance scores were no longer significantly improved in the treatment group when compared to the control group at the 6 week follow-up. However, this result also suggests that a period of no FES (to a maximum of 6 weeks) can be incorporated into the management plan for children with USCP without significant detriment to the satisfaction of users. This may be advantageous because of the potential to develop dependence on the external stimulus replacing the internal control of movement [6]. Given that self-perceived performance scores were no longer significantly higher in the treatment group than in the control group at follow-up, a non-use period greater than 6 weeks would not be recommended. Alternating between FES use and non-use, as adopted in this study, could be implemented to suit individual and family needs such as planning around holidays, school camps and seasons. Further study is warranted to determine whether extending this regimen would maintain the effects reported in the present study.

The secondary analysis of the priorities identified in the COPM demonstrated that the majority of occupational performance problems for children and parents were related to functional mobility activities, community mobility and active recreation participation. However in some instances, children and parents also identified specific impairments in body structure and function. Although the construct of the COPM facilitates the identification of priorities more relating to activities and participation, we included this data to reflect the priorities of children and their parents. The inclusion of priorities in this domain highlights that children

Table 3 Breakdown of the number (out of a total of 122) and percentage of ICF-CY domains (alongside the occupational performance components, areas and roles) in the identified priorities

Body Structure and Function Performance Components	N	%
Biomechanical		
Strength	15	
Balance	4	
ROM	1	
Sensory	1	
Leg pain	1	
	Sub Total	17 %
Activities Occupational Performance area		
Functional Mobility		
Improve walking mechanics	32	
Improve walking endurance	6	
Improve running	14	
Improve high level gross motor skills	7	
	Sub Total	49 %
Participation		
Occupational performance; role competence		
Community mobility		
Reduce falls	7	
Reduce trips	4	
Active Recreation		
Keep up with friends	10	
Improve sport performance	17	
	Sub Total	31 %
Environmental/Personal Factors		
Wear certain kinds of shoes	3	
Not need AFO	1	
	Sub Total	3 %

and their parents understand the body structure and function components that influence performance and for Physiotherapists, the value of addressing them in treatments. However, it also reinforces the importance of clear and sensitive communication from clinicians, realizing the influence of language on the priorities of children and their parents.

In some instances, multiple domains were included within each priority, reflecting the complexity and breadth of outcome measures that would be required in order to capture and quantify potential effects of treatment. Previous FES studies have reported discrepancies between the outcomes of objective clinical outcome measures and the more favourable parent reports [14, 20]. The complexity of priorities may explain the discrepancy between clinical objective measures and parent report, because the objective outcome measures emphasized body structure and function assessed within a clinical environment. Hence the outcome measures did not align closely with the priorities of children and parents, which often emphasized activities and participation in their own environment and community.

The self-report also provided some additional insights to (previously unreported) effects of FES after 8-weeks of use. These included reports of improved confidence, improved foot awareness, and improved range of footwear. The results of this study support the effectiveness of community applied FES to improve self-perceived individually identified priorities, particularly when they involve the performance of functional mobility, community mobility and active recreation in children with USCP.

Considerations and recommendations for the use of daily FES

Participants and their parents described some disadvantages to wearing the FES device. Their comments indicated that acceptance of the FES device goes beyond mere biomechanical physical and compliance requirements. Because the FES device needed to be strapped directly over skin, there were issues with clothing, in particular leggings or stockings for school uniforms. For younger children, the combination of the cuff and device were bulky, and parents struggled to find clothing to fit over it. Also for younger children, the cuff fitting was an issue, as it would slide down the leg during walking and running. Older children usually managed these problems, but younger children needed to have adequate support at home and school. When prescribing the Walk Aide®, it is important to consider the individually specific environmental factors that may affect treatment. Therefore, providing information and education to people involved in the child's care is essential. This highlights the importance of ensuring that community therapy services are available and in place prior to considering this intervention. However it should be noted that the Walk Aide® is still essentially a device that was specifically designed for adults. Though small cuffs have been recently available, the size of the Walk Aide® continues to be a potentially limiting factor for patient selection. Further investment into the technology and fit of this device is recommended.

Future studies should consider the cost effectiveness of this intervention. Although the cost-effectiveness of FES in the adult population has been supported [21], this has not been evaluated in children with USCP. For some children, it may be appropriate for FES to replace the use of AFOs. However, in other children, FES may be an adjunct to current therapy and AFO intervention. Evidently, this influences costs and should be evaluated further. Further work is also warranted to develop a questionnaire that would be appropriate for younger children to provide further perspectives on the effectiveness of FES treatments.

There are some limitations to note. Although qualitative self-report provided insights into the FES experience, it was unstandardized, and so the comments must be considered with some caution. Also, the outcomes of the intervention were dependent on family and school support. This could not be controlled and may have varied across the participants.

Conclusions

Daily FES during everyday walking activities improves self-perceptions of individually identified priorities, particularly involving the performance of activities, community mobility and active recreation in children with USCP. Alternating between a period of use and non-use may be appropriate without detriment to the satisfaction of the user, and this may be beneficial to suit family needs. The role of community therapy is also highlighted for the education and training of both families and teachers so that this intervention can be successfully implemented within each child's own relevant environments.

Abbreviations

FES: Functional Electrical stimulation; USCP: unilateral spastic cerebral palsy; COPM: Canadian Occupational Performance Measure; ICF-CY: International Classification of Functioning Child and Youth version; AFO: ankle foot orthosis; SD: Standard Deviation; CI: Confidence Interval; IQR: interquartile range; Rx: treatment; CP: cerebral palsy; GMFCS: Gross Motor Function Classification System.

Competing interests

The authors report no conflicts of interest. The authors alone are responsible for the content and writing of this article.

Authors' contributions

DP was the principle investigator and is a PhD student enrolled with The University of Western Australia. DP conceptualised and designed the study, drafted the initial manuscript. JC performed the Canadian Occupational Performance Measurement assessment. DP and AMB performed the International Classification of Functioning analysis on the priorities from the Canadian Occupational Performance Measurement and self-report. JV, KS and CE supervised the data collection and carried out the initial analysis. DP and NB performed the statistical analysis of the data. All authors read and approved the final manuscript.

Funding

This study was supported by the Princess Margaret Hospital Foundation, Perth Australia. In addition to 5 devices already owned by The Centre for Cerebral Palsy, Orthopaedic Appliances Pty Ltd (OAPL) donated 10 devices that were subsequently used for this trial.

Author details

[1]Department of Physiotherapy and Paediatric Rehabilitation, Princess Margaret Hospital for Children, Roberts Road, Subiaco, 6008 Perth, Australia. [2]Department of Paediatric Rehabilitation, Princess Margaret Hospital for Children, Perth, Australia. [3]The Centre for Cerebral Palsy, Perth, Australia. [4]Department of Occupational Therapy and Paediatric Rehabilitation, Princess Margaret Hospital for Children, Perth, Australia. [5]Department of Orthopaedics, Princess Margaret Hospital for Children, Perth, Australia. [6]Faculty of Health Science, Curtin University of Technology, Perth, Australia.

References

1. ACPR. Report of the Australian Cerebral Palsy Register, Birth years 1993–2003. 2009.
2. Carswell A, McColl MA, Baptiste S, Law M, Polatajko H, Pollock N. The Canadian occupational performance measure: a research and clinical literature review. Can J Occup Ther. 2004;71(4):210–22.
3. Cauraugh JH, Naik SK, Hsu WH, Coombes SA, Holt KG. Children with cerebral palsy: a systematic review and meta-analysis on gait and electrical stimulation. Clin Rehabil. 2010;24(11):963–78.
4. Chiu H-C, Ada L. Effect of functional electrical stimulation on activity in children with cerebral palsy: a systematic review: a systematic review. Pediatr Phys Ther. 2014;26(3):1–6.
5. Cusick A, McIntyre S, Novak I, Lannin N, Lowe K. A comparison of goal attainment scaling and the Canadian occupational performance measure for paediatric rehabilitation research. Pediatr Rehabil. 2006;9(2):149–57.
6. Damiano D. Effects of motor activity on brain and muscle development in cerebral palsy. In: Shepherd RB, editor. Cerebral palsy in infancy Targeted activity to optimize early growth and development. 1st ed. Sydney: Churchill Livingstone Elsevier; 2014. p. 205–15.
7. Damiano DL, Prosser LA, Curatalo LA, Alter KE. Muscle plasticity and ankle control after repetitive use of a functional electrical stimulation device for foot drop in cerebral palsy. Neurorehabil Neural Repair. 2013;27(3):200–7.
8. De Paiva A, Meunier FA, Molgó J, Aoki KR, Dolly JO. Functional repair of motor endplates after botulinum neurotoxin type A poisoning: biphasic switch of synaptic activity between nerve sprouts and their parent terminals. Proc Natal Acad Sci. 1999;96(6):3200–5.
9. Law M, Baptiste S, Carswell A, McColl MA, Polatajko H, Pollock N. Canadian Occupational Performance Measure. Thirdth ed. Ottawa: CAOT Publications ACE; 1999.
10. Law M, Baum C, Dunn W. Measuring occupational performance. Supporting best practice in occupational therapy. 2nd ed. Thorofare: SLACK Incorporated; 2005.
11. Meilahn JR. Tolerability and effectiveness of a neuroprosthesis for the treatment of footdrop in pediatric patients with hemiparetic cerebral palsy. PM R. 2013;5:503–9.
12. Merrill DR. Review of electrical stimulation in cerebral palsy and recommendations for future directions. Dev Med Child Neurol. 2009;51(Suppl 4(1)):154–65.
13. Palisano R, Rosenbaum P, Walter S, Russell D, Wood E, Galuppi B. Development and reliability of a system to classify gross motor function in children with cerebral palsy. Dev Med Child Neurol. 1997;39:214–23.
14. Pool D, Blackmore AM, Bear N, Valentine J. Effects of short-term daily community walk aide use on children with unilateral spastic cerebral palsy. Pediatr Phys Ther. 2014;26(3):308–17.
15. Prosser LA, Curatalo LA, Alter KE, Damiano DL. Acceptability and potential effectiveness of a foot drop stimulator in children and adolescents with cerebral palsy. Dev Med Child Neurol. 2012;54(11):1044–9.
16. Ranka J, Chapparo C. Definitions of terms. Occupational Performance Model (Australia): Monograph 1 [Internet]. 1997. p. 58–60. Available from: www.occupationalperformance.com/definitions. Accessed 16 July 2015.
17. Reed B. The physiology of neuromuscular electrical stimulation. Pediatr Phys Ther. 1997;9:96–102.
18. Rosenbaum P, Paneth N, Leviton A, Goldstein M, Bax M. The definition and classification of cerebral palsy contents foreword historical perspective definition and classification document. Dev Med Child Neurol. 2007;109:1–44.
19. Seifart A, Unger M, Burger M. Functional electrical stimulation to lower limb muscles after botox in children with cerebral palsy. Pediatr Phys Ther. 2010;22:199–206.
20. Sommerfelt K, Markestad T, Berg K, Saetesdal I. Therapeutic electrical stimulation in cerebral palsy: a randomized, controlled, crossover trial. Dev Med Child Neurol. 2001;43(9):609–13.
21. Taylor P, Humphreys L, Swain I. The long-term cost-effectiveness of the use of functional electrical stimulation for the correction of dropped foot due to upper motor neuron lesion. J Rehabil Med. 2013;45(2):154–60.
22. Wallen M, O'Flaherty SJ, Waugh M-C a. Functional outcomes of intramuscular botulinum toxin type a and occupational therapy in the upper limbs of children with cerebral palsy: a randomized controlled trial. Arch Phys Med Rehabil. 2007;88(1):1–10.

23. Wallen M, Ziviani JM. Canadian occupational performance measure: impact of blinded parent-proxy ratings on outcome. Can J Occup Ther. 2012;79(1):7–14.
24. Winters TF, Gage JR, Hicks R. Gait patterns in spastic hemiplegia in children and young adults. J Bone Jt Surg. 1987;69(3):437–41.
25. World Health Organisation. International Classification of Functioning, Disability and Health. Geneva, Switzerland: Children and Youth Version; 2007.

To sit or stand? A preliminary, cross sectional study to investigate if there is a difference in glenohumeral subluxation in sitting or standing in people following stroke

Nichola J. Hatton[1] and Rachel C. Stockley[2*]

Abstract

Background: Glenohumeral subluxation (GHS) is a common symptom following stroke. Many therapists postulate that GHS may be reduced if the base of support (BOS) is reduced and the centre of mass (COM) is raised as this requires greater postural muscle activity. However, there is little empirical evidence to support this practice.

Objective: The aim of this preliminary study was to investigate if the amount of GHS alters from sitting to standing.

Study design: A cross sectional, within-subject design in a convenience sample of 15 stroke patients with GHS was utilised.

Methods: A prospective design was used with a single blinded tester who assessed GHS using the calliper method in sitting, standing and on return to sitting. Friedman and post hoc Wilcoxon tests showed that GHS was significantly reduced in standing compared to sitting ($p < 0.05$) but this reduction was not maintained on return to sitting ($p = 0.25$).

Conclusions: The results of this study are limited by its small size. However, these results indicate that reducing BOS during rehabilitation may improve GHS after stroke. Whilst the maintenance of benefit is not established, these findings suggest that reducing BOS as part of treatment may help patients with GHS. Further research is now required to replicate these results in a larger sample and to directly examine shoulder muscle activity to investigate which muscles may influence GHS in response to changing BOS. Future work could also aim to determine whether the reduction in GHS was directly attributable to a reduced BOS or the effort associated with moving from sitting to standing.

Keywords: Stroke, Subluxation, Glenohumeral, Postural control, Rehabilitation

Background

Recovery of the upper limb has been described as 'notoriously poor' following stroke [1] (p1). Studies have shown that up to 75 % of individuals with upper limb deficits have ongoing symptoms preventing normal activities of daily living at six months post stroke [2]. Whilst weakness within any muscle group will affect recovery, it has been noted that glenohumeral subluxation (GHS) in particular, will reduce the rehabilitation potential of the whole arm [1] and has been significantly associated with poor functioning of the upper limb [3].

The stability of the shoulder joint is dependent upon an active system comprising the contractile tissues of the rotator cuff muscles and larger muscles such as deltoid, biceps brachii and pectoralis major [4]. Collectively the rotator cuff muscles pull the humeral head into the glenoid cavity to stabilise and centralise it [5]. However, this function requires an intact neuromuscular- system [6] which may be compromised after stroke due to alterations in descending neural excitation.

Inferior GHS is common after stroke and is estimated to affect between 17 and 81 % of all patients after stroke

* Correspondence: r.stockley@mmu.ac.uk
[2]Department of Health Professions, Birley Campus, Manchester Metropolitan University, Manchester M15 6GX, UK
Full list of author information is available at the end of the article

[7]. For the purposes of this study, we described inferior GHS to be an inferior glenohumeral joint displacement as a result of the gravitational pull of the humerus [8] which is observable and/or palpable, typically as a dip in the smooth contour under the acromion process. It can cause considerable pain and results in reduced upper limb function for many [6]. It is recognised that alignment of the GH joint can alter in both the flaccid and spastic stages of paralysis following stroke creating malalignment in a variety of directions however, this study was concerned only with inferior GHS as a consequence of gravity.

Current treatment of GHS includes the use of external supports such as strappings, slings and pillows, although there are no firm conclusions regarding their effectiveness [7, 8, 9]. The use of functional electrical stimulation has also been investigated but is currently only recommended as part of a clinical trial in the UK as its effectiveness and efficacy is not yet clear [10].

Many therapists postulate that a person positioned with a small supporting surface or base of support (BOS) and high centre of mass (COM) will require greater postural muscle activity than if they are in a position with a larger BOS and lower COM [11, 12]. Consequently, if the muscles that maintain normal glenohumeral alignment are considered to be tonic in function [13] then altering BOS and COM could influence GHS during therapy and could be a beneficial treatment strategy for people with GHS after stroke. Therefore, this small study aimed to gather preliminary data to explore whether changing the size of BOS influenced the amount of GHS in individuals with this symptom after stroke.

Methods

This study was a prospective, within subject, cross sectional uncontrolled study to measure the magnitude of GHS in sitting and standing. Participants were recruited from the local stroke population of a hospital in the North West of England, were above the age of 18, and met the following criteria:

- First stroke- identified on CT scan (ischaemic or haemorrhagic)
- Visible or palpable GHS in the affected shoulder in the sitting position (as identified by the individual's usual therapist.
- A score of less than 5 errors (from 10) on the Short Portable Mental Status Questionnaire, to ensure the individual had both the ability to consent and follow test procedures [14].
- Ability to sit unassisted on a plinth with feet on the floor and be able to stand with minimal assistance, sustaining an upright posture for several minutes (with standby supervision if required). This was determined by the individual being capable of completing the first four items on the Berg Balance Scale [15].

Participants were excluded if they had a diagnosis of dementia or other neurological deficits which may interfere with shoulder stability or speech problems which impaired their ability to understand instructions or give consent. Additionally, individuals with shoulder pain in the affected arm at rest, with the arm hanging dependent, or those unable to participate in usual physiotherapy because of shoulder pain were not included.

Participants completed the Barthel Index and details of the time since stroke, type and side of stroke, age and gender were recorded. Participants were seated at the end of a variable height plinth so that the affected arm could be lengthened at the side of the body without obstruction. The participants sat with their hips and knees at 90 degrees and their feet flat on the floor. The thighs were fully supported on the plinth and the posterior point of contact marked with tape to ensure the same position on returning to sitting. The amount of GHS was measured using the calliper technique which has been shown to be reliable and valid in stroke patients [13] by a physiotherapy technical instructor (BR) trained in its use but who was blind to the aim of the study. She marked the tip of the acromion process with a non-permanent pen and then located the superior aspect of the head of humerus using palpation. The distance between the two points was established using a standard school calliper. This was then placed on a standard ruler and the distance noted in millimetres.

All participants were measured in sitting, then asked to stand. The amount of GHS was re-measured in standing immediately and, as soon as the measurements had been taken, participants were asked to sit. The amount of GHS was measured for a third time immediately upon the participant returning to the original sitting position. In each position (sitting, standing and return to sitting) the measurement was repeated three times and the average of the three values was used for analysis.

Data analysis

To ascertain if there was a significant difference between the measures in each of the three positions (sitting, standing and return to sitting), a non-parametric repeated measures test (Friedman's test) was used. Post-hoc Wilcoxon tests were used to establish differences between GHS measurements in sitting and standing. A p value of <0.05 was used for all tests. All data were analysed using SPSS® version 17.

Ethical approval was obtained from the Manchester Metropolitan University Faculty of Health and Social Care and National and Local Research Ethics committees. The trial was reported according to STROBE guidelines.

Results

15 participants (6 males: mean age 61, range 46–83, SD 13 years) were recruited at a mean of 44 weeks following stroke (range 1–308: SD 79 weeks). Thirteen participants had been diagnosed with an ischaemic stroke, 8 had right sided weakness and 9 were out-patients.

Table 1 presents the participants' characteristics.

The Friedman test indicated that there was a significant difference in the amount of GHS between the three conditions (sitting, standing and return to sitting; $p = 0.009$). Wilcoxon tests showed that there was a significant reduction in GHS in standing compared to sitting ($p = 0.009$), with a significant increase in GHS when returning to sitting from standing ($p = 0.017$) as displayed in Table 2.

There was no significant difference in GHS between initial sitting and return to sitting ($p = 0.25$). Figure 1 shows the median values and interquartile ranges for GHS in each position.

Discussion

These results show that there was a statistically significant reduction in GHS in standing compared to sitting, suggesting that a reduction in the BOS also reduced the amount of GHS in participants after stroke.

There were several limitations to this study, most notably the small sample size. Nonetheless, the results support the practice of considering BOS of the patient when treating individuals following stroke [12, 16], as in standing there appears to be a greater potential for muscle recruitment and thus reduced GHS. However, these findings require verification in a larger study before clinical recommendations can be developed and therapists should balance the safety implications when reducing an individual's BOS against any possible benefits in muscle activity.

This small study was unable to demonstrate the cause of the reduced subluxation seen on standing, but it is likely that the changes observed are as a result of greater activity within the rotator cuff. These muscles, with some deltoid activity provide the main component of control at the GH joint [17-19, 20]. Indeed, paralysis of the supraspinatus muscle in particular has been suggested to be a predictor of a greater risk of GHS by some [21]. Marieb (2004) [15] describes the rotator cuff tendons as being kept taut by the resting tone within the muscle and Edwards (2002) [5] suggests that local stabilisers, comprising slow oxidative (tonic) fibres, are largely fatigue resistant with long lasting but weak contractions. The findings of the current study lend some support to the notion that the rotator cuff muscles appear to act as postural muscles. The results also suggest that they increase their activity on standing and thereby reduce GHS.

The effect of postural control on GHS has not been explored within the literature. The mechanical factors relating to aetiology and treatment have been outlined but few studies have considered the effect of changing the base of support upon muscle activity and GHS and so we can only hypothesise the mechanisms by which these changes have occurred [9]. It is possible that the activation of the rotator cuff and subsequent reduction

Table 1 Participant characteristics

Participant No.	Gender	Age	Affected side	Type of stroke	Time since stroke (Weeks)	Barthel Index score (/20)
1	F	46	R	Parietal lobe infarct	308	20
2	M	66	L	MCA infarct	105	19
3	M	69	L	Thalamic infarct	48	14
4	M	53	R	Parietal/internal capsule infarct	11	16
5	F	46	R	Basal ganglia infarct	75	15
6	F	53	L	Frontoparietal infarct	17	17
7	M	48	L	MCA infarct	1	11
8	F	48	R	Haemorrhage	18	11
9	F	69	L	MCA infarct	16	13
10	F	58	R	Basal ganglia infarct	25	14
11	M	82	L	MCA infarct	3	10
12	F	50	L	MCA infarct	3	8
13	F	66	R	Parietal infarct	29	14
14	F	83	R	Basal ganglia infarct	1	9
15	M	80	R	MCA infarct	2	9

R right, *L* left, *MCA* middle cerebral artery

Table 2 Glenohumeral subluxation (GHS) in sitting, standing and return to sitting

Position	GHS (mm)	Range (mm)	95 % CI of the change in GHS in different positions			
			Initial sitting	*P*	Standing	*P*
Initial sitting	13	12 (8-21)	-	-		
Standing	9	16 (0-16)	−1.29 to -6.98	0.009	-	-
Return to sitting	12	17 (4-21)	−0.91 to 3.8	0.25	5.36 to 0.24	0.017

A negative value indicates a reduction in GHS. *CI* confidence interval

in GHS within the standing position may occur because different neurological pathways are activated, for example, the medial reticulospinal tract [18, 19]. In comparison to sitting, standing elicits greater sensory input from the lower limbs, particularly the soles of the feet which can increase extensor muscle activity via synergistic muscle patterns [15]. This process is likely to utilise propriospinal neurons which are located within the spinal cord. The longest of axons of these nerve cells lie within the medial pathways and can innervate both proximal and axial muscles creating co-activation, even in the presence of a damaged central nervous system [22].

Another potential contributor to a reduction in GHS on standing is that some tracts which can influence muscle activity at the shoulder may originate on the ipsilateral side of the brain and so would maintain innervations to the affected side after stroke. Such tracts include the medial reticulospinal pathway which creates activity within the postural muscles and limb extensors and the lateral vestibulospinal tract which is activated by changes in response to gravity [18, 19].

An alternative explanation of why GHS may reduce as BOS and COM rises could be that it is purely the effect of the effort required to overcome the inertia of sitting to achieve standing. During movements that require effort it is normal to have a generalised increase in activity elsewhere in the body [11]. It is therefore a limitation of this study that the reason for the reduction in GHS cannot be determined; this could be further examined in future work by asking participants to stand for longer to determine if an initial increase in muscular activity reduces.

Further research could also seek to identify if muscular activity is related to shoulder pain in GHS [22] and to see which muscles increase their activity on standing, to determine the mechanism by which GHS was observed to decrease [21]. It is now also necessary to evaluate if treatment with a smaller BOS has lasting benefits to upper limb function in individuals who have GHS after a stroke.

Conclusions

Despite its limitations, the finding of the current study suggests that therapists should consider reducing a

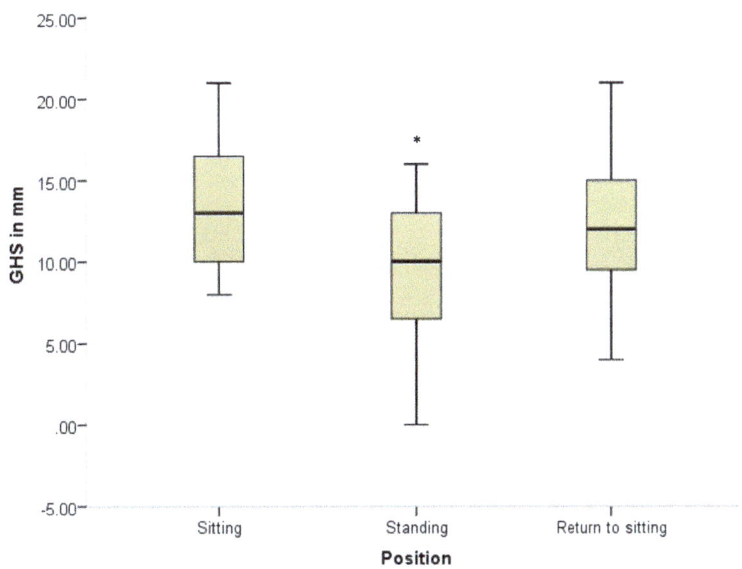

Fig. 1 Boxplot to show measurements of glenohumeral subluxation (GHS) in sitting, standing and upon return to sitting. Lines indicate median GHS in each position with the lower and upper margins of the box indicating the 25th and 75th centiles respectively. Error bars show the range. *denotes significant differences ($p < 0.05$) in GHS from both sitting and return to sitting

patient's BOS, where is safe to do so, during treatments in order to activate postural muscles and in turn reduce GHS. The use of internally generated mechanisms to reduce GHS in this way, rather than passive supports such as slings or cuffs, may promote more function within the arm and provide a low cost and simple method to augment treatment.

Further research is now needed in a larger trial to verify these findings and to determine whether it is the effort associated with standing or the reduction in BOS which leads to GHS reduction. Future research could also investigate if GHS reduction can be sustained when standing for longer periods to increase the clinical relevance of these results.

Competing interests

The authors declare that they have no competing interests.

Author's contribution

NH carried out data collection and initial analysis and drafted the early versions of the manuscript. RS assisted with the design of the study, completed further analysis and final drafting of the manuscript. All authors read and approved the final manuscript.

Author details

[1]Tameside General Hospital, Ashton-u-Lyne, Greater Manchester OL6 9RW, UK. [2]Department of Health Professions, Birley Campus, Manchester Metropolitan University, Manchester M15 6GX, UK.

References

1. Feys H, DeWeerdt W, Selz B, Steck G, Spichiger R, Vereeck L, et al. Effect of a therapeutic intervention for the hemiplegic upper limb in the acute phase after stroke: a single-blind, randomised, controlled multicentre trial. Stroke. 1998;29:785–92.
2. Cirstea M, Levin M. Improvement of arm movement patterns and endpoint control depends on type of feedback during practice in stroke survivors. Neurorehabilitation and Neural Repair. 2002;21:398–412.
3. Hanger H, Whitewood P, Brown G, Ball M, Harper J, Cox R, et al. A randomised controlled trial of strapping to prevent post-stroke shoulder pain. Clinical Rehabilitation. 2000;14:370–80.
4. Veeger H, van der Helm F. Shoulder function; the perfect compromise between mobility and stability. Journal of Biomechanics. 2007;40:2119–29.
5. Edwards S. Neurological Physiotherapy 2nd edition. Edinburgh: Churchill Livingstone; 2002.
6. Neumans D. Kinesiology of the musculoskeletal system – Foundations for physical rehabilitation. St Louis: Mosby; 2002.
7. Turner- Stokes L, Jackson D. Shoulder pain after stroke: A review of the evidence base to inform the development of an integrated care pathway. Clinical Rehabilitation. 2002;16:276–98.
8. Ada L, Foongchomcheay A and Canning C. (2005). Supportive devices for preventing and treating subluxation of the shoulder after stroke. *Cochrane database of systematic reviews. Issue 1.* Article number CD003863 doi:10-1002/14651858.
9. Morley A, Clarke A, English S, Helliwell S. Management of the subluxed low tone shoulder. Physiotherapy. 2002;88:208–16.
10. Intercollegiate Stroke Working Party. National clinical guideline for stroke. 4th ed. London: Royal College of Physicians; 2012.
11. Hess S. Functional stability of the glenohumeral joint. Manual Therapy. 2000;5:63–71.
12. Gjelsvik B. The Bobath Concept in adult neurology Stuttgart: Thieme. 2008.
13. Boyd E, Torrance G. Clinical measures of shoulder subluxation. Canadian Journal of Public Health. 1992;83(1 Suppl 2):524–8.
14. Paci M, Nannetti L, Taiti P, Baccini M, Pasquini J, Rinaldi L. Shoulder subluxation after stroke: relationships with pain and motor recovery. Physiotherapy Research International. 2007;12(2):95–104.
15. Berg K, Wood-Dauphinee S, Williams J. The Berg Balance Scale: Reliability assessment for elderly residents and patients with acute stroke. Scandinavian Journal of Rehabilitation Medicine. 1995;27:27–36.
16. Marieb S. Human Anatomy and Physiology. San Francisco: Pearson Benjamin Cummings; 2004.
17. Shumway-Cook A, Woollacott M. Motor control – translating research into clinical practice. Philadelphia: Lippincott, Williams and Wilkins; 2011.
18. Lundy-Eckman L. Neuroscience-Fundamentals for rehabilitation. Missouri: Saunders; 2007.
19. Linn S, Granat M, Lees K. Prevention of shoulder subluxation after stroke with electrical stimulation. Stroke. 1999;30:963–8.
20. Ghez C, Krakauer J. The organisation of movement in Kandel E, Schwartz J and Jessell T (eds) Principles of Neural Science 4th edition. New York: McGraw-Hill; 2000.
21. Kumar P, Kassam J, Denton C, Taylor E, Chatterley A. Risk factors for inferior shoulder subluxation in pts with stroke. Phys Ther Rev. 2010;15:3–11.
22. Ikai T, Tei K, Yoshida K, Miyano S, Yonemoto K. Evaluation and treatment of shoulder subluxation in hemiplegia: Relationship between subluxation and pain. American Journal of Physical Medicine and Rehabilitation. 1998;77:421–6.

Can experienced physiotherapists identify which patients are likely to succeed with physical therapy treatment?

Chad E Cook[1*], Thomas J Moore[2], Kenneth Learman[3], Christopher Showalter[4] and Suzanne J Snodgrass[5]

Abstract

Background: The purpose of the study was to determine if clinician predicted prognosis is associated with patient outcomes.

Methods: The study was a secondary analysis of data that were collected in 8 physiotherapy outpatient clinics. Nine physiotherapists with post-graduate training in manual therapy (mean 20.3 years of experience) were asked at baseline to project the outcome of the patients evaluated. In total, 112 patients with low back (74 %) or neck (26 %) pain were treated pragmatically with interventions consisting of manual therapy, strengthening, and patient-specific education. Outcomes measures consisted of percent change in disability (Oswestry or Neck Disability Index), self-reported rate of recovery (0–100 %), and percent change in pain (numerical pain rating scale). Hierarchical logistic regression determined potential factors (clinician predicted prognosis score (1–10) at baseline, dichotomised as poor (1–6) and good (7–10); symptom duration categorised as acute, subacute or chronic; same previous injury (yes/no); baseline pain and disability scores; within-session improvement at initial visit (yes/no); and presence of ≥ one psychological factor) associated with meaningful changes in each of the three outcomes at discharge (disability and pain > 50 % improvement, rate of recovery ≥82.5 % improvement).

Results: Clinician predicted prognosis (OR 4.15, 95%CI = 1.31, 13.19, $p = 0.02$) and duration of symptoms (OR subacute 0.24, 95%CI = 0.07, 0.89, $p = 0.03$; chronic 0.21, 95%CI = 0.05, 0.90, $p = 0.04$) were associated with rate of recovery, whereas only clinician predicted prognosis was associated with disability improvement (OR 4.28, 95 % CI 1.37, 13.37, $p = 0.01$). No variables were associated with pain improvement.

Conclusions: Clinician predicted prognosis is potentially valuable for patients, as a good predicted prognosis is associated with improvements in disability and rate of recovery.

Keywords: Prognosis, Prediction, Physiotherapist, Musculoskeletal, Spine

Background

Early prognosis is important for making clinical treatment decisions. Physiotherapists usually use a combination of decision making methods, including but not limited to hypothetico-deductive reasoning, intuition, and pattern recognition, when assessing prognosis and treatment [1, 2]. Pattern recognition is the categorization of patients based on exemplars from previous experience. It has been described as the non-analytic reasoning that contributes to clinical decision-making and it may increase clinician accuracy [3, 4]. Intuition or pattern recognition may assist physiotherapists in predicting patient prognosis early in the treatment process. This is supported by reports from physiotherapists that indicate they believe pattern recognition is an essential part of their decision-making [5, 6].

To our knowledge, the association between physiotherapist-predicted prognosis and various forms of patient outcomes has formally investigated in three studies. Hancock and associates [7] retrospectively examined the ability of physiotherapists to determine who was likely to have a quick resolution of pain in a population of patients with

* Correspondence: chad.cook@duke.edu
[1]Department of Orthopaedics, Duke University, 2200 Main Street, 27705 Durham, NC, USA
Full list of author information is available at the end of the article

acute low back pain ($N = 240$). Prognosis assessment was performed at baseline and prior to treatment, and based on an 11 point scale (0 = very slow resolution of pain, 10 = very fast resolution of pain). The authors found that physiotherapists were able to identify those who would have quicker resolution, although not with the same accuracy as a clinical prediction rule. Recently, Abbott and Kingan [8] prospectively investigated the prognosis of a physiotherapists' summative opinion on the long term functional outcome of individuals with a new episode of chronic or recurrent low back pain ($N = 138$). Physiotherapists formulated their opinion directly after performing a standardized physical examination and scored their prognoses on a 4 point Likert scale (1 = very good, very likely; 2 = good, moderately likely; 3 = poor, fairly likely; and 4 = very poor, very likely). Their investigation supported that physiotherapists were able to identify patients who had higher self-reported disability at 12 months.

Lastly, Dagfinrud and colleagues [9] examined the predictive ability of manual physiotherapists' prognostic assessment in identifying patients with neck and low back pain ($N = 157$) at risk for having persistent disability (high score on Oswestry Disability or Neck Disability Indices). The authors [9] also compared physiotherapists' findings to a standardized instrument (Orebro Musculoskeletal Pain Questionnaire, OMPQ). Although both the physiotherapists' prognosis and the OMPQ were significantly associated with 8-week outcome on the Oswestry Disability Index (ODI) for low back pain patients, associations were weak and neither predicted outcomes for the neck pain patients. The study differed from that of Hancock *et al.*, [7] and Abbott and Kingan [8], in that the authors did not allow physiotherapists to experience a typical clinician-patient encounter (physiotherapists in the study were blinded to the results of the patient questionnaires), and they included patients with neck pain whereas the other two studies did not.

The aforementioned studies [7–9] appear to support a physiotherapists' ability to identify the prognosis of patients with low back pain, specifically with respect to length of time for recovery for pain and disability scores. Mixed findings exist with respect to a physiotherapists' ability to predict prognosis better than a standardized instrument or clinical prediction rule. Only Dagnifrud *et al.*, [9] examined prognosis in a mixture of chronicity levels, and none of the previous studies investigated the concept of rate of recovery, which is a patient derived self-assessment that is neither solely affiliated with pain or disability. Subsequently, the primary purpose of the current study was to determine whether clinician prediction of patient prognosis was associated with changes in disability, changes in pain and self-reported rate of recovery, when all assessment information is available to the physiotherapist at the initial consultation. A secondary aim was to explore the relationships between a physiotherapists' predicted prognosis and other prognostic variables previously shown to be associated with patient outcomes.

Methods

Study design

This study was a secondary database analysis of a prospective cohort study [10] in which data were collected from May of 2011 to April of 2014. The prospective cohort study involved assessment of the concept of a "comparable sign", and was observational. Because the original design was observational and required no prospective assignment of human participants or groups of humans to one or more health-related interventions to evaluate the effects on health outcomes, clinical trials registration was not required. All patients enrolled in the study signed an informed consent statement that was approved by the Walsh University Human Ethics committee in North Canton, Ohio.

Eligibility criteria

Patients

All data were gathered in one of eight outpatient physical therapy clinics in the United States. For eligibility to participate in the primary study, patients were required to be 18 years of age or older with mechanically producible cervical or lumbar spine pain which occurred during clinical examination movements. All subjects also had to have required care beyond a single visit and had to speak English. Clinicians were instructed to target consecutive patients with spinal pain for inclusion into the study.

Exclusion involved the presence of any red flag (tumor, metabolic disease, rheumatoid arthritis, osteoporosis, prolonged history of steroid use) or signs consistent with nerve root compression that resulted in a radiculopathy (*i.e.*, diminished muscle stretch reflex, or diminished or absent sensation to pinprick in any upper or lower extremity dermatome). Additional exclusion criteria included a history of neck or low back related surgery or current pregnancy.

Physiotherapists

The study included 9 orthopedically-oriented physiotherapists, all of whom had rigorous, extensive training in manual therapy principles, orthopedic manual therapy certification, or were Fellows of the *American Academy of Orthopaedic Manual Physical Therapists*. The physiotherapists' experiences ranged from 12 to 30 years (mean = 20.3 years) and practice settings were either hospital-based or private outpatient facilities. All were familiar with data collection in research projects and had experience collecting and recording data in two previous randomized controlled trials [11, 12].

The examination and interventional process

Pre-study

Prior to involvement, all physiotherapists participated in a standardized, mandatory 30-minute educational webinar that explained the primary purpose of the study, the data collection methods, and the requirements for participation. Physiotherapists were also made aware of the secondary purpose of the study, which was to evaluate their ability to predict the projected outcome.

Initial visit

All physiotherapists performed a patient response-based examination [11] in which feedback was gathered with each targeted active or passive movement and subsequent treatment was a by-product of what was identified during the examination. A standardized examination process was used for all patients and the process involved analyzing movement patterns and pain during the examination phases of; 1) active physiological movements, 2) passive physiological movements and 3) passive accessory movements. All data captured during the initial visit was recorded immediately after completion of the encounter.

Week two and discharge

Throughout the bout of care, treatment interventions were performed pragmatically to ensure ecological validity and almost exclusively consisted of manual therapy, strengthening, and patient-specific education. Specific interventions were not the purpose of the study thus the components of each patient's treatment were not collected. The physiotherapists collected outcomes data for disability and pain at week two and at discharge collected these along with the rate of recovery. Patients were discharged when the physical therapist felt they had meet their maximal improvement, when the patients self-discharged, or when the two parties mutually agreed on discharge. Discharge was not delayed for the sake of the study, thus in rare cases patient-encounters were shorter than the 2 week follow up.

Variables captured

At baseline, each physiotherapist recorded demographics (*e.g.*, age, race, gender, and diagnosis), duration of symptoms (categorized by acute < 6 weeks, sub-acute 6 weeks to 12 weeks, and chronic > 12 weeks), baseline outcomes measures for pain (Numeric pain rating scale) and disability (ODI or Neck Disability Index), previous history of a similar injury/sameness of symptoms(Yes or No), presence of a within-session change in pain or movement strategies (Yes for improvement, or No for no change or worsening symptoms), and presence of baseline psychosocial concerns (Yes or No).

All variables used in the modeling for this study were selected based on their previously investigated relationships with prognosis for either neck or back pain [13]. Age has been associated with poorer prognosis for subjects with neck pain [14, 15]. Longer duration of symptoms has been associated with a poorer recovery [16], whereas higher intensity of baseline levels of pain and disability has been associated with delayed recovery for patients with neck pain [17] and low back pain [15, 18]. A previous injury has been identified as the most prominent variable associated with recurrent low back pain [18], for first-time low back pain [19], and for poor outcomes with neck and back pain [15, 18, 20, 21] although to our knowledge the similarity (sameness) of the symptoms to the previous injury has not been formally investigated. A within-session change is an improvement in the patient's pain or movement strategy that occurs during the initial visit [22]. A within-session change in either pain, movement, or both has been reported as a useful predictor of outcomes in previous studies [22–24].

Psychological factors have been associated with negative outcomes for subjects with neck [25] and back pain [26]. Presence of baseline psychosocial concern was based on any single positive answer from seven questions associated with enjoyment of employment, presence of a relationship with spouse or partner, depression, anxiety, social support systems, relationship with work colleagues, and use of medications for an unmentioned mental health condition. The tool used was novel and was created to provide a comprehensive assessment of psychosocial problems without overly burdening the patient with multiple psychological scales. The tool has not been analyzed for reliability or validity. Any positive finding from the seven was coded as "yes" whereas negative findings were coded as "no".

At the initial clinical encounter, each physiotherapist was asked to estimate each patient's potential for a successful outcome, based on their professional appraisal. Operationally, the physiotherapists were instructed to evaluate *all component parts* of their evaluation in their prediction of prognosis for the patient. Similar to the method used by Dagfinrud and colleagues [9], physiotherapists were instructed to score each patient on a continuum of 1 (suggesting a very poor projected outcome) to 10 (suggesting an excellent projected outcome) during the initial assessment. Each therapist was asked to score each patient following their complete encounter with the patient, including patient history, physical examination, treatment and reassessment. Upon examining the distribution of physiotherapists' scores and using a receiver operating curve(ROC), the physiotherapist prediction of prognosis was dichotomised as a *good projected prognosis*(scores that range from 7 to 10), or a *poor projected prognosis* (scored as 1–6).

Outcome measures

Primary disability measures included the ODI [27] or the Neck Disability Index (NDI) [28], whereas the primary pain measure was the numeric pain rating scale (NPRS). At discharge, the self-reported Rate of Recovery (RoR) was captured [11].

Oswestry disability index and the neck disability index

The ODI was used to measure patient disability in the patients with back pain. The ODI is a scale of 10 questions with scoring of 0–5 for each question, and the ODI defines disability as the higher the score, the greater the disability [27]. We used percentage change to determine the change score for each patient. This was calculated as [(baseline ODI score–final ODI score)/(baseline ODI score)] × 100 [29]. The NDI was used for the patients with neck pain, as it was designed for measuring pain related disability in this population [28]. The NDI contains ten focused sections. Seven items focus on activities of daily living. Each item is scored on a 6 point scale and can reach a maximum score of 5; therefore, the maximum score is 50 [28]. Content and construct validity and reliability of the NDI have been previously shown in patients with neck pain [30]. As with the ODI, we used percentage change to determine the change score for each patient. This was calculated as [(baseline NDI score–final NDI score)/(baseline NDI score)] × 100. Others have used a 50 % change from baseline as an appropriate discriminative threshold for disability scores in previous studies [29]. Thus, for analysis, the percent change in ODI/NDI was dichotomised as ≥ 50 % change (successful outcome) and <50 % change (not successful).

Numeric pain rating scale

The NPRS was used for patient perception of pain intensity using a scale of 0 ("no pain") to 10 ("worst pain imaginable"). The NPRS has been found to be reliable and responsive [31]. We also used a percentage change as our outcome measure. This was calculated as: [(baseline NPRS score–final NPRS score)/(baseline NPRS score)] × 100. Greater than or equal to a 50 % improvement has been used by others [32] in different populations as an acceptable level of change indicating successful outcome. Thus for analysis, we categorized the percent change in NPRS as ≥ 50 % change (successful outcome) and <50 % change (not successful).

Rate of recovery

Self-reported rate of recovery was scored as (0–100 %) [11]. Patients responded to the physiotherapists asking them whether they were recovered and by how much by scoring their recovery on a scale from 0 % (meaning no recovery at all) to 100 % (meaning totally recovered). This scoring procedure is a variant of the single alpha-numeric evaluation, and has been previously used with patients with shoulder pain [31, 33] and low back pain [11]. Previous work [34] has identified scores >82.5 % are related to global improvements in outcome. Thus, for analysis, we categorized the % recovery as ≥ 82.5 % improved (successful outcome) and < 82.5 % improvement (not successful).

Number of observations per variable

Number of observations per variable was determined by using the recommendations of Homer and Lemeshow [35]. For simple univariate multinomial or logistic regression analyses, a minimum observation-to-variable ratio of 10 is recommended, although a number this low will likely overfit a model [35]. For this study, only eight variables were targeted.

Data analysis

All analyses completed were performed using Statistical Package for the Social Sciences (SPSS), version 21.0 (IBM Corp, Armonk, NY). Intention to treat analysis was used, and for missing data at any follow-up time point, the last observation was carried forward. Descriptive statistics were used to describe the full patient sample. Frequencies of physiotherapists' prediction of prognosis scores were evaluated for each physiotherapist to determine variations among practitioners. Linearity of effect of continuous variables was evaluated by plotting to identify potential curvilinear relationships. If curvilinear relationships were found, categories were created and were entered as ordinal data with a set of indicators (dummies). Individual estimates were then plotted to visualize linearity and checked if there are significant differences in the individual estimates.

To assess multicollinearity in the modeling and relationships among the 8 predictor variables, a correlation matrix was calculated for all independent variables. A correlational finding of $r > 0.7$ between independent variables was used to assess the potential of multicollinearity [36]. Analyses of continuous measures were performed with a Pearson Product Correlation. Analyses of dichotomous or categorical measures were performed with Cramer's V whereas analyses of continuous to dichotomous or categorical variables were performed with a Biserial correlation. Cohen [37] characterized a correlation of 0.10 as depicting a small relationship, a correlation of 0.30 as a moderate relationship, and a correlation of 0.50 as a large/strong relationship. P values of <0.05 were considered significant.

Distinct hierarchical logistic regression analyses were performed for each of the dependent variables: percent improvement on patient-reported rate of recovery, ODI or NDI, and NPRS. Hierarchical models were used instead of stepwise modeling because automated stepwise models may sometimes lead to potential illogical conclusions and because the modeling used in this study was exploratory. For each analysis, individual P values, odds ratios and 95 % confidence intervals, and Nagelkerke values were reported. A Nagelkerke is a pseudo R square measure that investigates the usefulness of the model [38]. The value is similar in concept to the coefficient of determination (R^2) in linear regression. The R^2 statistics do not measure the goodness of fit of the model but indicate how useful the explanatory variables are in predicting the response variable and can be referred to as measures of effect size.

Results

The study enrolled 83 (74.1 %) patients with low back pain and 29 (25.9 %) with neck pain. Of the 112, nearly all were Caucasian (95.5 %), a majority were female ($N = 64$; 57 %), and the mean age was 54.3 years (SD = 13.4 years). Slightly fewer than 50 % (48.6 %) reported a previous history of this same spinal condition. The baseline ODI was 32.8/100 (SD = 17.8) whereas the baseline NDI was 32.7/100 (SD = 16.8). The baseline pain scores were a mean of 5.76 (SD = 2.1) and individuals were seen for a mean of 10.4 total visits (SD = 8.3). The average duration of symptoms reported at baseline was 11.9 weeks (SD = 19.3). Fifty-two (46.8 %) of the individuals qualified as acute spinal pain, 31.5 % were sub-acute and 21.6 % were chronic. Slightly over 41 % (41.4 %) responded yes to one or more of the seven psychosocial questions. A total of 86.6 % of the individuals exhibited a within-session change during the examination. The mean raw physiotherapist prediction of prognosis value was 6.94 (SD = 2.02). For individual physiotherapists, mean raw prediction of prognosis values ranged from a low of 2.3 (SD = 0.57) to a high of 7.7 (SD = 1.15). Using the dichotomised variables discussed earlier (a score of 7–10), physiotherapists projected that 74.8 % of the patients would have a good prognosis.

Average ODI percentage change scores for patients with LBP were 64.6 % (SD = 35.9), average NDI percentage change scores for those with neck pain were 64.1 % (SD = 37.8), and average NPRS percentage change scores were 71.2 % (SD = 28.8) for those with LBP and 63.4 % (SD = 36.6) for those with neck pain. Rate of recovery percentages were 83.5 % (SD = 19.6) for LBP and 79.7 % (SD = 23.9) for neck pain.

When evaluating linearity of effect, only baseline pain demonstrated a non-normally distributed composition. However, when categorized, associations did not improve. Because there is a lack of an appropriate threshold within the literature for the categorization of the baseline measures used in the current study, the continuous variables collected at baseline were entered into the models without transformation.

For the correlation matrix (Table 1), small to moderate significant correlations were present among a number of variables. Physiotherapists' prediction of prognosis was statistically significantly associated with pain at baseline, disability at baseline, age, and the presence of a within session change (all with small to moderate relationships). There were no instances in which multicollinearity was present and variable modification was not required prior to regression modeling.

Table 2 outlines the results for the logistic regression analysis with an outcome variable of rate of recovery. Physiotherapist prediction of a good prognosis and duration of symptoms were both associated with rate of recovery. Patients identified by the physiotherapists as predicted to have a good prognosis were 4.15 (95 % CI = 1.3, 13.19) times more likely to report a rate of recovery of greater than or equal to 82.5 % at discharge than those who were identified to have a poor prognosis. Further, compared to patients with acute pain, those with sub-acute and chronic conditions were less likely to report a rate of recovery score greater than 82.5 %.

The physiotherapists' prediction of prognosis was also the only significant variable associated with a 50 % change in the disability status (ODI or NDI) with use of the logistic regression analysis. Patients identified by the physiotherapists to have a good prognosis were 4.28 (95 % CI = 1.4, 13.37) times more likely to report a 50 % improvement in disability at discharge than those who were identified to have a poor prognosis (Table 3).

There were no variables that were significantly associated with a 50 % reduction of pain (Table 4). Physiotherapist prognostic prediction provided an odds ratio of 3.96 (95 % CI of 0.99, 15.75) but the odds ratio crossed 1.0 and was not statistically significant.

Discussion

Our purpose for the present study was to determine whether the physiotherapists' prediction of prognosis during the initial clinical encounter for the projected outcome of patients they treated was associated with the actual clinical outcome. In addition, we examined the relationship of physiotherapists' prediction of prognosis to other prognostic variables that have been associated with clinical outcomes in previous literature, and modeled the overall relationship of these variables with the physiotherapists' predicted prognosis. The findings suggest that experienced physiotherapists can project a recovery and disability outcome in patients with back and neck pain. This lends support to the value of a clinical judgment during prognostic assessment. In our study, physiotherapists' prediction of prognosis was the only significant predictor variable associated with disability and one of two variables associated with rate of recovery. Although our primary finding is similar to that of others, our results are unique in several notable ways.

We selected a number of prognostic variables that were not included in the previous three studies [7–9], such as within session changes, sameness of previous

Table 1 Correlation Matrix evaluating Association of predictor variables: nominal measures were calculated using Cramer's V, continuous to nominal measures were calculated using a Biserial correlation, whereas continuous measures were analyses using Pearson Product correlations

Variables	Clinician prediction of prognosis	Duration	Previous injury	Pain baseline	Oswestry/Neck disability baseline	Age	Within session change	Psychological factor
Clinician prediction of prognosis								
Duration	0.41 $P = 0.51$							
Previous injury	0.28 $P = 0.36$	0.31 $P = 0.95$						
Pain baseline	0.20 $P = 0.03$	−0.09 $P = 0.30$	−0.20 $P = 0.84$					
Oswestry/Neck disability baseline	0.27 $P < 0.01$	−0.03 $P = 0.75$	−0.46 $P = 0.64$	0.46 $P < 0.01$				
Age	0.19 $P = 0.03$	−0.20 $P = 0.84$	−0.05 $P = 0.61$	−0.04 $P = 0.69$	0.17 $P = 0.08$			
Within session change	0.48 $P < 0.01$	0.47 $P = 0.18$	0.01 $P = 0.94$	0.28 $P < 0.01$	0.29 $P < 0.01$	−0.06 $P = 0.55$		
Psychological factor	0.18 $P = 0.87$	0.41 $P = 0.49$	0.05 $P = 0.59$	0.10 $P = 0.29$	0.09 $P = 0.34$	0.02 $P = 0.85$	0.01 $P = 0.91$	

injury, and a novel psychological instrument. However, none of these variables were significant in any of the models. Past work has suggested that a between session change is a much stronger predictor of outcomes than a within session change and lends support to the concerns that an immediate effect is truly a valuable finding within an examination [24]. Within session findings were related to the physiotherapists' prediction of prognosis and it is likely that these findings are used to guide the physiotherapists' the prognostic assessment but further study is needed. The concept of sameness of a previous episode is different than prior episodes (or number of prior episodes) in that we required patients to report a familiarity with their current bout of spine pain. Our novel psychological measure was an untested instrument and it may have failed to appropriately capture the most important constructs associated with delayed prognosis. It is worth noting that the previously investigated studies did find significance with measures such as the modified somatic pain questionnaire, catastrophizing, and fears avoidance beliefs, all of which were represented by specific questionnaire items within the novel tool.

The current study found that physiotherapists' prognosis was a stronger predictor of clinical outcome (disability and rate of recovery) that the other prognostic variables used in our models. In contrast, Hancock *et al.*, [7] found that a clinical prediction rule of a) baseline pain, b) duration of current episode, and c) number of previous episodes was a stronger predictor than clinician judgment. One reason for the difference may be because we opted not to include number of previous episodes. Further, because this was a secondary analysis, the current study omitted several of the prognostic variables that have been investigated by others [7–9]. These include: work-related

Table 2 Final logistic regression model for factors associated with Rate of Recovery (patient report of ≥82.5 % improvement at discharge; $N = 112$, Nagelkerke = 0.32)

Predictor variable	Odds ratio (95 % confidence interval)	*P* value
Clinical prediction of prognosis	4.15 (1.31, 13.19)	**0.02**
Duration of symptoms		
Subacute	0.24 (0.07, 0.89)	**0.03**
Chronic	0.21 (0.05, 0.90)	**0.04**
Same previous injury	0.68 (0.24, 1.93)	0.47
Pain scale at baseline	0.98 (0.72, 1.31)	0.89
Oswestry/Neck disability index at baseline	1.01 (0.97, 1.04)	0.68
Age (years)	1.02 (0.98, 1.08)	0.29
A within session change during the initial visit	2.03 (0.42. 9.79)	0.38
Presence of at least one psychological factor	1.67 (0.59, 4.73)	0.33

Bold indicates statistical significance

Table 3 Final logistic regression model for factors associated with disability (≥50 % change on the Oswestry Disability Index or Neck Disability Index, $N = 112$, Nagelkerke = 0.18)

Predictor variable	Odds ratio (95 % confidence interval)	*P* value
Clinical prediction of prognosis	4.28 (1.37, 13.37)	**0.01**
Duration of symptoms		
Subacute	0.60 (0.18, 2.67)	0.60
Chronic	0.88 (0.28, 4.38)	0.88
Same previous injury	1.42 (0.51, 4.01)	0.51
Pain scale at baseline	1.20 (0.88, 1.63)	0.25
Oswestry/Neck disability index at baseline	0.98 (0.95, 1.02)	0.36
Age (years)	1.01 (0.97, 1.05)	0.58
A within session change during the initial visit	1.61 (0.39, 6.68)	0.51
Presence of at least one psychological factor	1.08 (0.38, 3.07)	0.88

Bold indicates statistical significance

Table 4 Final logistic regression model for factors associated with pain outcome (≥50 % improvement on the numerical pain rating scale, $N = 112$, Nagelkerke = 0.26)

Predictor variable	Odds ratio (95 % confidence interval)	*P* value
Clinical prediction of prognosis	3.96 (0.99, 15.76)	0.05
Duration of symptoms		
Subacute	0.38 (0.78, 1.81)	0.22
Chronic	0.75 (0.17, 3.40)	0.71
Same previous injury	2.61 (0.76, 9.01)	0.13
Pain scale at baseline	0.74 (0.53, 1.05)	0.09
Oswestry/Neck disability index at baseline	1.03 (0.98, 1.07)	0.22
Age (years)	0.96 (0.92, 1.01)	0.11
A within session change during the initial visit	1.82 (0.35, 9.39)	0.47
Presence of at least one psychological factor	0.70 (0.20, 2.44)	0.58

requirements, depression indices, and pain drawings [8]; spinal mobility measures [8, 9]; influence of catastrophizing, number of previous episodes, coping skills, or pain distal to the knee [7]; and the Örebro Musculoskeletal Pain Questionnaire [9]. Similar to previous studies, we did include duration of symptoms and it was the only variable other than the physiotherapists' prediction of prognosis that was associated with outcome in any of the models; significantly associated only with the rate of recovery. Conversely, neither Dagnifrud *et al.*, [9] nor Abbott and Kingan [8] found significant associates with duration of symptoms and their outcomes.

The effect size of the physiotherapists' prognosis in our study was larger than those previously reported. This may be reflective of 1) the differences in thresholds we used to determine success in our trial, 2) the skill set of our physiotherapists, or 3) the fact that we did not include a number of variables previously included in other studies. For the disability measures (ODI and NDI) we required a 50 % change from baseline measures to qualify as a success; a value that requires a notable overall improvement from baseline. Dagnifrud *et al.*, [9] required only a change of 10 points or greater in ODI and NDI scores (*i.e.*, 20 % improvement) from the raw baseline score. It is difficult to assess the comparability of our findings with Abbott and Kingan [8] and Hancock *et al.*, [7] because their selections for thresholds for disability and pain are notably different than those used in our study. Abbott and Kingan [8] retained the linearity of the Roland Morris Disability Index for their computational modeling. Hancock and associates [7] used number of days until a successful outcome (defined as a 1–10 pain score of 0 or 1 for seven consecutive days). The physiotherapists in our study were highly trained and were very experienced with a mean of 20.3 years of clinical practice and were similar in skills and experience to those of Abbott and Kingan [8] (17 years, all with postgraduate training in manual therapy). Hancock *et al.*, [7] and Dagnifrud *et al.* [9] did not report the skill level of their study clinicians. The additional training and years of experience of the physiotherapists in the current study may have contributed to their ability to make an accurate prognosis. However other factors, such as the variables selected for the models or the information available to the therapists at the time of prognosis may have been the key reasons for a larger effect size for physiotherapist prognosis.

Unlike Dagnifrud *et al.*, [9] but consistent with Abbott and Kingan [8] and Hancock *et al.*, [7] the physiotherapists in our study had complete information when making their prognostic assessment. Physiotherapists were told to take into account all aspects of the patient's presentation, including demographics, patient history, the physical examination and results and their own experiences with similar patient presentations in the past. We were interested in the physiotherapists' decision making ability when all these factors were present because this is similar to what occurs during a traditional patient-clinician encounter. Our findings suggest that outside of duration of symptoms, physiotherapist prognosis was a stronger predictor of outcome than the other variables that were investigated in our study. Further, variables that have demonstrated they are prognostic in previous studies were not significantly associated with our three different outcome constructs. We were somewhat surprised by these findings, especially since past works [14–24] have reported rather robust relationships. Nonetheless, by constructing a prognosis, potentially through use of comprehensive clinical information collected, the physiotherapists were able to determine the probable outcomes.

One other area of difference was that pain and disability scores at baseline were not related to the outcomes in the modeling we performed, which is a finding that is different from Hancock *et al.*, [7] and Dagnifrud *et al.* [9] (in Model B of their modeling scheme). Abbott and Kingan [8] did not formally investigate these measures. This difference may again be related to how we identified success for our outcome measures. By using percentage change from baseline, we marginalized the influence of the baseline raw score (severity), a confounding issue recognized previously [39].

Limitations

There are number of limitations in this study. First, the same physiotherapists who made the prognostic estimates were also the individuals who provided care. There is a risk that physiotherapists could have subconsciously influenced the outcomes (resulting in a poorer or better outcome) based on the initial assessment of each patient. The current study incorporated prognostic findings that were represented in past literature; however, it is possible that other factors not represented in the models influenced outcomes. Another limitation is the experience and skill sets of each physiotherapist. All physiotherapists had similar, structured training and it is possible that the prognosis prediction was actually a by-product of a structured decision making model used by clinicians from a similar background or training. Although the tool we used for measuring prognosis was the same as the tool used by Dagfinrud *et al.* [9] we were slightly less restrictive on what qualified as a good prognosis (7–10 scores were considered to be associated with a good prognosis). Further, the generalisability of the findings from this study is questionable since the majority of physiotherapists have not had the same level of postgraduate training of those in this study.

Conclusions

Physiotherapist prediction of prognosis is based on the theory that the physiotherapist can use previous knowledge obtained from multiple sources and experiences to come to an appropriate decision about the likely outcome of care. This study suggests that experienced physiotherapists' prediction may be useful for determining prognosis.

Competing interests

The authors declare that they have no competing interests.

Authors' contributions

CC generated the study idea. CC and KL received ethics approval. CC and TM generated the initial draft. CC and KL performed the statistical analyses. CS assisted in collection of data. CC and SS heavily edited the initial drafts. All authors read and approved the final manuscript.

Author details

[1]Department of Orthopaedics, Duke University, 2200 Main Street, 27705 Durham, NC, USA. [2]Department of Physical and Occupational Therapy, Duke University Medical Center, Clinic 1E, Trent Drive and Erwin Road, 27710 Durham, NC, USA. [3]Department of Physical Therapy, One University Plaza, 44555 Youngstown, Ohio, USA. [4]Maitland-Australian, Physiotherapy Seminars, PO Box 1244, 11935 Cutchogue, NY, USA. [5]Department of Physiotherapy, University Drive, 2308 Callaghan, NSW, Australia.

References

1. Jones MA, Rivett DA. Clinical Reasoning for Manual Therapists. Edinburgh: Butterworth-Heinemann; 2004.
2. Miller P. Pattern recognition is a clinical reasoning process in musculoskeletal physiotherapy. (MMedSc(Physiotherapy) Masters thesis), University of Newcastle. 2009. Retrieved from http://hdl.handle.net/1959.13/44629.
3. NormanGR EKW. Diagnostic error and clinical reasoning. Med Educ. 2010;44(1):94–100.
4. Norman GR, Young M, Brooks L. Non-analytical models of clinical reasoning: the role of experience. Med Educ. 2007;41(12):1140–5.
5. Haskins R, Osmotherly PG, Southgate E, Rivett DA. Physiotherapists' knowledge, attitudes and practices regarding clinical prediction rules for low back pain. Man Ther. 2014;19(2):142–51.
6. Slade SC, Molloy E, Keating JL. Dilemma of diagnostic uncertainty when treating people with chronic low back pain: a qualitative study. Clin Rehabil. 2012;26(6):558–69.
7. Hancock MJ, Maher CG, Latimer J, Herbert RD, McAuley JH. Can rate of recovery be predicted in patients with acute low back pain? Development of a clinical prediction rule. Eur J Pain. 2009;13(1):51–5.
8. Abbott JH, Kingan EM. Accuracy of physical therapists' prognosis of low back pain from the clinical examination: a prospective cohort study. J Man ManipTher. 2014;22(3):154–61.
9. Dagfinrud H, Storheim K, Magnussen LH, Ødegaard T, Hoftaniska I, Larsen LG, et al. The predictive validity of the Örebro Musculoskeletal Pain Questionnaire and the clinicians' prognostic assessment following manual therapy treatment of patients with LBP and neck pain. Man Ther. 2013;18(2):124–9.
10. Cook C, Learman K, Showalter C, O'Halloran B. The relationship between chief complaint and comparable sign in patients with spinal pain: an exploratory study. Man Ther. 2015;20(3):451–5.
11. Cook C, Learman K, Showalter C, Kabbaz V, O'Halloran B. Early use of thrust manipulation versus non-thrust manipulation: a randomized clinical trial. Man Ther. 2013;18(3):191–8.
12. Cook C, Learman K, Houghton S, Showalter C, O'Halloran B. The addition of cervical unilateral posterior-anterior mobilisation in the treatment of patients with shoulder impingement syndrome: a randomised clinical trial. Man Ther. 2014;19(1):18–24.
13. Bialosky JE, Bishop MD, Price DD, Robinson ME, George SZ. The mechanisms of manual therapy in the treatment of musculoskeletal pain: a comprehensive model. Man Ther. 2009;14(5):531–8.
14. Hoving JL, de Vet HC, Twisk JW, Devillé WL, van der Windt D, Koes BW, et al. Prognostic factors for neck pain in general practice. Pain. 2004;110(3):639–45.
15. Walton DM, Macdermid JC, Giorgianni AA, Mascarenhas JC, West SC, Zammit CA. Risk factors for persistent problems following acute whiplash injury: update of a systematic review and meta-analysis. J Orthop Sports PhysTher. 2013;43(2):31–43.
16. Indahl A. Low back pain: diagnosis, treatment and prognosis. Scand J Rheumatol. 2004;33(4):199–209.
17. Sterling M, Hendrikz J, Kenardy J, Kristjansson E, Dumas JP, Niere K, et al. Assessment and validation of prognostic models for poor functional recovery 12 months after whiplash injury: a multicentre inception cohort study. Pain. 2012;153(8):1727–34.
18. Karjalainen K, Malmivaara A, Mutanen P, Pohjolainen T, Roine R, Hurri H. Outcome determinants of subacute low back pain. Spine (Phila Pa 1976). 2003;28(23):2634–40.
19. Taylor JB, Goode AP, George SZ, Cook CE. Incidence and risk factors for first-time incident low back pain: a systematic review and meta-analysis. Spine J. 2014;14(10):2299–319.
20. Hill J, Dunn K, Lewis M, Mullis R, Main C, Foster NE, et al. A primary care back pain screening tool: identifying patient subgroups for initial treatment. Arthritis Care Research. 2008;59(5):632–64.
21. Hayden JA, Dunn KM, van der Windt DA, Shaw WS. What is the prognosis of back pain? Best Pract Res ClinRheumatol. 2010;24(2):167–79.
22. Tuttle N. Do changes within a manual therapy treatment session predict between-session changes for patients with cervical spine pain? Aust J Physiother. 2005;51(1):43–8.
23. Hahne AJ, Keating JL, Wilson SC. Do within-session changes in pain intensity and range of motion predict between-session changes in patients with low back pain? Aust J Physiother. 2004;50:17e23.
24. Cook CE, Showalter C, Kabbaz V, O'Halloran B. Can a within/between-session change in pain during reassessment predict outcome using a manual therapy intervention in patients with mechanical low back pain? Man Ther. 2012;17(4):325–9.
25. Carroll LJ, Hogg-Johnson S, van der Velde G, Haldeman S, Holm LW, Carragee EJ, et al. Bone and Joint Decade 2000–2010 Task Force on Neck Pain and its Associated Disorders. Course and prognostic factors for neck pain in the general population: results of the Bone and Joint Decade 2000–2010 Task Force on Neck Pain and Its Associated Disorders. Spine (Phila Pa 1976). 2008;33(4 Suppl):S75–82.
26. van der Windt DA, Dunn KM. Low back pain research–future directions. Best Pract Res ClinRheumatol. 2013;27(5):699–708.
27. Fairbank J, Couper J, Davies J, O'Brien JP. The Oswestry low back pain questionnaire. Physiother. 1980;66:271–3.
28. Vernon H, Mior S. The Neck Disability Index: a study of reliability and validity. J Manipulative Physiol Ther. 1991;14(7):409–15.

29. Fritz JM, Hebert J, Koppenhaver S, Parent E. Beyond minimally important change: defining a successful outcome of physical therapy for patients with low back pain. Spine (Phila Pa 1976). 2009;34:2803–9.
30. Cleland JA, Childs JD, Whitman JM. Psychometric properties of the Neck Disability Index and Numeric Pain Rating Scale in patients with mechanical neck pain. Arch Phys Med Rehabil. 2008;89(1):69–74.
31. Childs JD, Piva SR, Fritz JM. Responsiveness of the numeric pain rating scale in patients with low back pain. Spine. 2005;30:1331–4.
32. Parsons B, Sanin L, Yang R, Emir B, Juhn M. Efficacy and safety of pregabalin in patients with spinal cord injury: a pooled analysis. Curr Med Res Opin. 2013;29(12):1675–83.
33. O'Halloran B, Wright A, Cook CE. Criterion validation of the rate of recovery, a single alphanumeric measure, in patients with shoulder pain. Int J Sports PhysTher. 2013;8(6):784–92.
34. Wright AA, Cook CE. Criterion validation of the rate of recovery, single alphanumeric measure, in patients with low back pain. Physiother Res Int. 2013;18(2):124–9.
35. Hosmer DW, Lemeshow S. Applied Logistic Regression. 2nd ed. New York: Wiley; 2000.
36. Shen J, Gao SA. Solution to separation and multicollinearity in multiple logistic regression. J Data Sci. 2008;6(4):515–31.
37. Cohen J. Statistical Power Analysis for the Behavioral Sciences. 2nd ed. New Jersey: Lawrence Erlbaum; 1988.
38. Nagelkerke NJD. A note on a general definition of the coefficient of determination. Biometrika. 1991;78:691–2.
39. Wang YC, Hart DL, Stratford PW, Mioduski JE. Baseline dependency of minimal clinically important improvement. PhysTher. 2011;91(5):675–88.

Proprioceptive Based Training for stroke recovery. Proposal of new treatment modality for rehabilitation of upper limb in neurological diseases

Pawel Kiper[1*], Alfonc Baba[1], Michela Agostini[1] and Andrea Turolla[1,2*]

Abstract

Background: The central nervous system (CNS) has plastic properties allowing its adaptation through development. These properties are still maintained in the adult age and potentially activated in case of brain lesion. In the present study authors hypothesized that a significant recovery of voluntary muscle contraction in post stroke patients experiencing severe upper limb paresis can be obtained, when proprioceptive based stimulations are provided. Proprioceptive based training (PBT) is based on performing concurrent movements with both unaffected and affected arm, with the aim to foster motor recovery through some mutual connections of interhemispheric and transcallosal pathways. The aim of this pre-post pilot study was to evaluate the feasibility of PBT on recovery of voluntary muscle contraction in subacute phase after stroke.

Methods: The treatment lasted 1 h daily, 5 days per week for 3 weeks. The PBT consisted of multidirectional exercises executed synchronously with unaffected limb and verbal feedback. The Medical Research Council scale (MRC), Dynamometer, Fugl-Meyer Upper Extremity scale (F-M UE), Functional Independence Measure scale (FIM) and modified Ashworth scale were administered at the beginning and at the end of training. Statistical significance was set at $p < 0.05$.

Results: Six patients with severe paresis of the upper limb within 6 months after stroke were enrolled in the study (5 ischemic and 1 hemorrhagic stroke, 3 men and 3 women, mean age 65.7 ± 8.7 years, mean distance from stroke 4.1 ± 1.5 months) and all of them well tolerated the training. The clinical changes of voluntary muscle contraction after PBT were statistically significant at the MRC scale overall ($p = 0.028$), and dynamometer assessment overall ($p = 0.028$). Each patient improved muscle contraction of one or more muscles and in 4 out of 6 patients voluntary active movement emerged after therapy. The functional outcomes (i.e. F-M UE and FIM) did not show significant change within group.

Conclusions: The findings of this preliminary research revealed that PBT may be a feasible intervention to improve the motricity of upper limb in stroke survivors.

Keywords: Stroke, Neurorehabilitation, Upper limb, Bilateral arm training, Intracortical inhibition

* Correspondence: pawel.kiper@ospedalesancamillo.net; andrea.turolla@ospedalesancamillo.net
[1]Laboratory of Kinematics and Robotics, IRCCS San Camillo Hospital Foundation, via Alberoni 70, Venice 30126, Italy
[2]Department of Neuroscience, University of Sheffield, Glossop Road, Sheffield S10 2JF, UK

Background

The impairment of motor function represents one of the major causes of disability after stroke. More than 69 % of cerebrovascular lesions provokes impairment of motor function to the upper limb, moreover about 56 % of subjects experience severe hemiparesis even after 5 years from stroke [1, 2]. The functional impairment of the upper limb can impact negatively on quality of life and limit the autonomy in many activities of daily living (ADL). The recovery process occur through neural mechanisms mediating spontaneous cortical reorganization, but evidence indicates that intensive stimulation is essential to improve motor recovery either [3–7]. Several studies, both in animals and humans, have shown different reorganization of the central nervous system (CNS), at molecular as well as synaptic connectivity levels, dependent on the type of behavioral interactions with the external environment [4, 7]. The possibility to estimate as early as possible the outcomes achievable due to rehabilitation is one of the most meaningful clinical point to address, with the aim to promote the best recovery after stroke. This information is important for prognosis and personalization of rehabilitation programs for every individual patient [8, 9]. Several modalities for upper limb motor rehabilitation after stroke were proposed recently, among that the bilateral training has received outstanding attention. The bilateral training is a method based on the execution of repetitive tasks with both (affected and non–affected) upper extremities, with the aim of regaining a better motor function. This approach is based on the rationale that bilateral movements allow to optimize the activation/inhibition balance between the two hemispheres. The bilateral motor training emphasizes the importance of bilateral approach, intended as the involvement of both limbs in daily life practice (e.g. dressing, bathing, feeding, driving, cooking). Several studies on healthy subjects showed that when a motor task is performed the dominant arm has the goal to reach the target, whereas the non-dominant arm play a role in stabilizing adjacent musculoskeletal districts [10]. Evidence from studies with transcranial magnetic stimulation (TMS) in stroke survivors showed that both hemispheres induce a reduction of intracortical inhibition, when bilateral movements were performed. On the contrary, if only one arm was activated the increased inhibition was observed in the ipsilateral hemisphere [10, 11]. However, it is not clear whether the modifications in cortical excitability are attributable to the non-use of the affected limb or to compensatory overuse of the healthy limb [12]. These findings raise the hypothesis that the reduction of excitability of the healthy hemisphere can help to improve motor function of the paretic limb after stroke.

The conventional neuromotor rehabilitation for upper limbs early after stroke in case of complete plegia, consists mainly of passive mobilization or electrical stimulation, since most of the current available therapies require that residual voluntary activation of muscles or partial movements are present [13, 14]. Most of the studies on bilateral arm training focused their attention on the functional improvement of the affected limb and in most of them the motor training is provided by robotic devices, performing passive movement of affected arm and active movement of non-affected limb [15, 16]. The current findings did not report a meaningful advantage on functional outcomes for the affected limb treated with bilateral training [17]. However, clinical studies with functional magnetic resonance imaging (fMRI) seemed to confirm the importance of bilateral exercises to improve motor learning [5]. Therefore, to understand exhaustively which recovery mechanisms occur after stroke it is fundamental that new therapeutic modalities are tested in clinical settings. The proprioceptive based training (PBT) aims to stimulate the emergence of voluntary contraction and is based on motor learning principles, such as the repetition of tasks with concurrent use of feedbacks. The proposed concept is based on the concurrent repetitions of movements performed with the non-affected limb and with the affected one, passively mobilized by physiotherapist in charge of guaranteeing the optimal kinematic execution. Executing the intention to move in the affected limb, supported by physiotherapist, aims to re-educate the proprioceptive sensitivity coherently to each movement phase. Proprioception is the capacity of CNS to determine where all of body parts are positioned at any given time. Proprioceptors located in soft tissues can sense changes and pass afferent information to the brain. Hypothetically PBT can reinforce proprioception through simple movement executed in one plane where any compensatory movements (e.g. shoulder rotation) are abolished. Furthermore, the treatment modality requires recognition of position of both limbs which can act on affected arm proprioception. The common application of bilateral arm training (BAT), is based only on passive movements supported by robotic devices and the potential active movement of affected limb is not permitted. Therefore the difference between PBT and BAT is that the movement in the unaffected limb is performed synchronously with patient's efferent motor command to both limbs, as assisted by physiotherapist on affected side. Thus, the treatment requires generation of voluntary activation from patient, as reference for both limbs, moreover physiotherapist is asked to adapt passive mobilization of affected limb simultaneously with voluntary active movements of unaffected one. The recognition of position of both limbs, therefore, is always requested. The advantage of the proposed approach relies on the possibility to be applied since the early acute phase after stroke, when several therapeutic modalities (e.g. Constraint-Induced Movement Therapy) cannot be provided because of the absence of residual voluntary muscular activation. Moreover, according to Whitall et al. the involvement of unaffected limb in bilateral training represents a fundamental component for training, based on the rationale of the interlimb coupling theory, where stimuli from two limbs concur to create a "neurofunctional" unit [18].

The purpose of this pre-post pilot study was to evaluate the feasibility of PBT for fast recovery of voluntary muscle contraction, after stroke. The end-point of the proposed treatment modality was based on mean force increase of at least 20 % of all the muscles considered for the PBT treatment.

Methods

Recruitment

All the patients were informed about the aim and procedures of the study and written informed consent was obtained from all the participants. The pre-post pilot study group included inpatients affected by a first stroke (i.e. ischemic or hemorrhagic) occurred no longer than 6 months before the enrolment (mean distance from onset 4.1 ± 1.5 months). Presence of severe upper limb paresis (0 to 1 point according to the Medical Research Council scale) of the following muscles: deltoid, biceps brachii, triceps brachii, flexor carpi radialis, flexor carpi ulnaris, extensor carpi radialis, extensor carpi ulnaris, flexor digitorum and extensor digitorum; passive range of motion (ROM) completely free; absence of primary joint trauma of the wrist, elbow and shoulder, were considered as inclusion criteria. All patients who refused to participate were excluded from the study together with ones presenting: increased muscle tone defined as a score higher than 1 point (modified Ashworth scale) in at least one of the treated muscles described above for MRC assessment, apraxia (De Renzi test < 62 points) [19], global sensory aphasia (clinical notes), neglect (clinical notes), cognitive impairments (Mini Mental State Examination MMSE < 24 points) [20], sensitivity disorders (defined as < 2 points in items shoulder, elbow, wrist and thumb at the proprioceptive sensitivity section of the Fugl-Meyer scale), stroke lesion located in the cerebellum (clinical notes). The institutional review board of the IRCCS San Camillo Hospital Foundation (Italy) approved the study protocol (Prot. 2012.07 BAT v.1.2) and the study have been conducted in accordance with the Declaration of Helsinki.

Interventions

During the treatment patient was lying supine with the upper limbs positioned in symmetric posture. The subject was asked to move both limbs with the same frequency performing bilateral flexion-extension of one of the upper limb districts according to the available free ROM of the target joint. The movement execution of the affected arm was supported by the physiotherapist performing the passive movement at the same rhythm, as the one executed with the unaffected side. During the therapeutic session patient was asked to focus his/her attention on the movement performed against gravity, which was reinforced by a verbal command. Afterwards, the physiotherapist fully supported movement execution coherently with the patient's movement initialization. The active movements performed voluntarily by the patient with unaffected limb were considered as the reference movement, that the physiotherapist has to emulate passively, by synchronization of passive movement executed in phase with the affected side. The treatment lasted one hour and was divided as follows: 2 proprioceptive based stimulation sessions per 3 min for each movement, with a rest of 2 min between every session. Every patient received 15 treatments, 5 days a week, for 3 weeks. The PBT was introduced as additional hour to conventional neuromotor treatment (CNT). Each patient received CNT, based on tailored individual exercises (passive, active-assisted or active), in accordance with the patient's functional status and with the aim to: reduce degree of disability, improve quality of life. The patients performed exercises for postural control in sitting and standing position, exercises for coordination with and without physiotherapist assistance and gait training, whether appropriate.

However, the upper limb motion were trained providing only PBT and passive mobilization, to maintain mechanical properties of soft tissues.

Clinical outcome measures

The assessment was conducted by two physiotherapists not involved in providing the experimental treatment. The following domains were assessed at the beginning and at the end of treatment: muscles strength, motor impairment and functional activities. The primary outcomes were: the Medical Research Council (MRC) scale [21] and force measured by dynamometer. The following muscles were considered: deltoid, biceps brachii, triceps brachii, flexor carpi radialis, flexor carpi ulnaris, extensor carpi radialis, extensor carpi ulnaris, flexor digitorum and extensor digitorum. The secondary outcomes were: the Fugl-Meyer upper extremity (F-M UE) scale [22] for upper limb motor function, the Functional Independence Measure (FIM) scale for global independence [23], the modified Ashworth scale for spasticity [24]. Positions for dynamometer test were standardized as requested for MRC scale assessment. Data were recorded on study case report sheet form, which contained the patient's study number, date of enrolment, pre and post assessment results, adverse events, and clinical data. Completed form was registered on study management database.

Statistical analysis

The descriptive results were reported as mean and standard deviation. Moreover, distribution skewness was assessed by Shapiro-Wilk test and due to the small sample size non-parametric test for paired measures (Wilcoxon) was used to determine the differences before and after treatment. Statistical significance level was set at $p < 0.05$ and IBM SPSS 20.0 package software was used for the analysis.

Results

A group of 28 eligible patients was screened between July 2013 and October 2014. Among them 21 did not meet the inclusion criteria and 1 did not complete the full training session. According to the inclusion/exclusion criteria 6 patients were enrolled for PBT (3 men and 3 women), to evaluate the feasibility of treatment. The group consisted of 5 ischemic and 1 hemorrhagic stroke, the mean age was 65.7 ± 8.7 years, and the mean distance from stroke was 4.1 ± 1.5 months. All patients reported to be comfortable throughout the training. Table 1 represents motor and functional mean score of the affected arm of the 6 patients before and at the end of PBT treatment. The voluntary muscle contraction of the biceps brachii, flexor carpi radialis and flexor digitorum (MRC scale) significantly improved after PBT. Furthermore, as measured by dynamometer the muscle strength of biceps brachii significantly increased after PBT. The results of the study showed that each patient improved muscle contraction in one or more muscles and in 4 out of 6 patients the full range of voluntary active movement emerged after therapy, mainly in elbow flexion and extension (Table 2). Moreover, in 4 out of 6 patients the active movement relieved by physiotherapist appeared for following movements: shoulder flexion, elbow flexion, wrist flexion and extension. The F-M UE scale, the FIM scale and the modified Ashworth scale did not change significantly after treatment.

Discussion

To our knowledge, this study is the first one assessing the effect of specific proprioceptive stimulation provided for one hour of training, in stroke patients. Both, results achieved and patients' positive feedback after experimental treatment suggest the feasibility of proposed intervention modality. Moreover, patients in this study showed improvement of muscle force after intervention. The significant changes observed mainly in the biggest muscles (e.g. elbow flexion/extension, actuated by biceps and triceps brachii, respectively) could be due to the easiness of stimulating large muscles acting in one main axis than small muscles involved in many complex movements. Our findings showed that PBT may induce a recovery of voluntary muscle contraction in the subacute phase after stroke. Moreover, several muscles (i.e. deltoid, triceps brachii, flexor carpi radialis and ulnaris) showed clinical improvement. The lack of reaching statistical significance could be due to the small sample of patients, as well as to the many outcomes collected. The functional scales (i.e. F-M UE and FIM) did not show differences within group, however, the functional outcomes of common used bilateral training were tested before and previous evidence showed mixed results for them [17]. This finding sustains our hypothesis that PBT could play a role in the first phase after stroke, by promoting a better background for following rehabilitation therapies. These preliminary results are important for sustaining the possibility to treat patients beneficially soon after stroke, in fact muscle contraction is the basic prerequisite for expressing an effective motor behavior. Our preliminary findings indicate that motor training, whether enriched by proprioceptive exercises involving unaffected arm, should be introduced in the subacute phase of rehabilitation after stroke, as a clinical tool to elicit physiological muscular contraction. Furthermore, the absence of changes at the modified Ashworth scale suggests that the training did not increase pathological muscle tone. As mentioned previously, the largest repertoire of known rehabilitation therapies require the presence of minimum voluntary motor activation which is a limitation for their application in the acute or subacute phase after stroke. The possibility to approach patients experiencing an almost complete paralysis of the limb, with PBT may provide a motor background useful for future functional and complex rehabilitation modalities. Results of this study allow to hypothesize that simultaneous stimulation of both afferent and efferent pathways enriched by verbal feedback may play a role in the creation of new connections in the affected brain structures [5]. Indeed, during the treatment patient create efferent command action, conversely afferent information is provided through the execution of assisted movement, in the affected limb. On this basis, concomitant movements may act on both signals concurrently and might act directly on some of the mechanisms exploiting the transcallosal pathways.

Table 1 Effect of proprioceptive based training on overall outcomes

Clinical outcomes	Pre-test	Post-test	*p*-value
MRC	0.16 ± 0.15	0.98 ± 0.36	.028*
Dynamometer	1.36 ± 1.81	6.72 ± 3.48	.028*
F-M UE	4.50 ± 1.22	5.16 ± 1.32	.285
FIM	68.33 ± 32.26	75.16 ± 27.05	.066
MAS	3.00 ± 4.28	3.16 ± 4.26	.564

Data are displayed as mean and standard deviation
MRC Medical Research Council, *F-M UE* Fugl-Meyer Upper Extremity, *FIM* Functional Independence Measure, *MAS* Modified Ashworth Scale
*$p < 0.05$; Wilcoxon test

Table 2 Effect of proprioceptive based training on single muscles

Clinical outcomes	Patient 1		Patient 2		Patient 3		Patient 4		Patient 5		Patient 6		Overall		p
	Before	After	Before	After	Before	After	Before	After	Before	After	Before	After	Before	After	
MRC															
Deltoid	0	2	1	2	0	0	1	1	0	2	0	1	0.33 ± 0.51	1.33 ± 0.81	.063
Biceps brachii	0	3	1	2	0	1	1	2	0	3	1	3	0.50 ± 0.54	2.33 ± 0.81	.026*
Triceps brachii	0	3	1	3	0	0	0	0	0	3	0	1	0.16 ± 0.40	1.16 ± 1.50	.066
Flexor carpi radialis	0	2	0	1	0	1	1	1	0	1	0	1	0.16 ± 0.40	1.16 ± 0.40	.034*
Flexor carpi ulnaris	0	2	0	1	0	0	0	0	0	0	0	1	0.00 ± 0.00	0.66 ± 0.81	.102
Extensor carpii radialis	0	0	0	0	0	0	0	1	0	0	0	1	0.00 ± 0.00	0.33 ± 0.51	.157
Extensor carpi ulnaris	0	0	0	0	0	0	0	0	0	0	0	1	0.00 ± 0.00	0.16 ± 0.40	.317
Flexor digitorum	0	1	0	1	1	1	0	1	0	0	0	1	0.16 ± 0.40	0.83 ± 0.40	.046*
Extensor digitorum	0	0	0	0	1	1	0	0	0	0	0	1	0.16 ± 0.40	0.33 ± 0.51	.317
Dynamometer															
Deltoid	0	15	7	17	0	0	0	0	0	12	0	8	1.16 ± 2.85	8.60 ± 7.37	.068
Biceps brachii	0	31	7	19	0	7	13	21	0	27	8	16	6.26 ± 7.48	20.21 ± 8.49	.028*
Triceps brachii	0	26	12	31	0	0	0	0	0	39	0	7	3.33 ± 8.16	17.26 ± 17.0	.068
Flexor carpi radialis	0	14	0	0	0	6	0	0	0	12	0	9	0.00 ± 0.00	6.88 ± 5.97	.068
Flexor carpi ulnaris	0	14	0	0	0	0	0	0	0	0	0	6	0.00 ± 0.00	3.26 ± 5.71	.180
Extensor carpi radialis	0	0	0	0	0	0	0	0	0	0	0	4	0.00 ± 0.00	0.66 ± 1.63	.317
Extensor carpi ulnaris	0	0	0	0	0	0	0	0	0	0	0	4	0.00 ± 0.00	0.66 ± 1.63	.317
Flexor digitorum	0	5	0	0	5	5	0	0	0	0	0	4	0.83 ± 2.04	2.26 ± 2.53	.180
Extensor digitorum	0	0	0	0	4	4	0	0	0	0	0	0	0.66 ± 1.63	0.66 ± 1.63	1.000

Data are reported as mean and standard deviation (m ± SD)
MRC Medical Research Council, *$p < 0.05$; Wilcoxon test

Several studies suggest that inter-hemispheric connection between M1s plays a main role for the control of hand movements [25, 26]. Studies on stroke patients reported that the excitability of M1 in unaffected hemisphere is augmented after stroke, because of a lack of inhibition from the stroke affected hemisphere [25, 27, 28]. The bilateral movement studied with fMRI showed increased activation in both side of the cerebellum and some plastic changes in both hemispheres. Conversely, decreased activation has been noted in cerebellum when unilateral movement was provided. Moreover, the fMRI studies showed that the cerebellum could be a critical site involved in bilateral movement [5].

In multicenter study from Platz et al., authors compared unilateral approach for impairment-oriented training, with conventional therapy. Authors showed that the patients can benefit from highly structured therapeutic intervention and they concluded that specificity of training can be more important for arm motor recovery, than intensity [29].

The results of our study showed that the PBT could be a favorable approach for motor recovery, after stroke. Future studies are needed with the aim to optimize the technical aspects of the intervention, moreover the implications in a larger cohort of patients enrolling various clinical pictures has to be explored.

Limitations of the study and further research perspectives

Some limitations as to be acknowledged, the changes observed within outcomes perhaps were due to the combination of CNT and PBT, because both were introduced in this study. The time since stroke could be an issue inasmuch the spontaneous recovery is the main driving factor in subacute phase, after stroke. The voluntary muscle contraction observed after training was statistically significant, however, the results were not clinically meaningful for functional outcomes as resulted with absence of statistical significance. Therefore, both small sample size and absence of a control group are further limitations of this study. The authors' future work will be focused to increment the sample and to compare results with a control group, with the aim to test the potential effectiveness of PBT.

Conclusions

With respect to previous proposals of bilateral arm training, this study extended its application to subacute phase after stroke, including a highly structured program enriched by proprioceptive exercises. Furthermore, the modality proposed aims to underline the importance of muscles contraction for upper limb recovery. Therefore, it is important to provide to clinicians an useful tool, which could be easily introduced into rehabilitation programme. Despite the small group, results has shown an effect of the PBT in improving muscle contraction and some aspects of motor control on the biggest muscles of the upper limb. These preliminary results on PBT feasibility need to be addressed in future larger controlled studies, to consider its implementation in real clinical settings.

Competing interests

The authors declare that they have no competing interests.

Authors' contributions

PK conceived the project and is leading the trial. PK, AT wrote the manuscript, designed the study and provided training to the enrolled participants. AB, MA were assessors on the project. All authors read and approved the final manuscript.

References

1. Roth EJ, Heinemann AW, Lovell LL, Harvey RL, McGuire JR, Diaz S. Impairment and disability: their relation during stroke rehabilitation. Arch Phys Med Rehabil. 1998;79:329–35.
2. Urton ML, Kohia M, Davis J, Neill MR. Systematic literature review of treatment interventions for upper extremity hemiparesis following stroke. Occup Ther Int. 2007;14:11–27.
3. Bolognini N, Pascual-Leone A, Fregni F. Using non-invasive brain stimulation to augment motor training-induced plasticity. J Neuroeng Rehabil. 2009;6:8.
4. Ward NS, Cohen LG. Mechanisms underlying recovery of motor function after stroke. Arch Neurol. 2004;61:1844–8.
5. Wu CY, Hsieh YW, Lin KC, Chuang LL, Chang YF, Liu HL, et al. Brain reorganization after bilateral arm training and distributed constraint-induced therapy in stroke patients: a preliminary functional magnetic resonance imaging study. Chang Gung Med J. 2010;33:628–38.
6. Buschfort R, Brocke J, Hess A, Werner C, Waldner A, Hesse S. Arm studio to intensify the upper limb rehabilitation after stroke: concept, acceptance, utilization and preliminary clinical results. J Rehabil Med. 2010;42:310–4.
7. Nudo RJ. Plasticity. NeuroRx. 2006;3:420–7.
8. Dimyan MA, Cohen LG. Neuroplasticity in the context of motor rehabilitation after stroke. Nat Rev Neurol. 2011;7:76–85.
9. Rossini PM, Calautti C, Pauri F, Baron JC. Post-stroke plastic reorganisation in the adult brain. Lancet Neurol. 2003;2:493–502.
10. McCombe Waller S, Whitall J. Bilateral arm training: why and who benefits? NeuroRehabilitation. 2008;23:29–41.
11. McCombe Waller SJW. Fine Motor Control in Adults With and Without Chronic Hemiparesis: Baseline Comparison to Nondisabled Adults and Effects of Bilateral Arm Training. Arch Phys Med Rehabil. 2004;85:1076–83.
12. Hummel FC, Cohen LG. Non-invasive brain stimulation: a new strategy to improve neurorehabilitation after stroke? Lancet Neurol. 2006;5:708–12.
13. NICE. Stroke rehabilitation. Long-term rehabilitation after stroke. Manchester: National Institute for Health and Care Excellence; 2013.
14. Kiper P, Turolla A, Piron L, Agostini M, Baba A, Rossi S, et al. Virtual Reality for Stroke Rehabilitation: assessment, training and the effect of virtual therapy. Med Rehabili. 2010;14:15–23.
15. van Delden AL, Peper CL, Nienhuys KN, Zijp NI, Beek PJ, Kwakkel G. Unilateral versus bilateral upper limb training after stroke: the Upper Limb Training After Stroke clinical trial. Stroke. 2013;44:2613–6.
16. Wu CY, Yang CL, Chen MD, Lin KC, Wu LL. Unilateral versus bilateral robot-assisted rehabilitation on arm-trunk control and functions post stroke: a randomized controlled trial. J Neuroeng Rehabil. 2013;10.
17. Coupar F, Pollock A, van Wijck F, Morris J, Langhorne P. Simultaneous bilateral training for improving arm function after stroke. Cochrane Database Syst Rev. 2010;14(4):CD006432.
18. Whitall J, Waller SM, Sorkin JD, Forrester LW, Macko RF, Hanley DF, et al. Bilateral and unilateral arm training improve motor function through differing neuroplastic mechanisms: a single-blinded randomized controlled trial. Neurorehabil Neural Repair. 2011;25:118–29.
19. De Renzi E, Motti F, Nichelli P. Imitating gestures. A quantitative approach to ideomotor apraxia. Arch Neurol. 1980;37:6–10.
20. Folstein MF, Folstein SE, McHugh PR. "Mini-mental state". A practical method for grading the cognitive state of patients for the clinician. J Psychiatr Res. 1975;12:189–98.
21. Council MR. Aids to Examination of the Peripheral Nervous System. London, England: HMSO; 1976.
22. Fugl-Meyer AR, Jaasko L, Leyman I, Olsson S, Steglind S. The post-stroke hemiplegic patient. 1. a method for evaluation of physical performance. Scand J Rehabil Med. 1975;7:13–31.
23. Keith RA, Granger CV, Hamilton BB, Sherwin FS. The functional independence measure: a new tool for rehabilitation. Adv Clin Rehabil. 1987;1:6–18.
24. Bohannon RW, Smith MB. Interrater reliability of a modified Ashworth scale of muscle spasticity. Phys Ther. 1987;67:206–7.
25. Avanzino L, Bassolino M, Pozzo T, Bove M. Use-dependent hemispheric balance. J Neurosci. 2011;31:3423–8.
26. Stevens JA, Stoykov ME. Using motor imagery in the rehabilitation of hemiparesis. Arch Phys Med Rehabil. 2003;84:1090–2.
27. Murase N, Duque J, Mazzocchio R, Cohen LG. Influence of interhemispheric interactions on motor function in chronic stroke. Ann Neurol. 2004;55:400–9.
28. Luft AR, McCombe-Waller S, Whitall J, Forrester LW, Macko R, Sorkin JD, et al. Repetitive bilateral arm training and motor cortex activation in chronic stroke: a randomized controlled trial. JAMA. 2004;292:1853–61.
29. Platz T, van Kaick S, Mehrholz J, Leidner O, Eickhof C, Pohl M. Best conventional therapy versus modular impairment-oriented training for arm paresis after stroke: a single-blind, multicenter randomized controlled trial. Neurorehabil Neural Repair. 2009;23:706–16.

22

What is the clinical course of transient synovitis in children: a systematic review of the literature

Sylvana S Asche[1], Rogier M van Rijn[1,3], Johannes HJM Bessems[2], Marjolein Krul[1] and Sita MA Bierma-Zeinstra[1*]

Abstract

Background: Transient synovitis of the hip (TS) is considered to be a self-limiting disease in childhood. However, because the etiology is unclear and some cases precede Legg-Perthes' disease, data on follow-up are important. Our aim was to summarize the knowledge on the clinical course of TS in children.

Methods: The study design was a systematic review and a literature search was conducted in Medline and Embase. Studies describing short and/or long-term follow-up of TS in children were included. Case reports, reviews and studies describing traumatic hip pain were excluded. Study quality was scored and data extraction was performed. The main outcome measures were short-term and long-term clinical course, and recurrence of symptoms.

Results: A total of 25 studies were included of which 14 were of high quality. At two-week follow-up, almost all children with TS were symptom free. Those with symptoms persisting for over one month were more prone to develop other hip pathology, such as Legg-Perthes' disease. The recurrence rate of TS ranged from 0–26.3%. At long-term follow-up, 0-10% of the children diagnosed with TS developed Legg-Perthes' disease. Hip pain after intensive physical effort and limited range of motion of the hip at long-term follow-up was reported in 12-28% and in 0-18% of the children, respectively.

Conclusions: The majority of the studies indicate that children with TS recover within two weeks; recurrence was seen in 0-26% of the cases. Children with TS should be followed at least six months to increase the likelihood of not missing Legg-Perthes' disease.

Keywords: Child, Hip, Transient synovitis, Coxitis fugax, Legg-Perthes' disease, Course, Prognosis, Follow-up

Background

Transient synovitis of the hip (TS) in children is a relatively common disorder with an average annual incidence of 0.2% in the general population [1]. There is a male-to-female ratio of slightly more than 2:1. The disease typically presents at a mean age of 6 (3–8) year [1].

TS is characterized by pain and limited motion of the hip [1]. This hip pain and limited range of movement is caused by reactive effusion, leading to a position of the hip in flexion and external rotation [2]. TS is confirmed by excluding potentially more severe causes for hip symptoms, such as septic arthritis, osteomyelitis, Legg-Perthes' disease, juvenile idiopathic arthritis, fractures and tumors [1]. These conditions can be verified by imaging and laboratory investigations [3]. However, the mainstay of diagnosis for TS remains that of clinical findings [3]. For detection of hip effusion, ultrasound is considered to be the best non-invasive technique [2]. The etiology of TS remains largely unknown. Infections of the upper respiratory tract may be a predisposing factor, although identifiable causes or agents have not yet been found [4]. Treatment generally consists of rest and anti-inflammatory agents [5].

In many countries, the majority of children with non-traumatic hip symptoms will initially present to the general practitioner (GP). Krul *et al.* [6] reported an incidence rate for TS in general practice of 76.2 per 100,000 person-years [6]. According to Vijlbrief *et al.* [7], GPs prefer to adopt a wait-and-see approach to TS rather than referring patients for additional diagnostics [7]. However, TS has been associated with the risk of developing other diseases, such as Legg-Perthes' disease [1].

Increased understanding of the short and long-term course of this disease will help medical doctors to better

* Correspondence: s.bierma-zeinstra@erasmusmc.nl
[1]Department of General Practice, Erasmus MC-University Medical Centre Rotterdam, PO Box 2040, 3000 CA, Rotterdam, The Netherlands
Full list of author information is available at the end of the article

determine follow-up policy and better inform patients about the prognosis. Early recognition of subsequent disorders may also lead to timely referral and more optimal treatment. Therefore, this study presents a systematic review of the literature on TS, focusing on its short-term symptomatic course, long-term clinical course, and recurrences.

Methods

Searches

A literature search using Medline and Embase was performed from Januari 1966 (Medline) and Januari 1947 (Embase) till September 2013. Medical subject headings (mesh) terms and corresponding entry terms for the diagnosis, age group and outcome were used (Additional file 1: Table S1).

Study inclusion and exclusion criteria

Studies describing recurrence or clinical follow-up (either on the short or long-term) of TS in children were included. Studies describing children with traumatic hip problems were excluded, as were reviews and case reports. Randomized controlled trials, and cohort and case–control studies were included. Relevant articles in English, German, French, Swedish, Norwegian, Danish and Dutch were included. The abstract of the article had to be available in order to select relevant studies. First, two reviewers (SA, RvR) selected relevant articles by title and abstract. All articles selected by either reviewer were ordered in full text. One reviewer (SA) made the final selection by reading the full text of the selected articles. In case of doubt, a second reviewer (SB) read the full text to ensure that no studies were excluded unjustly.

Study quality assessment

Three reviewers assessed the quality of the selected articles independently. One reviewer (SA) assessed the quality of all studies and two reviewers (SB, JB) each assessed the quality of half of the studies. Seven criteria were used, which were rated as positive, negative or inconclusive. These criteria were based on the quality assessment used by van Rijn *et al.* [8] and adjusted for the purpose of investigating TS. Disagreements were resolved by consensus. The initial agreement was measured by using the Kappa value (k). Agreement is considered poor if $k \leq 0.20$; fair if $0.21 \leq k \leq 0.40$; moderate if $0.41 \leq k \leq 0.60$; substantial if $0.61 \leq k \leq 0.80$; good if $k > 0.80$ [9]. Summing the positive criteria, a quality score was calculated ranging from 0 to 7 points. Studies with five or more positive criteria were considered to be of 'high quality'.

Data extraction strategy

One reviewer (SA) performed data extraction for all the studies, which was subsequently checked by two other reviewers (RvR and MK) each checking half of the studies. Data extraction included number of patients with TS; characteristics of patients with TS (age, male/female ratio, primary or secondary care, duration of symptoms prior to admission); study design; tests done before diagnosing TS; treatment for TS; length of follow-up period; and outcomes (short-term symptomatic course, recurrence, long-term course). Disagreements were resolved by consensus.

Data synthesis and presentation

Included articles were classified in three groups based on their outcome: short-term symptomatic course, recurrence and/or long-term course. Short-term symptomatic course implied clinical follow-up < 3 months. Studies classified as *recurrence* reported a recurrence rate and/or clinical course of patients with recurrent TS. Long-term course was defined as clinical course of TS > 3 months; this also included the development of other diseases subsequent to TS.

Results

Review statistics

After removal of duplicates, our search strategy resulted in 153 potentially relevant studies. Of these, 25 met the inclusion criteria (Figure 1). Study selection by title and abstract reached an initial agreement of 90.4%; after further consultation 100% agreement was achieved. Details of the study characteristics are listed in Table 1. We found no randomised clinical trials or case–control studies. Fifteen cohort studies [3,4,10-22] were prospective and 10 [1,2,23-30] were retrospective. All studies were written in English except for three, of which two were written in German [11,21] and one in French [26]. The number of patients with TS ranged from 13 [17] to 475 [24]. Patients with TS were followed either after admission to hospital or as outpatients.

All studies included patients treated for TS, of which three studies [17,29,30] had a specific target group. One study [30] focused on patients with recurrences of TS, defined as at least two separate episodes of TS at least two months apart. One study [17] included patients with recurrent or prolonged TS, defined as recurrence of symptoms within one month after initial resolution, or symptoms that lasted more than one month. Another study [29] compared patients with no recurrence of TS with patients who had one or more recurrence(s).

Study quality assessment

Table 2 presents the methodological quality assessment of the included studies. Of the 25 studies, 15 were considered to be of high quality (i.e. 5 or more criteria were rated positive). The initial agreement of the total quality assessment was 84% (147 of 175 items). The kappa score calculated on the total quality assessment was 0.65, which is considered to be a substantial agreement. Critical items were 'same duration of follow-up' and 'follow-up data

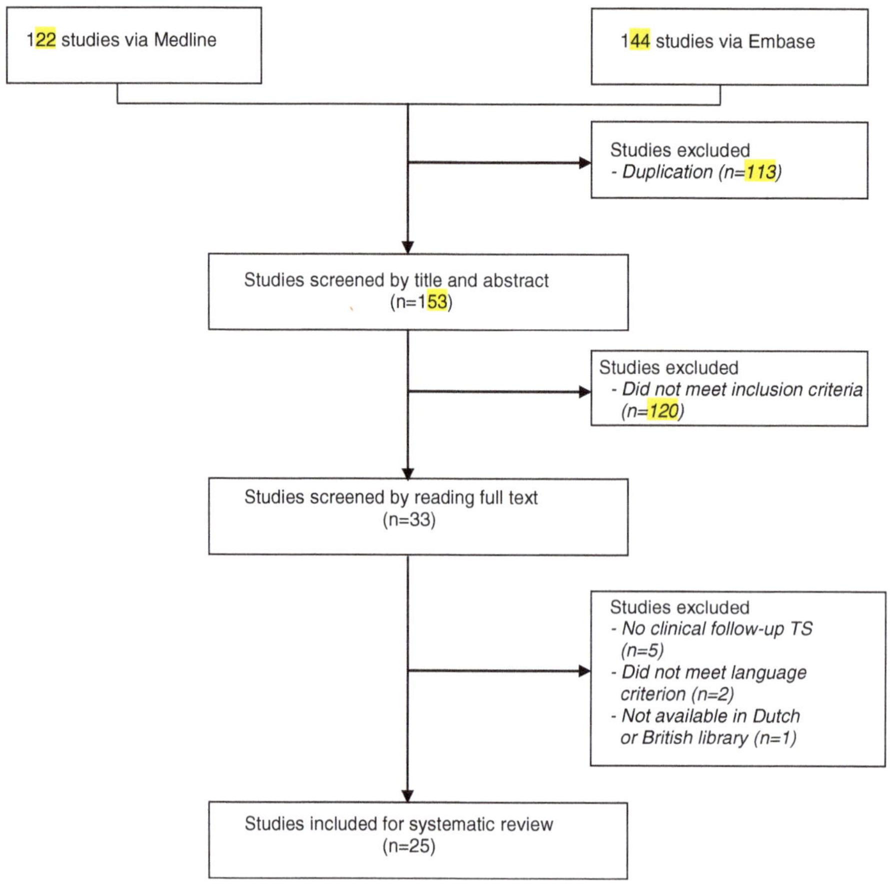

Figure 1 **Flow chart of the selection process.**

available from at least 80% of the study population' which were present in 48% and 52% of the studies, respectively. All initial disagreements were resolved by discussion.

Synthesis

Short-term symptomatic course

Eleven studies [3,11,12,18,21-24,27-29] described the short-term course of TS, of which five are of high quality and six of low quality. The outcomes are shown in Additional file 2: Table S2.

An overview of six studies [3,18,21,22,24,28], which exclusively reported the percentage of patients with symptoms on short-term follow-up, is shown in Figure 2. Of these, three are of high quality and three of low quality.

In the high quality studies, the length of symptoms (hip pain, limp, limited range of motion and/or refusal to bear weight), ranged from 2.5 days to 3 months [3,12,18,22]. In three of these studies [12,18,22], between 3-8% of patients had symptoms persisting for over one month.

In one high quality study [12], all nine patients with persisting symptoms for over one month developed Legg-Perthes' disease.

In the low quality studies, the length of symptoms ranged from 1 week to 3 months [21,24,28]. Between 4-12% of patients had persisting symptoms for over one month [21,24,28].

Recurrence

Thirteen studies [1,2,16,20,22-30] described recurrences of patients with TS (Additional file 2: Table S2). Of these, four are of high quality and nine of low quality.

All four high quality studies [16,20,22,23] calculated a recurrence rate, ranging from 0%[20] to 18.3%[16] in a follow-up period ranging from 3 months to 15 years (Figure 3).

According to one high quality study by Terjesen *et al.* [22], 75% of the recurrences occur in the first six months after the initial episode of TS. Also, in 25% of the cases in this study the opposite hip was involved at recurrence.

The recurrence rate was calculated in six low quality studies [2,24,26-29], varying from 4.1% [24] to 26.3% [26] in a follow-up period ranging from 6 months to 20 years.

According to five low quality studies [2,25,26,29,30], recurrences usually appear within the first two years after the initial episode of TS. Five low quality studies

Table 1 Study characteristics

Source	No. TS[a]	Prospective/ Retrospective	Patient characteristics	Tests before diagnosing TS[b]	Age mean ± SD (range)	M/F ratio	Treatment	Follow-up period mean (range)
Uziel 2006 [30]	39	Retrospective	Patients with at least 2 separate episodes of transient synovitis, at least 2 months apart, seen by pediatric rheumatologists.	- Lab: ESR, WCC, ANA, RF, FMF, HLA-E27 - Plain radiographs of the hip, ultrasound, MRI, technetium bone scans	6 ± 2.6 years	2:1	13 pt: NSAIDs, 5 pt: skin traction.	4.2 ± 2.5 years
Skinner 2002 [3]	25	Prospective	Patients with TS with proven hip joint effusions detected on ultrasound, managed in the accident and emergency department as outpatients. The median duration prior to presentation was 2 days.	- History, full clinical examination, temperature - Lab: FBC, ESR - Ultrasound, radiography of the hip	6 (4–11) years	4:1	Rest at home, paracetamol.	1–2 weeks
Kermond 2002 [18]	36	Prospective	Patients with clinical diagnosis of TS with a median duration of symptoms prior to presentation of 1 day.	- Clinical examination of the hip - Lab full blood examination, ESR, CRP - Radiography of the hip in AP + frog leg lateral views	1–11 years	4.1:1	17 pt. ibuprofen/ paracetamol19 pt. placebo/paracetamol.	Time till symptom free
Fischer 1999 [4]	65	Prospective	Patients with a history of atraumatic limp who presented to a paediatric accident and emergency department either by self referral or from their general practitioner, with a median duration of symptoms of 1 day at presentation.	- History, full clinical examination, temperature - Lab: FBC, ESR - Ultrasound, plain radiographs of the hip	4.35 years[c]	1.7:1[c]	Unclear	18–21 months
Mattick 1999 [27]	103	Retrospective	Patient with hip pain or suspected hip pathology presenting to a Children's Hospital.	- Range of movement of the hip, temperature - Lab: ESR, WBC - Radiography of the hip	0.9-15 years (median age of 5 years)	3:1	Rest at home.	7 years
Eggl 1999 [12]	106 hips	Prospective	Patients with hip pain and a preliminary diagnosis of TS referred to an outpatient clinic.	- History, clinical examination - Lab: CRP, ESR, blood count, ASLO, electrophoresis - Ultrasound	5.7 (1.8–10.1) years	2.8:1	Bed rest, positioning hip in flexion and oral application of naproxen.	42 days
De Pellegrin 1997 [11]	100	Prospective	Patient with hip pain presenting to the orthopedic department with duration of symptoms prior to admission of 1 to 60 days.	- History - Lab: full blood examination - Ultrasound, scintigraphy, radiography of the hip, MRI	4.14 ± 2.2 (1–10) years	1.8:1	Positioning hip in flexion/ abduction and external rotation and analgesics.	Unclear

Table 1 Study characteristics *(Continued)*

Kesteris 1996 [19]	21	Prospective	Patients with TS admitted to the Department of Orthopedics, treated in two consecutive groups. The mean duration of symptoms before admission was 2.6 days.	Unclear	7.1 (4–12) years	9.5:1	12 pt: arthrocentesis, 9 pt: no arthrocentesis All children were kept in bed in the supine position with the hips in a few degrees of flexion.	6–12 months
Keenan 1996 [17]	13	Prospective	Children with a recurrent or prolonged irritable hip syndrome, defined as those with symptoms >1 month or in whom symptoms recurred within 1 month after initial resolution.	- Clinical examination of the hip - Radiography of the hip in Lauenstein + frog lateral views, ultrasound	(4–8 years)	Not given	Restriction sporting activities, bed rest with positioning hip in flexion/ abduction and external rotation.	3 months
Taylor 1995 [29]	426	Retrospective	Patients with an irritable hip admitted to hospital with a mean duration of symptoms before admission ranging from 3.7 to 4.9 days.	- History, temperature, range of movement - Lab: FBC, ESR - Radiography of the hip in AP + frog lateral views, bone isotope scans, MRI	A: 5.7 years B: 6.6 years C: 6.4 years[d]	A: 2.3:1 B: 2.4:1 C: 2:1	Unclear	Unclear
Gopakumar 1992 [2]	181	Retrospective	Patients with suspected irritable hip syndrome admitted to hospital with a mean duration of symptoms prior to presentation of 3 days.	- Clinical examination of the hip - Lab: WBC, ESR - Radiography of the hip in AP, ultrasound, bone isotope scan	7 (0.9–14) years	2:1	Bed rest followed by early mobilization.	7 (6–24) months
Terjesen 1991 [22]	58	Prospective	Patients with TS treated in the Department of Orthopedic Surgery with a mean duration of symptoms prior to admission of 3 days.	- Ultrasound, radiography of the hip in AP	5.8 (2–15) years	3.1:1	Bed rest, bilateral skin traction and moderate flexion of the hip.	11 (6–26) weeks
Briggs 1990 [23]	286	Retrospective	Children with TS presented to a Children's Hospital.	- Clinical examination - Lab: FBC, ESR, serum urea, electrolyte estimations, bacteriological investigations: by throat swabs, urine cultures and blood cultures, agglutinins against Salmonella, brucellosis, viral antibodies, Paul Beunnell test, RA Latex and Rose-Waaler titers, antinuclear factor, Tine test or Mantoux test. - Radiography of the hip in AP and Lauenstein views	(2–13 years)	2:1	Bed rest with or without traction applied to the affected leg with the hip in extension.	Unclear

Table 1 Study characteristics *(Continued)*

Hasegawa 1988 [14]	55	Prospective	Children with the clinical diagnosis TS admitted for examination at hospital, with duration of symptoms prior to examination of 18 days.	- Range of movement - Radiography of the hip in AP + Lauenstein views	7 (2–13) years	2.4:1	Unclear	4–9 months
Kallio 1988 [16]	109	Prospective	Children with TS admitted to hospital, with duration of symptoms prior to admission of 3 days in 75% of the cases.	- Clinical examination - Hematologic and serologic examinations, bacterial cultures from the throat, blood, urine and synovial fluid - Radiography of the hip in AP + Lauenstein views, ultrasound, hip aspiration with intraarticular pressure	5.6 years	2:1	Unclear	1 year
Landin 1987 [1]	275	Retrospective	Children with TS admitted to hospital or treated as outpatients with a 1 to 7 day history of symptoms prior to treatment.	- Range of movement, temperature - Lab: Hb, WBC, antistreptolysin, CRP, antibodies against Yersinia enterocolitica and Shigella, bacterial cultures from throat swab and urine - Radiography of the hip in AP + frog lateral views	(1–13 years)	2.6:1	Skin traction with the affected hip placed in extension and/or bed rest.	3 months–9 years
Egund 1987 [13]	70	Prospective	Children with TS admitted to the Department of Diagnostic Radiology and Orthopedics.	- History, clinical findings - Radiography of the hip in AP + Lauenstein, CT, ultrasound	6 (1–12) years	2.7:1	Unclear	6.5 (5–9) months
Kallio 1986 [15]	119	Prospective	Children with TS seen at a Children's Hospital.	- Clinical examination - Hematology, serology and bacterial culture from throat, blood, urine and synovial fluid - Radiography of the hip in AP + Lauenstein views, ultrasound, hip aspiration	Not given	Not given	Bed rest.	1 year
Haueisen 1986 [24]	475	Retrospective	Children with TS who have been hospitalized.	- Physical examination, temperature - Lab RF, ANA, WBC, ESR - Radiography of the hip, hip aspiration	6.2 (0.8–18) years	2.2:1	Bed rest, Buck's traction, antibiotics, spica casting.	6 months–4 years
Mukamel 1985 [20]	41	Prospective	Children with TS followed as outpatients.	- History, physical examination - Lab: ESR, WBC - Radiography of the hip	Average of 3.8 (1.3–12.5) years	3:1	Bed rest and analgesics.	9.3 months (3 months–3 years)

Table 1 Study characteristics *(Continued)*

Illingworth 1983 [25]	54	Retrospective	Children with a first episode of TS or with a recurrence of TS who attended hospital.	- Range of hip movement - Lab: ESR, WBC, CRP, ASO, RF, bacterial culture from throat and stool, monospot test for infectious mononucleoisis - Radiography of the hip	6.4 (2–12) years	4.4:1	Unclear	Unclear
Sharwood 1981 [28]	101	Retrospective	Children with TS admitted to a Children's Hospital with a period of symptoms prior to admission <7 days in 82% of the cases.	- Clinical examination of the gait, range of hip movement and leg length - Lab: ESR, WBC - Radiography of the hips in AP + frog lateral positions.	5.6	Unclear	Unclear	Average of 8.2 (5–15) years
Calver 1981 [10]	50	Prospective	Children with TS presented at a Children's Hospital with a mean duration of symptoms prior to admission of 4.5 days.	- Range of hip movement - Lab: blood count, blood film, ESR, RA latex agglutination, Widal and anti-staphylococcal titre, bacterial cultures from the throat and urine - Radiography of the hip in AP + frog lateral views, radioisotope scans.	6.1 (3–12) years	2:1	Bed rest and skin traction followed by slow mobilization.	1 year
Mallet 1981 [26]	38	Retrospective	Children admitted to hospital, with duration of symptoms prior to admission between 0 and 45 days.	- Radiography of the hip	6 (2–13) years	1.1:1	Skin traction, plaster.	7 (2–20) years
Stock 1977 [21]	34	Prospective	Children treated for TS at the Orthopedic Department, with duration of symptoms prior to admission mostly less than 1 week.	- History, physical examination - Lab: WBC, AST, CRP - Radiography of the hip	7.9 (4–14) years	1.6:1	Bed rest, relievement of hip, antibiotics, plaster, Tanderil, remedial therapy.	4.3 (0.5–15) years

[a]Number of children with transient synovitis of the hip included in the study; [b]Not all tests were performed on every patient; some tests were only done if certain diseases were suspected; [c]Given of the whole studied group of 243 children with a limp; [d]A: No recurrence B: 1 recurrence C: >1 recurrence; TS: children with transient synovitis of the hip; ESR: erythrocyte sedimentation rate; Hb: haemoglobin concentration; WBC: white blood cell count; ANA: antinuclear antibodies; RF: rheumatoid factor; FMF: familial Mediterranean fever; FBC: full blood count; CRP: C-reactive protein; ASO: antistreptolysin O titre.

Table 2 Quality scores of the included studies

Authors	Criteria								
	1	2	3	4	5	6	7	Score	Quality
Uziel 2006 [30]	–	–	–	+	–	–	–	1	Low
Skinner 2002 [3]	+	+	+	+	–	+	–	5	High
Kermond 2002 [18]	+	+	+	+	+	+	+	7	High
Fischer 1999 [4]	+	+	+	–	+	+	–	5	High
Mattick 1999 [27]	–	–	+	–	–	+	+	3	Low
Eggl 1999 [12]	+	+	+	+	+	+	–	6	High
De Pellegrin 1997 [11]	+	+	–	+	+	–	–	4	Low
Kesteris 1996 [19]	+	+	+	+	+	–	+	6	High
Keenan 1996 [17]	–	+	–	+	+	+	+	5	High
Taylor 1995 [29]	+	–	+	–	–	–	–	2	Low
Gopakumar 1992 [2]	+	–	+	+	–	–	–	3	Low
Terjesen 1991 [22]	+	+	+	+	+	–	+	6	High
Briggs 1990 [23]	+	–	+	+	–	+	+	5	High
Hasegawa 1988 [14]	+	+	+	–	+	–	+	5	High
Kallio 1988 [16]	+	+	+	–	+	+	+	6	High
Landin 1987 [1]	+	–	+	+	–	–	+	4	Low
Egund 1987 [13]	–	+	+	–	+	+	+	5	High
Kallio 1986 [15]	–	+	+	+	+	+	+	6	High
Haueisen 1986 [24]	+	–	+	+	–	+	–	4	Low
Mukamel 1985 [20]	+	+	+	+	+	–	–	5	High
Illingworth 1983 [25]	+	–	–	–	–	–	–	1	Low
Sharwood 1981 [28]	–	–	–	–	–	–	+	1	Low
Calver 1981 [10]	+	+	+	+	+	+	+	7	High
Mallet 1981 [26]	+	–	+	+	–	–	+	4	Low
Stock 1977 [21]	+	+	–	+	–	–	+	4	Low

+ the criterion was satisfied; – the criterion was not satisfied or it was unclear. Quality criteria: 1) Sample definition given (at least 4 of: age, male–female ratio, in-and exclusion criteria, duration of symptoms prior to submission, diagnostic criteria for transient synovitis), 2) Prospective design, 3) Inception cohort 4) Treatment subsequent to inclusion in cohort is described, 5) Follow-up data available from at least 80% of study population, or reason for loss of follow-up is known, 6) Same duration of follow-up for all patients (maximum range of 30%), or if patients have been followed by a protocol that defines end of follow-up, 7) Same tests used for all patients with transient synovitis during follow-up.

[24-26,29,30] showed that in 20-50% of the cases, the opposite hip is involved at recurrence.

Long-term course

Nineteen studies [1,2,4,10,13-17,23,24,26-30] observed the long-term course of TS (Additional file 2: Table S2). Of these, ten are of high quality and nine of low quality.

Three high quality studies reported clinical follow-up of TS on the long-term. Limited range of motion was found in 7% to 8% of the patients with TS [15,16].

Ten high quality studies [4,10,13-17,19,20,23] reported development of Legg-Perthes' disease subsequent to TS, ranging from 0% [15,16,19] to 38% [17]. In a study by by Kallio *et al.* [15] two patients with TS in one hip had recent symptom-free Legg-Perthes' disease in the opposite hip. Also, in this study all patients initially diagnosed with TS who developed Legg-Perthes' disease on long-term follow-up had early signs of Legg-Perthes' disease on the original radiographs. Early signs of Legg-Perthes' disease on radiographs were defined as signs of avascular necrosis and/or increased joint space.

Two high quality studies mentioned the long-term prevalence of coxa magna subsequent to TS ranging from 0%[23] to 32% [16].

Five low quality studies reported clinical follow-up of TS on the long-term. Hip pain after intensive physical effort ranged from 12% to 28% [21,26,30]. Limited range of motion of the hip was found in 0% to 18% of the patients with TS [21,28].

Seven low quality studies [1,2,21,24,28-30] reported development of Legg-Perthes' disease subsequent to TS, ranging from 0% [21,30] to 4% [1].

Two low quality studies reported that patients initially diagnosed with TS who developed Legg-Perthes' disease on long-term follow-up, had early signs of Legg-Perthes' disease on the initial radiographs in 67% [2] and 80% [1] of the cases.

Discussion

As no prognostic review of TS has yet been published, this systematic review is the first to provide an overview of the short and long-term clinical course of children with TS. Both high and low quality studies show that most children with TS experience symptoms for less than two weeks. Recurrence ranged from 0% to 18.3% in the high quality studies and from 4.1% to 26.3% in the low quality studies. In 20% to 50% of the children with a second episode of TS the opposite hip is affected. On long-term follow-up of high quality studies, limited range of motion was found in 7% to 8% of children with TS. Legg-Perthes' disease subsequent to TS, which was reported most frequently on long-term follow-up, ranged from 0% to 38% in the high-quality studies and from 0% to 4% in the low-quality studies.

Although all the studies followed patients with TS over time their objective(s) sometimes differed, leading to heterogeneity and adversely affecting comparability. With 40% of the included studies having a retrospective design, selection bias may have interfered with the overall outcomes. All included studies described children with TS who were hospitalised or treated as outpatients, none of the patients were seen by a GP only. This might imply that potentially useful information is lost, since many children with TS will be followed only in primary care. Also noteworthy is that the follow-up of children with TS began from the moment of inclusion in the study. This means that the numbers of symptomatic days prior to inclusion are not included in the

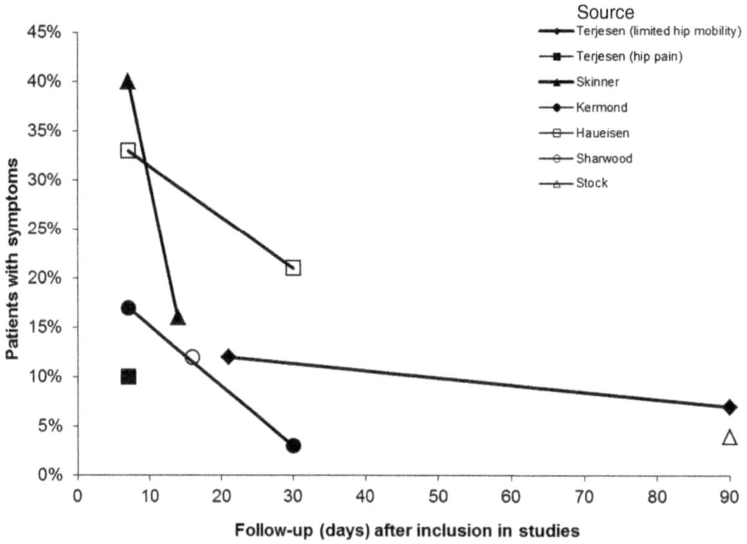

Figure 2 Data on short-term symptoms reported in six studies arranged by high (black) and low (white) methodological quality of the studies.

follow-up period, which might have led to underestimation of the duration of symptoms on short-term follow-up.

The scoring system we used for methodological quality assessment was adopted from an earlier review on assessing clinical course [8], but has not yet been validated. Furthermore, a distinction into high and low quality studies may be too black-and-white a representation of the quality of the included studies. Nevertheless, according to our rating, the methodological quality was high for more than 50% of the included studies. Critical items were criteria 5 and 6 ('same length of follow-up' and 'follow-up available from at least 80% of the study population'). Both these criteria induced loss of patient information during follow-up and might have influenced the outcomes of the present review. It showed that even within high quality studies large differences in outcomes were seen. The percentage of children with persistent symptoms after one to three weeks of follow-up in Figure 2 ranged from 10% to 40%. The studies' that showed the extreme values of 33% [24] and of 40% [3] did neither use the same test for all patients nor did they have a follow-up larger than 80%. The other studies showed a more homogeneous percentage of 10-17% for persistent symptoms after one to three weeks of follow-up.

For recurrence rate the largest differences was 0% after 9.3 months [20] and 19% after one year [16]. In this last study an extensive systematic re-examination in all patients was used, while the other study re-examined only some of the patients at three months based on initial findings and just reported that there was no recurrence between three months and three years of follow-up. A low quality study also showed a large recurrence rate after seven months of follow-up, but this study was retrospective and had more than 20% loss to follow-up [2].

The relatively high recurrence rate of TS at the opposite hip supports the hypothesis that TS is due to a systemic

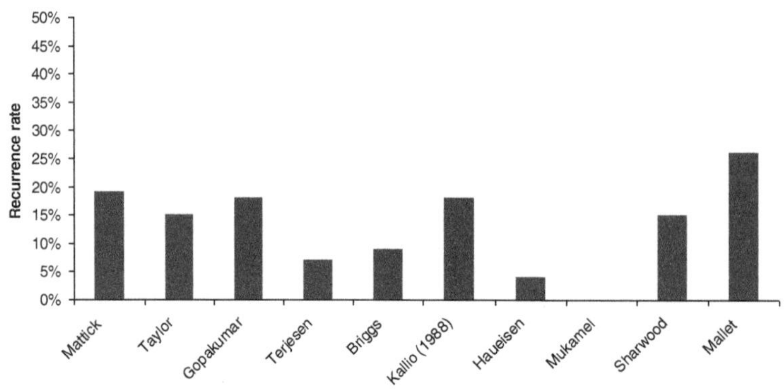

Figure 3 Recurrence rate reported in ten studies.

factor rather than being a local problem. A review by Do [5] includes various studies suggesting that a viral agent (causing respiratory tract infection or other flu-like syndromes) may also lead to the development of TS in children; elevated viral titers have been found in children with TS, although an infectious agent has not yet been identified.

The prevalence of Legg-Perthes' disease subsequent to TS (reported in nine high-quality studies) [4,10,13-16,19,20,23] ranged from 0% to 10%. One high-quality study by Keenan *et al.* [17] reported that 38% of the cases initially diagnosed as TS subsequently developed Legg-Perthes' disease. The aim of this latter study differs from the rest since only 13 patients with either prolonged or recurrent TS were studied. Five of them had a delay of more than two years in bone age and all five developed changes of Legg-Perthes' disease at three-months follow-up. These outcomes are consistent with the earlier mentioned hypothesis of a higher risk of Legg-Perthes' disease in children with prolonged symptoms of TS [1]. However, due to the low number of included patients and the preselected group of children with TS, the prevalence of 38% should not be generalized to the risk of developing Legg-Perthes' disease subsequent to TS.

Gaughan *et al.* describe an estimated prevalence rate of Legg-Perthes' disease (reported in the general pediatric population in the USA) of 0.023% [31]. The high quality studies in our review report a prevalence of Legg-Perthes' disease subsequent to TS of 0-10%. The question remains whether Legg-Perthes' disease is a direct consequence of TS in children. Symptoms of TS could also represent early signs of Legg-Perthes' disease. Children initially diagnosed with TS and (after ongoing symptoms) subsequently diagnosed with Legg-Perthes' disease fit this hypothesis. Early signs of Legg-Perthes' disease found at retrospective analysis of initial radiographs of patients with TS [15], also support this theory. Moreover, subtle radiologic changes of Legg-Perthes' disease are easily overlooked. In the literature, Gopakumar *et al.* found an absence of early radiologic signs in about 20% of the patients at first presentation, and in about 50% of the patients diagnosed with Legg-Perthes' disease [2].

Regrettably, some studies excluded children with Legg-Perthes' disease whereas information about the medical history of these patients might have revealed a misdiagnosis in TS. The reported follow-up periods after the initial diagnosis of TS in which subsequent Legg-Perthes' was diagnosed ranged between 1 and 6 months [1,10,11,17,20,24,28]. This might indicate that some studies did not follow their patients long enough to detect this.

Conclusions

The majority of the studies indicate that children with TS recover within two weeks; recurrence was seen in 0-26% of the cases. In the future, a long-term cohort study would be useful to more precisely evaluate the course of TS. Meanwhile, given the knowledge so far, it seems warranted to follow children with TS for at least 6 months to ensure that no hip symptoms are present that might indicate Legg-Perthes' disease.

Additional files

Additional file 1: Detailed search strategy.
Additional file 2: Outcomes of the studies.

Abbreviation

TS: Transient synovitis of the hip.

Competing interests

All authors declare no competing of interest. This article was commissioned and peer-reviewed.

Authors' contributions

RvR, MK, JB, and SB initiated the study. SA designed and performed the search, and wrote the manuscript. SA and RvR selected relevant articles from the titles and abstracts. SA and SB included final from the selected full text articles. SB, JB, and SA assessed quality, and SA and MK extracted data from the selected articles. All authors were involved in critically summarising the evidence and writing the article, and agreed with the final version.

Acknowledgments

The authors thank Dr. Hans van der Wouden (Dept. of General Practice, Erasmus MC) for translating and assessing the quality score of the French study by Mallet *et al.* We also thank Louis Volkers (Medical Library, Erasmus MC) for his assistance in the design of our search strategy.

Author details

[1]Department of General Practice, Erasmus MC-University Medical Centre Rotterdam, PO Box 2040, 3000 CA, Rotterdam, The Netherlands. [2]Department of Orthopedic Surgery, Erasmus MC-Sophia Children's Hospital Rotterdam, Dr. Molewaterplein 60, 3015 GJ, Rotterdam, The Netherlands. [3]Department of Public Health, Erasmus MC-University Medical Centre Rotterdam, PO Box 2040, 3000 CA, Rotterdam, The Netherlands.

References

1. Landin LA, Danielsson LG, Wattsgard C: **Transient synovitis of the hip. Its incidence, epidemiology and relation to Perthes' disease.** *J Bone Joint Surg Br* 1987, **69**(2):238–42.
2. Gopakumar TS, Vaishya R, Klenerman L, Carty H: **The role of ultrasound and isotope scanning in the management of irritable hips.** *Eur J Radiol* 1992, **15**(2):113–7.
3. Skinner J, Glancy S, Beattie TF, Hendry GM: **Transient synovitis: is there a need to aspirate hip joint effusions?** *Eur J Emerg Med* 2002, **9**(1):15–8.
4. Fischer SU, Beattie TF: **The limping child: epidemiology, assessment and outcome.** *J Bone Joint Surg Br* 1999, **81**(6):1029–34.
5. Do TT: **Transient synovitis as a cause of painful limps in children.** *Curr Opin Pediatr* 2000, **12**(1):48–51.
6. Krul M, van der Wouden JC, Schellevis FG, van Suijlekom-Smit LW, Koes BW: **Acute non-traumatic hip pathology in children: incidence and presentation in family practice.** *Family practice* 2010, **27**(2):166–70.
7. Vijlbrief AS, Bruijnzeels MA, van der Wouden JC, van Suijlekom-Smit LW: **Incidence and management of transient synovitis of the hip: a study in Dutch general practice.** *Br J Gen Pract* 1992, **42**(363):426–8.
8. van Rijn RM, van Os AG, Bernsen RM, Luijsterburg PA, Koes BW, Bierma-Zeinstra SM: **What is the clinical course of acute ankle sprains? A systematic literature review.** *Am J Med* 2008, **121**(4):324–31. e6.

9. Petrie A, Sabin C: *Medical Statistics at a Glance*. 2nd edition. Oxford: Blackwell Publishing; 2005.
10. Calver R, Venugopal V, Dorgan J, Bentley G, Gimlette T: **Radionuclide scanning in the early diagnosis of Perthes' disease.** *J Bone Joint Surg Br* 1981, **63-B**(3):379–82.
11. de Pellegrin M, Fracassetti D, Ciampi P: **[Coxitis fugax. The role of diagnostic imaging] Coxitis fugax. Die Rolle der bildgebenden Verfahren.** *Orthopade* 1997, **26**(10):858–67.
12. Eggl H, Drekonja T, Kaiser B, Dorn U: **Ultrasonography in the diagnosis of transient synovitis of the hip and Legg-Calve-Perthes disease.** *J Pediatr Orthop B* 1999, **8**(3):177–80.
13. Egund N, Hasegawa Y, Pettersson H, Wingstrand H: **Conventional radiography in transient synovitis of the hip in children.** *Acta Radiol* 1987, **28**(2):193–7.
14. Hasegawa Y, Wingstrand H, Gustafson T: **Scintimetry in transient synovitis of the hip in the child.** *Acta Orthop Scand* 1988, **59**(5):520–5.
15. Kallio P, Ryoppy S, Kunnamo I: **Transient synovitis and Perthes' disease. Is there an aetiological connection?** *J Bone Joint Surg Br* 1986, **68**(5):808–11.
16. Kallio PE: **Coxa magna following transient synovitis of the hip.** *Clin Orthop Relat Res* 1988, **228**:49–56.
17. Keenan WN, Clegg J: **Perthes' disease after "irritable hip": delayed bone age shows the hip is a "marked man".** *J Pediatr Orthop* 1996, **16**(1):20–3.
18. Kermond S, Fink M, Graham K, Carlin JB, Barnett P: **A randomized clinical trial: should the child with transient synovitis of the hip be treated with nonsteroidal anti-inflammatory drugs?** *Ann Emerg Med* 2002, **40**(3):294–9.
19. Kesteris U, Wingstrand H, Forsberg L, Egund N: **The effect of arthrocentesis in transient synovitis of the hip in the child: a longitudinal sonographic study.** *J Pediatr Orthop* 1996, **16**(1):24–9.
20. Mukamel M, Litmanovitch M, Yosipovich Z, Grunebaum M, Varsano I: **Legg-Calve-Perthes disease following transient synovitis. How often?** *Clin Pediatr (Phila)* 1985, **24**(11):629–31.
21. Stock D, Diezemann E, Birnesser H: **Late sequelae of transient coxitis in childhood.** *Z Kinderchir* 1977, **20**(3):270–4.
22. Terjesen T, Osthus P: **Ultrasound in the diagnosis and follow-up of transient synovitis of the hip.** *J Pediatr Orthop* 1991, **11**(5):608–13.
23. Briggs RD, Baird KS, Gibson PH: **Transient synovitis of the hip joint.** *J R Coll Surg Edinb* 1990, **35**(1):48–50.
24. Haueisen DC, Weiner DS, Weiner SD: **The characterization of "transient synovitis of the hip" in children.** *J Pediatr Orthop* 1986, **6**(1):11–7.
25. Illingworth CM: **Recurrences of transient synovitis of the hip.** *Arch Dis Child* 1983, **58**(8):620–3.
26. Mallet JF, Rigault P, Padovani JP, Touzet P: **[Transient synovitis of the hip in childhood. "observation hip" (author's transl)] La synovite aigue transitoire de hanche de l'enfant et son avenir a long terme. Le "rhume de la hanche".** *Rev Chir Orthop Reparatrice Appar Mot* 1981, **67**(8):791–803.
27. Mattick A, Turner A, Ferguson J, Beattie T, Sharp J: **Seven year follow up of children presenting to the accident and emergency department with irritable hip.** *J Accid Emerg Med* 1999, **16**(5):345–7.
28. Sharwood PF: **The irritable hip syndrome in children. A long-term follow-up.** *Acta Orthop Scand* 1981, **52**(6):633–8.
29. Taylor GR, Clarke NM: **Recurrent irritable hip in childhood.** *J Bone Joint Surg Br* 1995, **77**(5):748–51.
30. Uziel Y, Butbul-Aviel Y, Barash J, Padeh S, Mukamel M, Gorodnitski N, Brik R, Hashkes PJ: **Recurrent transient synovitis of the hip in childhood. Longterm outcome among 39 patients.** *J Rheumatol* 2006, **33**(4):810–1.
31. Gaughan DM, Mofenson LM, Hughes MD, Seage GR 3rd, Ciupak GL, Oleske JM: **Osteonecrosis of the hip (Legg-Calve-Perthes disease) in human immunodeficiency virus-infected children.** *Pediatrics* 2002, **109**(5):E74–4.

The natural course of low back pain: a systematic critical literature review

Nadège Lemeunier[1,2*], Charlotte Leboeuf-Yde[1,3] and Olivier Gagey[1]

Abstract

Background: Most patients in the secondary care sector consulting for low back pain (LBP) seem to have a more or less constant course of pain during the ensuing year. Fewer patients with LBP in the primary care sector report continual pain over a one-year period. However, not much is known about the long-term course of LBP in the general population. A systematic critical literature review was undertaken in order to study the natural course of LBP over time in the general population.

Methods: A search of articles was performed in Pubmed, Cinahl and Psychinfo using the search terms 'epidemiology'; 'low back pain' or 'back pain'; 'prospective study' or 'longitudinal study'; 'follow-up', 'natural course', 'course' or 'natural history'; 'general population' or 'working population'. Inclusion criteria were that one of the objectives was to study the course of (L)BP in the adult population, that the period of follow-up was at least 3 months, and that there were three points of observation or more. The review was undertaken by two independent reviewers using three checklists relating to description of studies, quality and outcomes. The course of LBP was established in relation to those who, at baseline, were reported not to have LBP or to have LBP. Would this course be stable, fluctuating, worsening, or improving over time? A synthesis of results in relation to common patterns was presented in a table and interpreted in a narrative form.

Results: Eight articles were included. Articles were different on time span, the number of surveys, and the definition of LBP. In six of the seven relevant studies, for those with no LBP at baseline, relatively substantial stable subgroups of people who continued to be LBP free were identified. In six of the seven relevant studies, definite stable subgroups of continued LBP were noted and improvement (becoming pain free) was never reported to be a common finding.

Conclusion: The status of LBP in individuals of the general population appears to be relatively stable over time, perhaps particularly so for those without LBP at baseline.

Keywords: Low back pain, Course, General population, Prospective study, Review

Introduction

Low back pain (LBP), which is a common disorder in the general population, was previously considered a generally short lasting disease with spontaneous recovery the most likely outcome. Because it is difficult to provide specific diagnoses to this condition, it became common to classify it according to the duration of the pain (i.e. acute, subacute or chronic) [1] with chronicity being considered relatively uncommon [2]. Nowadays, LBP is considered, rather, to be a recurring or persistent condition with a fluctuating course over time [3,4]. Yet, patients in the secondary care sector consulting for LBP seem to have a more or less constant course of pain during the ensuing year [5]. In contrast, fewer patients with LBP in the primary care sector report continual pain over a one-year period [6]. However, not much is known about the long-term course and different course patterns of LBP in the general population.

Our objective was to conduct a systematic critical literature review to improve our understanding of the natural course of LBP in the general population.

* Correspondence: nlemeunier@ifec.net
[1]Complexité, Innovation et Activités Motrices et Sportives, Bâtiment 335, UFR STAPS, Université Paris Sud-11, Orsay Cedex 91405, France
[2]Institut Franco-Européen de Chiropratique, 72 Chemin de la Flambère, Toulouse 31300, France
Full list of author information is available at the end of the article

Specifically, we wanted to find out the proportions of people with LBP at baseline who, when studied over prolonged periods of time, got better, worse, remained unchanged or fluctuated between LBP and no LBP. Similarly, we wanted to identify the most common course patterns for people without LBP at baseline; would they remain LBP free, develop LBP over time, or fluctuate between LBP and no LBP?

Method

Search strategy

A search for articles was performed in Pubmed, Cinahl and Psychinfo (until May 2012) using the search terms: 'epidemiology'; 'low back pain' or 'back pain'; 'prospective study' or 'longitudinal study'; 'follow-up', 'natural course', 'course' or 'natural history'; 'general population' or 'working population'. None of our two universities had access to Embase. An additional citation search was performed of reference lists of the retrieved articles. We used no restrictions for date of publication or language.

Inclusion and exclusion criteria

Selection of articles were made by NL and verified by CLY according to predetermined criteria for inclusion and exclusion that were defined by NL and CLY in relation to the objectives of the review.

Articles were included if (one of) their stated objective(s) was to study the course of (L)BP in the general population, i.e. no studies concerning clinical populations or pregnancy were included. Further inclusion criteria were that LBP should be measured at baseline and at a minimum of 2 subsequent follow-ups. Studies should report on the same individuals ($n > 100$) for a minimum of 3 months and participants should be ≥ 18 years old.

Because we expected to find only few studies of the general population, we also included studies of specific working populations if they did not represent hard physical work (e.g. construction workers) or extreme postures (e.g. painters, vineyard workers). Studies from the army or on compensation cases were also not accepted.

Checklists

Three checklists were created especially for this subject. These checklists related to the description of studies (Additional file 1: Appendix 1), their methodological quality (Additional file 1: Appendix 2), and their results. The criteria for methodological quality have been listed under three main headings: 1) representativeness of the study sample, 2) quality of data and 3) clear definition of LBP (Additional file 1: Appendix 2). The quality grid consisted of a slightly modified list of items previously used for prevalence studies of LBP [7]. All check-lists were tested by the reviewers for relevance and user friendliness on two articles, modified as needed to fit the purpose of the review, and tested once more prior to use.

Review process and interpretation of findings

Each article that fitted the criteria was independently and blindly reviewed by NL and CLY. In case of disagreement, the third author would be consulted. For all studies, the presence or absence of criteria was noted and the response rates were sought out or, if necessary, calculated. Only information mentioned in the methods or results sections was taken into account. A quality score was then calculated for each article according to the total number of acceptable criteria divided by the total number of relevant criteria. Each article was scrutinized for methodological quality, using the previously described scoring system but without determining an à priori cut-point for a minimal score, using it as an informative rather than a prescriptive score.

Results were taken into account only in relation to the pain aspect such as presence of LBP, duration, severity, or pattern; i.e. disability and consequences of LBP were not considered. The result sections were scrutinized for description of the course over time in relation to those who, at baseline, were reported a) not to have LBP or b) to have LBP. Results in each study were sought out in relation to whether absence or presence of LBP was stable, fluctuating, worsening, or – in the case of those having LBP at baseline -improving over time. The findings were reported in a table and interpreted in a narrative fashion. In addition, results were analyzed in relation to type of population and the number and spacing of surveys.

Results

Number of articles

Initially in Pubmed, 18 articles were considered suitable based on their title and study objectives (Additional file 1: Appendix 3). Of these, only 8 were retained after scrutiny of their text for all inclusion and exclusion criteria [8-15]. The 9 articles found with the search in Cinahl database overlapped with those already found in Pubmed. No relevant articles were found in the Psychinfo database. The additional citation search did not result in any relevant publications. An additional article was found in one of the authors' archives.

Some discussion between the reviewers was necessary for most articles, not because of disagreement but in order to clarify points that were unclear in the text; particularly in relation to the definition of LBP and the various response rates. There was no need to call in the third author for arbitration.

Description of the articles

The eight accepted articles had all been published since 1997, reporting on studies having been conducted between 1991 and 2005. Three had been carried out in the Nordic countries (Finland and Denmark), two in Switzerland and the rest in Northern Europe (UK, Netherlands and Germany).

As seen in Table 1, there were four articles on the general population [9,12-14] and four on specific working population (nurses [8,15], hospital employees [10] and employees of factories [11]). One article [12] included only people with previous LBP. In all but one of the reports, participants were between 20 and 60 years, the eight article only provided the mean age with the SD (23.2(5.1) [15]. In no two articles was the duration of the entire study period or the numbers of surveys identical, ranging from 52 surveys over one year [12] to 4 surveys over 28 years [11]. Four of the studies used the Nordic Back Pain Questionnaire either in postal surveys [9,10], through the internet or via postal diaries [12], or by computer assisted telephonic interview [14]. For the remaining four [8,11,13,15], questionnaires of unknown source were used. Although the exact wording of the LBP question was not always the same, definitions of LBP were generally relatively similar (usually LBP in the past year) with only two concentrating on LBP in the past month [8,12]. One reported also on longstanding LBP [14] and another used the description 'severity', which we renamed 'duration', as it related to number of days in the past year and not severity of symptoms [12]. One of the articles related the recall period to the duration since the last survey [15].

Furthermore, LBP was not always described in the same way between studies. In four articles [8,11,13,15], the presence or absence of LBP in the past year was measured at each survey without further specification; in two articles [9,10], LBP was classified in relation to duration during the past year; one article [12] categorized LBP according to severity and persistence of symptoms, whereas another article [14] used two different definitions for longstanding LBP in the past year (>3 months in two surveys and >1 month in one survey).

Quality of studies

Table 2 shows that all articles had a fairly high score according to the quality checklist; none scored less than 7/11. For this reason we took no further notice of the quality score, as we considered all articles to be credible. Nevertheless, it is worth noticing that two of the articles did not clearly deal with the issue of representativeness [8,10]. Other quality issues of interest are described below.

Not all reported the response rate in percentages [8,10-12,15] but when reported these ranged from 34% [13] to 96% [9]. In the article in which data were collected 52 times (every week) during one year [12], participants who completed at least 50% of these questionnaires were defined as 'responders', resulting in a total response rate of 90%. However, as is often the case in prospective studies, not everybody reported response rates for each subsequent survey clearly in relation to either those invited to participate in the first survey or (if that number was unknown) at least in relation to the number of participants at baseline. A calculation based on these figures reduced the response rates to a range from 21% [10] to 65% [14]. Furthermore, only five reports [9-11,14,15] discussed the potential impact that the non-responders may have on the results and in only one article were data modeled for this group [9].

Course of LBP

Table 3 gives the results on the course of absence or presence of LBP for each article. Interpretation of the natural course of LBP is reported below both for those without and those with LBP at baseline, in relation to stability, fluctuation, worsening or improvement.

No LBP at baseline

As shown in Table 3, in six of the seven relevant studies, relatively substantial stable stable subgroups were identified of people who continued to be LBP free. In one study [8], absence of LBP at baseline was said to be predictive of continued absence of LBP. In another study [13], absence of LBP was noted to be the most common subgroup of 32 possible combinations and in another [9], almost 50% belonged to this category. According to one of these six studies, approximately 10% with no LBP at baseline reported long standing LBP five and ten years later [14]. Further, at the 28 years follow-up, LBP was reported by 2/3 of those initially free of LBP [11].

LBP at baseline

The course over time in those who reported LBP at baseline seemed to be somewhat more heterogeneous (Table 3). In all of the seven relevant studies, definite stable subgroups of continued LBP were noted and improvement (becoming pain free) was never reported to be a common finding. According to one article [11], LBP was a stable occurrence five, ten and 28 years down the track, and also when surveyed weekly over one year [12], persistence of symptoms was noted in the majority of participants.

When fluctuation occurred (n = 4), it seemed most common between neighboring groups [9,10,14,15]. One study identified also a relatively small subgroup of people that worsened over time [10].

Additional analyses

There were no obvious differences in our results in relation to type of study population or number and spacing of surveys, with the possible exception of the results for

Table 1 Descriptive checklist

Reference number	I[st] author Year Country	Type of population (Age range)	Specific inclusion criteria in relation to LBP	Method of data collection	Definition of relevant LBP outcome variable (Anatomical site, recall periods, duration, severity, consequence)	Years or time of surveys	Numbers of surveys over the study period/years
[8]	Smedley 1998 UK	University hospital-based nurses, all types (19–64 years)	NA	Q^{aire}	LBP > 1 day in the past month	1993 Every 3 month Until 1995	8/2
[9]	Hestbaek 2003 Denmark	Men and women living in a Danish municipality (30–50 years)	NA	Q^{aire}	Number of days with LBP in the past year (0; 1–7; 8–30; >30) days	1991 1992 1995	3/5
[10]	Maül 2003 Germany	University hospital-based nurses (?)	NA	Q^{aire}	Number of days with LBP past year (0; 1–7; ≥8)* days	1991 1992 1999	3/9
[11]	Kääriä 2006 Finland	The employees in factories, all types (at least 47 yrs)	NA	Q^{aire}	LBP in the past year	1973 1978 1983 2000	4/28
[12]	Tamcan 2010 Switzerland	General population (?)	Those who report LBP in 2002–03 and who still report LBP in 2005	Internet-based diaries or postal diaries	LBP past month at week 1 and week 53 Intensity of pain each week between	2005 Every week	53/1
[13]	Kolb 2011 Switzerland	General population (?)	NA	Computer assisted telephonic interviews	In past year >1 month of bad BP or LBP	1999 2000 2001 2002 2003	5/5

Table 1 Descriptive checklist *(Continued)*

[14]	Van Oostrom 2011 The Netherlands	General population (20–60)	NA	Q^{aire}	Persistent LBP past year	1993-97	3/10
					Defined as more than three months (study 1 and 3) and more than one month (study 2)	1998-02 2003-07	
[15]	Videman 2005 Finlande	Nursing students	NA	Q^{aire}	BP past 4 month, past year and past 4 years	Baseline	9/7.5
					(0; 1–7; 8–30; >30) days but not daily, and daily	Every 4 month during 2 years 1 year after school 5 year after school	

*Mentionned in methods. Reclassified from 'severity' to duration.
NA: Not applicable.

Table 2 Quality checklist

Ref N°	Representativeness					Quality of data			Definition of LBP			
	Response rates in relation to invited study sample at baseline. If new study subjects invited, response rates calculated based on number of invited participants at each survey	Sample sizes	N/% response at all surveys based on number of participants at first survey	At least one of the following: Whole target population; Randomly selected sample; or Sample stated to represent general population (Yes/No)	At least one of the following: Reasons for non response described; Non-responders described; Comparison responders-non-responders; or Comparison of sample and target population (Yes/No)	Same mode of data collection for all subjects, and all surveys (Yes/No)	Same definition(s) of LBP outcome variable used for all subjects at all survey (Yes/No)	At least one of the following: Questionnaires, diaries, or interviews validated; Tested for reproductibility or Tested in pilot study (Yes/No)	Precise anatomical delineation of lumbar area; or Reference to easily obtainable article that contains such specification (Yes/No)	Further specification of definition of LBP; Questions put to study subjects quoted; or Reference to easily obtainable article that contains such specification (Yes/No)	Recall periods specified (Yes/No)	Quality score: Number of 'Yes'/ Number of relevant items
[8]	1088/2405 = 45 %	1088	470/1165	No	Yes	Yes	Yes	No	Yes	Yes	Yes	9/11
	999/2405 = 41%	999	40%									82%
	878/2405 = 36%	878										
	827/2405 = 34%	827										
	758/2405 = 31%	758										
	700/2405 = 29%	700										
	614/2405 = 25%	614										
	599/2405 = 25%	599										

Table 2 Quality checklist *(Continued)*

[9]	1309/2000 = 65%	1309	765/1309	Yes	Yes	Yes	Yes	Yes	Yes	Yes	Yes	11/11
	1198/2000 = 60%	1198	58%									100%
	813/2000 = 41%	813										
[10]	1307/1963 = 67%	1307	269/1307	No	Yes	Yes	Yes	Yes	Yes	Yes	Yes	10/11
	1159/2185 = 53%	1159	21%									91%
	1584/2744 = 58%	1584										
[11]	902/1057 = 85%	902	418/902	Yes	No	Yes	Yes	No	No	Yes	Yes	8/11
	748/1057 = 71%	748	46%									73%
	654/1057 = 62%	654										
	546/1057 = 52%	546										
[12]	340/400 = 85%	340	206/340	Yes	Yes	Yes	Yes	Yes	Yes	Yes	Yes	11/11
	participated		76%									100%
	Used in analysis: 305/340 = 90%		(95-100% responses)									
[13]	?	7791	3881/7791	Yes	Yes	Yes	Yes	No	No	Yes	Yes	8/11
		6335	50%									73%
		5755										
		4885										
		4354										
[14]	6118/7769 = 79%	6118	4007/6118	Yes	Yes	Yes	No	Yes	Yes	Yes	Yes	10/11
	4917/7769 = 63%	4917	65%									91%
	4520/7769 = 58%	4520										

Table 2 Quality checklist *(Continued)*

[15]	?/308	?	108/308	No	Yes	Yes	Yes	No	Yes	Yes	Yes	7/11
	?/308	?										64%
	?/308	?										
	?/308	?										
	?/308	?										
	?/308	?										
	?/308	?										
	?/308	?										
	197/308	197										
	174/308	174										

Table 3 Results

At Baseline	Reference N°	Development of LBP over time				Comments
		Stable	Fluctuating	Worsening	Improving	
No LBP	[8]	No LBP at BL was highly predictive of future absence of pain throughout 8 surveys over 2 years			NA	
	[9]	45% with no pain at 3 surveys over 5 years			NA	
	[10]	70% no pain at second survey and 57% at 3rd survey over 8 years			NA	
	[11]	67% and63% respectively no pain at 2nd and 3rd survey over 28 years		64% had LBP at the 4th survey (28 years later)	NA	
	[12]	NA	NA	NA	NA	Not applicable: all participants were chosen because they had LBP
	[13]	The most frequent course was no BP each year over 5 years (35%)			NA	
	[14]	- 29% of the population was free of LBP at 3 surveys over 10 years - 62% never had long standing LBP at 3 surveys over 10 years		- 11% developed long standing LBP at 2nd and 3rd survey over 10 years	NA	
	[15]	Stable (visual analysis)				
Presence of LBP	[8]	Presence of LBP at BL was highly predictive of future pain throughout 8 surveys over 2 years				
	[9]	If >30 days of LBP at BL: 39% in the same category after 1 and 5 years	If 1–30 days of LBP at BL 62% fluctuated to the neighboring groups over 5 years			
	[10]	38% have the same intensity of LBP at 3 surveys over 8 years	27% of LBP (intensity) fluctuated; movements between extremes groups were rare (12%) at 3 surveys over 8 years	17% of LBP (intensity) increased at 3 surveys over 8 years	19% of LBP (intensity) decreased at 3 surveys over 8 years	
	[11]	75, 73 and 88% were symptomatic at 3 FUs over 28 years 31% of the subjects reported LBP in all 4 surveys				
	[12]	Stability of severity and frequency of LBP was high in 4 periods over 1 year			3% reported no pain after BL throughout the weekly surveys over one year	

Table 3 Results *(Continued)*

	[13]	The most frequent course was BP each year over 5 years (14%)			
	[14]	6% had long standing LBP at 3 surveys over 10 years	11% had long standing LBP only at some surveys over 10 years		10% had recovered from long lasting low back pain at 2nd and 3rd survey
	[15]	For those who had more than 8 days of BP during that first year (visual analysis)	For those who have between 1–7 days of BP the first year of the 5-yr study period (visual analysis)		

LBP: Low back pain; *FU*: Follow-up; *BL*: Baseline; *NA*: Not Applicable.

the 28-year follow-up that indicated that LBP will occur in the end among the previously 'protected' non-sufferers [11].

Discussion

The purpose of this review was to gain an understanding of the natural course of LBP. The conclusion is that the LBP status at baseline is predictive of the future course and, probably, in particular for those who do not have LBP at baseline.

The eight studies that were identified were all of relatively high quality, judging by their quality scores, but their study approaches were dissimilar in relation to definition of LBP, method of data collection, number of surveys, time between surveys, and type of population. That the results nevertheless pointed in the same direction, strengthens the validity of these findings. However, it would have been helpful if studies could have reported their data more clearly and systematically, as otherwise it is difficult to extract the relevant information from the text.

In particular, it would have been more informative if researchers could have reported more clearly the percentage of drop-outs at the various surveys and attempted to take into account the possible effect of missing data. Although several authors [9-11,14,15] considered potential differences between responders and non-responders, only one [9] visualized them in their result section and even took them into account in a best case and worst case analysis, which obviously can be important in studies with large dropout rate numbers, as is often the case in studies with multiple follow-ups over long periods of time.

This systematic and critical review was done independently by two readers with no particular interest in the outcome of the review. Nonetheless, it suffers the same potential weaknesses as many other similar reviews. For example, it is not sure that all relevant articles were retrieved, if checklists were relevant, or if the information was properly interpreted.

However, this topic is fairly new, indicating that there would not be numerous studies and those that have been published were easily noticed. Further, our thorough citation search did not result in any additional publications, although, admittedly, one retrieved article [15] failed to be captured in our search procedure. Still, it is possible that this type of data can be found interspersed between the main messages of articles with other specific objectives than describing the natural course of LBP. It is possible that we may have missed those. The grids for systematic data collection were designed to meet our needs and the quality checklist was a previously published and used checklist for this type of studies with only minor adjustments to fulfill the needs of the present review. Another type of quality checklist could of course have resulted in a different view of which articles to accept for analysis. Although the literature sometimes was difficult to extract and interpret, partly because not all articles had the same primary research objectives as we had, it was never necessary to seek arbitration from the third author, indicating good consensus between reviewers although, of course, not guaranteeing accuracy.

Another potential shortcoming could be that we included studies also from the working population. Such studies could have biased study samples either through a healthy worker effect [16] or the opposite, in the case of physically undemanding jobs. In our case, a healthy worker effect would probably not be pronounced, as we on purpose did not include working populations representing heavy manual labor. Also, there were no obvious differences in outcomes between studies of the general and working populations.

Conclusion

The results of this survey indicate that, in the general population, absence of LBP at one time in life is a blessing, in that it will indicate also a pain-free future at last for a fairly large number of years. On the other hand, those with LBP will fairly consistently report LBP again.

Additional file

Additional file 1: Appendices. 1: Descriptive checklist for a systematic literature review on the natural course of low back pain (LBP). **2:** Quality checklist for a systematic literature review on the natural course of LBP. **3:** List of 10 articles that were excluded from the literature review in concordance with our inclusion and exclusion criteria.

Competing interests

One of the authors (CLY) was co-author on one of the reviewed articles. However, the review was performed by two of the authors, and there were no discrepancies between these two on the findings from that article. Otherwise, the authors state that they have no competing interest.

Authors' contributions

All authors helped to plan the review. NL and CLY performed the literature review. NL and CLY interpreted the findings. NL wrote the first draft. All authors participated in completing the manuscript. All authors read and approved the final manuscript.

Author details

[1]Complexité, Innovation et Activités Motrices et Sportives, Bâtiment 335, UFR STAPS, Université Paris Sud-11, Orsay Cedex 91405, France. [2]Institut Franco-Européen de Chiropratique, 72 Chemin de la Flambère, Toulouse 31300, France. [3]Research Department, Spine Center of Southern Denmark, Hospital Lillebaelt and Institute of Regional Health Services Research, University of Southern Denmark, Ostre Hougvej 55, Middelfart, Denmark.

References

1. Spitzer WO, LeBlanc RE, Dupuis MS: **Scientific approach to the assessment and management of activity-related spinal disorders. In monograph for clinicians: report of the Quebec task force on spinal disorders.** *Spine* 1987, **12:**s16–s21.
2. Waddell G: **A new clinical model for the treatment of low back pain.** *Spine* 1987, **12**(7):632–641.
3. Stanton TR LJ, Maher CG, Hancock MJ: **How do we define the condition 'recurrent low back pain'? A systematic review.** *Eur Spine J* 2010, **19:**533–539.
4. Von Korff MDK: **Chronic pain reconsidered.** *Pain* 2008, **138**(2):267–276.
5. Leboeuf-Yde C, Jensen RK, Axen I: **Absence of low back pain in patients followed weekly over one year with automated text messages.** *Chiropr & Man Th* 2012, **20:**9.
6. Dunn K, Jordan K, Croft P: **Characterizing the course of low back pain: a latent class analysis.** *Am J Epidemiol* 2006, **163**(8):754–761.
7. Leboeuf-Yde C, Lauritzen JM: **The prevalence of low back pain in the literature.** *Spine* 1995, **20**(19):2112–2118.
8. Smedley J, Inskip H, Cooper C, Coggon D: **Natural history of low back pain: a longitudinal study in nurses.** *Spine* 1998, **23**(22):2422–2426.
9. Hestbaek L, Engberg M, Lauritzen T, Bruun NH, Manniche C: **The course of low back pain in a general population. Results from a 5-year prospective study.** *J Manipulative Physiol Ther* 2003, **26**(4):213–219.
10. Maul I, Läubli T, Klipstein A, Krueger H: **Course of low back pain among nurses: a longitudinal study across eight years.** *Occup Environ Med* 2003, **60:**497–503.
11. Kääriä S, Luukkonen R, Riihimäki H, Kirjonen J, Leino-Arjas P: **Persistence of low back pain reporting among a cohort of employees in a metal corporation: A study with 5-, 10-, and 28-year follow-ups.** *Pain* 2006, **120:**131–137.
12. Tamcan O, Mannion AF, Eisenring C, Horisberger B, Elfering A, Müller U: **The course of chronic and recurrent low back pain in the general population.** *Pain* 2010, **150**(3):451–457.
13. Kolb E, Canjuga M, Bauer GF, Läubli T: **Course of back pain across 5 years.** *Spine* 2011, **36**(4):E268–E273.
14. van Oostrom SH, Verschuren VMM, de vet HCW, Picavet HS: **Ten year course of low back pain in an adult population-based cohort - The Doetinchem Cohort Study.** *Eur Journal of Pain* 2011, **15:**993–998.
15. Videman T, Ojajärvi A, Riihimäki H, Troup JDH: **Low back pain among nurses.** *Spine* 2005, **30**(20):2334–2341.
16. McMichael A: **Standardized mortality ratios and the "healthy worker effect": Scratching beneath the surface.** *J Occup Med* 1976, **18**(3):165–168.

24

Body mass index and musculoskeletal pain: is there a connection?

David R Seaman

Abstract

Background: Back pain is one of the most common complaints that patients report to physicians and two-thirds of the population has an elevated body mass index (BMI), indicating they are either overweight or obese. It was once assumed that extra body weight would stress the low back and lead to pain, however, researchers have reported inconsistencies association between body weight and back pain. In contrast, more recent studies do indicate that an elevated BMI is associated with back pain and other musculoskeletal pain syndromes due to the presence of a chronic systemic inflammatory state, suggesting that the relationship between BMI and musculoskeletal pains be considered in more detail.

Objective: To describe how an elevated BMI can be associated with chronic systemic inflammation and pain expression. To outline measurable risk factors for chronic inflammation that can be used in clinical practice and discuss basic treatment considerations.

Discussion: Adiposopathy, or "sick fat" syndrome, is a term that refers to an elevated BMI that is associated with a chronic systemic inflammatory state most commonly referred to as the metabolic syndrome. The best available evidence suggests that the presence of adiposopathy determines if an elevated BMI will contribute to musculoskeletal pain expression. It is not uncommon for physicians to fail to identify the presence of adiposopathy/ metabolic syndrome.

Conclusion: Patients with an elevated BMI should be further examined to identify inflammatory factors associated with adiposopathy, such as the metabolic syndrome, which may be promoting back pain and other musculoskeletal pain syndromes.

Keywords: Back pain, Body mass index, Obesity, Metabolic syndrome, Inflammation

Introduction

An elevated BMI, due to an increase in adipose tissue mass, is rapidly becoming the norm of our modern society. In the United States, approximately sixty-five percent of adults aged 20 years or older are either overweight or obese [1]. Despite the associations between obesity and diabetes, heart disease, and other chronic diseases, adiposity or fatness, can be misinterpreted to merely represent an excess calorie storage depot due to overeating, rather than an overactive immune/endocrine organ that can generate chronic systemic inflammation [2].

Historically, studies have suggested a weak association between body weight and low back pain [3], and guidelines for the treatment of low back pain have not included diet and weight loss as recommendations [4,5]. Updating this view appears to be in order as an elevated body mass index is considered a risk factor for low back pain chronicity [6,7], and recent studies have indicated that overweight and obese patients are at a higher risk for musculoskeletal pain expression, as are patients with the metabolic syndrome and type 2 diabetes. For example, overweight and obese individuals are more likely to suffer from tension-type or migraine headache, fibromyalgia, abdominal pain, and chronic widespread pain [8,9]. Studies have implicated an elevated by BMI as a promoter of low back pain [10-12]. Obese subjects with hsCRP levels above 3 mg/dL are more likely to report low back pain, compared to obese subjects with normal levels [13].

Correspondence: dseaman@nuhs.edu
National University of Health Sciences, SPC-Health Education Center, 7200 66th St, Pinellas Park, FL 33781, USA

Studies have demonstrated that local and widespread musculoskeletal pains are more common in patients with the metabolic syndrome [14-16]. Prevalence of neck pain is higher in patients with metabolic syndrome [17]. Shoulder pain is associated with the metabolic syndrome [18]. Achilles, patella, and elbow tendinopathy are associated with the metabolic syndrome [19-21]. Risk of lumbar disc herniation is increased by the metabolic syndrome [22]. Low back and radiating pain is associated with elevated serum lipids and cardiovascular disease risk factors [23-31]. Osteoarthritis is also promoted by the metabolic syndrome [32-35]. Patients with type 2 diabetes have reduced mobility across all joints tested compared to age/weight matched controls [36], and are more likely to develop lumbar stenosis compared to non-diabetics [37,38]. Type 2 diabetes also increases the risk of expressing disc herniation in both the cervical and lumbar spines [39,40].

The term "adiposopathy" has been proposed to describe a "sick fat" inflammatory state versus an overweight state without inflammation [2,41,42]. In other words, not all patients suffer from chronic inflammation when adipose tissue mass increases. This may be the reason for the previous inconsistent correlations between an elevated BMI and low back pain. The emerging interpretation is that adiposopathy and the related metabolic syndrome leads to pain chronicity because the associated non-resolving systemic inflammation is a pathophysiologic state that promotes nociception in injured/dysfunctional musculoskeletal tissues and prevents healing and pain resolution [10,14,35]. This view is consistent with the evidence that chronic non-resolving inflammation is associated with a diversity of seemingly unrelated chronic diseases, such as low back pain, arthritis, atherosclerosis, cancer, chronic obstructive pulmonary disease, asthma, inflammatory bowel disease, neurodegenerative disease, multiple sclerosis, psoriasis, and rheumatoid arthritis [43-51].

Thus, understanding the nature of chronic inflammation, adiposopathy, and the metabolic syndrome is relevant to understanding and treating low back pain and other conditions commonly seen by chiropractors. The remainder of this commentary will discuss these topics.

What is chronic systemic inflammation?

Chronic systemic inflammation is a "state" of body chemistry that develops over time, which gradually leads to the expression of chronic disease. While this view of inflammation is not novel [52-65], it has yet to be emphasized in the pages of physiology and pathology texts where inflammation is still typically perceived in the context of local physical injury or infection [66,67]. In the traditional context, inflammation is viewed as a normal response to the acute injury/infection, which leads to tissue healing and the resolution of inflammation. As chronic inflammation is typically not a consideration in physiology texts (66), this can lead to a misunderstanding about the nature of common musculoskeletal diseases, of which osteoarthritis is the best example.

Osteoarthritis (OA) is still characterized as a "non-inflammatory, wear and tear" condition [35,67], despite the evidence over the last several decades indicating that it is a chronic inflammatory condition [35,68-73]. In fact, OA joints are inflamed and express the same inflammatory chemistry as found in atherosclerotic vessels [74,75]. And contrary to what might be expected, chondrocytes participate in cartilage degradation by releasing inflammatory mediators [76,77]. Mounting evidence suggests that as with atherosclerosis, OA is a local manifestation of systemic inflammation [32-35,78]. Interestingly, the metabolic syndrome is associated with the expression of OA [35].

Although difficult to visualize, compared with a an injury or infection, the body responds in a similar fashion to "non-overtly injurious" homeostatic challenges. Reduced sleep, stress, sedentary living, and high glycemic index foods, promotes cellular release of inflammatory mediators, most notably are the pro-inflammatory cytokines such as interleukin-1β (IL-1), interleukin-6 (IL-6), and tumor necrosis factor-α (TNF). In other words, immune cells release the same mediators whether there is overt tissue injury or noxious homeostatic challenges, such as inadequate sleep, stress, and a high glycemic meal [62,63,74,79-82].

The clinical expression of the systemic pro-inflammatory state takes time to develop and varies among patients, which makes specific cause-effect relationships difficult to identify. Nonetheless, it is known that chronic inflammation, while nonspecific in terms of symptoms, is the pathophysiological state found in most chronic diseases, such as depression, asthma, atherosclerosis, rheumatoid arthritis, diabetes, osteoporosis, Alzheimer's disease, cancer, and osteoarthritis [75,83,84].

While the clinical expression of the systemic pro-inflammatory state varies among patients, they commonly report poor self-rated health and a depressed affect [85-91], which are risk factors for pain chronicity [6,7]. This inflammatory "state" of ill-health and depression can be induced in many patients when they are given interferon, which causes immune cells to release pro-inflammatory cytokines [91]. The outcome can be a depressed mood, severe fatigue, lethargy, irritability, emotional lability, social withdrawal, lack of concentration and full-blown major depression in a considerable number of patients, which remits when cytokine therapy is withdrawn [91,92]. The direct administration of IL-1 and TNF in animals acts in a dose-dependent manner to generate symptoms of sickness, depression, and pain [93].

Measurements of circulating levels of high sensitivity C-reactive protein (hsCRP) support the contention that the average patient in the United States is inflamed to moderate or high degrees [56], which may explain why depression, fatigue, poor health, and pain are such common symptoms. Levels of hsCRP of <1, 1 to 3, and >3 mg/L denote lower, moderate, and higher relative risk for future vascular events; however, on a practical basis these values should be interpreted as low, moderate, and high systemic inflammation. With this in mind, the average middle-aged American is moderately inflamed with an hsCRP level at about 1.5 mg/L; however, approximately 25% of the US population is highly inflamed with levels of hsCRP greater than 3 mg/L [56]. The recommended anti-inflammatory behavioral changes to reduce hsCRP include diet, exercise, losing weight, and cessation of smoking [56].

Adiposopathy and chronic inflammation

Multiple interrelated factors lead to weight gain and the development of obesity, the most commonly articulated is a positive caloric balance coupled with sedentary living [41,42]. Inadequate sleep and stress also promote obesity by increasing palatable food consumption, due to increased release of ghrelin and other hormones [94-100]. Less than 6 hrs of sleep per night can undermine dietary efforts to reduce obesity [101] and less than 6 hours or greater than 9 hours of sleep is associated with increased next day pain [102]. Additionally, inadequate sleep and stress independently promote systemic inflammation [103-105]. Sedentary living is also associated with systemic inflammation, which can be modulated with exercise [106-110]. Lees and Booth have gone so far as to call a lack of exercise the "sedentary death syndrome" [111]. A lack of exercise leads to an increase in BMI [112], poorer self-rated health [113,114], and depression [108,115], each of which is a risk factor for developing chronic low back pain [6,7].

The current American diet consists largely of refined, nutrient-free foods, such as sugar, flour, and refined oils. The current American diet is approximately 20% refined sugar, 20% refined grains, 20% refined oils, 15-20% fatty meat, and 10% dairy by calories [1]. Notice that the average American eats virtually no vegetables and fruit and the vast majority of calories (40%) come from refined sugar and flour. Not well known is that high calorie meals consisting of refined carbohydrates and lipids leads to an immediate postprandial response that manifests as hypercoagulability, sympathetic hyperactivity, endothelial dysfunction and the release of inflammatory mediators, such as cytokines and C-reactive protein [62,63]. Postprandial inflammation can occur before substantial elevations in BMI; however, eating in this fashion eventually leads to adipose tissue expansion.

As adiposity increases, there is a fundamental change in the metabolic activity of adipose tissue. In lean individuals, adipocytes exert an anti-inflammatory function by releasing adiponectin and anti-inflammatory interleukin-10, which are associated with health promotion and body repair [116,117]. Adiponectin supports insulin sensitivity and mitochondrial biogenesis in skeletal muscle and interleukin-10 has analgesic and anti-inflammatory immune modulating properties [118-121].

In contrast, as adipocytes increase in size, which is associated with an increase in BMI, a metabolic shift can occur in adipose tissue, such that a systemic chronic inflammatory state develops in certain patients. Indeed, circulating inflammatory mediators, such as hsCRP, TNF and IL-6, were measured in obese individuals and non-obese controls. In obese individuals, an increase in weight, BMI, waist circumference, hip circumference, and waist-hip ratio was correlated to increased levels of inflammatory mediators [122]. These non-invasive measurements can be readily used in clinical practice to get an impression of a patient's potential inflammatory or pain status.

There is normally a small population of macrophages in lean adipose tissue and they exist in their "M2" or non-activated state [116,117]. However, as adipocytes grow in size, mast cells, lymphocytes, and macrophages can actively enter adipose tissue [123,124], which leads to the transformation of macrophages from M2 to the "M1" or activated state [116,117]. This combination of immune cells causes adipose tissue to behave as an overactive immune organ that promotes chronic systemic inflammation [2,42,116,117,123-127]. Indeed "adiposopathy" is a state in which adipose tissue immune cells are behaving in a fashion that mimics a bacterial infection and autoimmune disorders [123,124]. Thus, it should not be a surprise that overweight individuals are more likely to suffer from pain, malaise and depression.

Adiposopathy, the metabolic syndrome, and pain expression

As an individual's waistline continues to increase in size due to gains in adipose tissue mass, additional health/disease markers can change, such as elevations in fasting blood glucose, fasting triglycerides, and blood pressure, as well as reductions in high density lipoprotein (HDL) cholesterol. These five markers reflect the presence of adiposopathy [42], and comprise risk factors for the metabolic syndrome, of which at least three must be present to apply the diagnosis [128-130]. Table 1 is an example of how predictors of the metabolic syndrome and other pro-inflammatory markers can be followed in the clinical setting.

With metabolic syndrome values in mind, the interpretation of glucose and triglyceride values can be further refined to reflect important postprandial inflammatory responses [62]. Population studies have shown that a fasting glucose as low as 90 mg/dL can be associated with a 2-

Table 1 Markers of chronic inflammation

Markers		Date	Date	Date	Date
Metabolic syndrome	**Abnormal value**				
1. Fasting blood glucose	≥ 100 mg/dL				
2. Triglycerides	≥ 150 mg/dL				
3. HDL cholesterol	< 50 for women; < 40 men				
4. Blood pressure	≥ 130/85				
5. Waist circumference	> 35″ women; > 40″ men				
Pro-inflammatory markers	**Parameters**				
2-hour postprandial glucose	<140 mg/dl = normal				
	140–199 = prediabetes				
	200+ = diabetes				
Fasting triglycerides	<90 mg/dl predicts controlled postprandial response				
hsCRP in mg/L (marker of chronic inflammation)	<1.0 = normal				
	1.0-3.0 = moderate				
	>3.0 = high				
25(OH)D (vitamin D)	32-100 ng/ml (goal >40 ng)				
Body mass index (BMI)	18.5-24.9 = normal				
	25–29.9 = overweight				
	≥30 = obese				
Waist/hip ratio women (risk factor for diabetes)	<0.80 = low risk				
	0.81-.85 = moderate risk				
	>0.85 = high risk				
Waist/hip ratio men (risk factor for diabetes)	<0.95 = low risk				
	0.96-1.0 = moderate risk				
	>1.0 = high risk				
Lack of sleep	Less than 6 hrs				
Stress	Associated with systemic inflammation				
Sedentary living	Associated with systemic inflammation				
Depression	Associated with systemic inflammation				
Self-rated health	Associated with systemic inflammation				

hour post-prandial glucose of >200 mg/dL, which is diagnostic for type 2 diabetes. A 2 hour post-prandial blood glucose level less than 140 mg/dL suggests normal glucose handling; however, data are emerging suggesting that the ideal value may be less. While a fasting triglyceride 150 mg/dl is the cut off for metabolic syndrome, a fasting triglyceride value 90 mg/dl or less is more predictive of postprandial responses [62].

A reduced level of circulating HDL cholesterol is typically viewed as an atherosclerotic plaque risk factor. However, HDL also plays a key role in role in binding absorbed endotoxin to ensure low basal circulating levels, such that reduced HDL cholesterol levels can promote chronic endotoxemia and systemic inflammation [131]. Furthermore, when HDL is burdened by endotoxin, there are multiple pro-inflammatory atherogenic consequences including a suppression of lecithin: cholesterol acyltransferase activity and cholesterol ester transfer protein mass, and a reduced capacity to efflux cholesterol [132], which impact musculoskeletal pain. As mentioned in the introduction, several studies have found a relationship between serum lipids, cardiovascular disease risk factors, and the expression of low back and radiating pain [23-31]. Vitamin D deficiency is also associated with chronic inflammation [133], the metabolic syndrome [134], and low back pain [135].

Approximately 25% of individuals age 40–49, 35% of those age 50–59, and 45% of those over 60 year of age may have the pro-inflammatory metabolic syndrome [136]. In other words, 25-40% of the adult population is chronically inflamed in the fasted state, which is further augmented by repeated consumption of meals that leads to the acute postprandial inflammatory state that was described earlier. When the metabolic syndrome is identified in a patient, the interpretation should be that the patient has transformed into a state of chronic inflammation as evidenced by a host of inflammatory changes [125,137,138] (see Table 2).

Table 2 Pro-inflammatory chemistry of the metabolic syndrome

Hyperglycemia	↑ NF-κB
Hyperinsulinemia	↑ CRP
Hypertriglyceridemia	↑ TNF
Hyperuricemia	↑ IL-6
↓ HDL	↑ Increased white blood cell count
↓ protein synthesis	↑ plasminogen activator inhibitor
↑ protein catabolism	↑ Fibrinogen
↑ gluconeogenesis	↑ Leptin
↑ serum amyloid A	↑ Resistin
↑ angiotensinogen	↓ adiponectin

The pro-inflammatory metabolic syndrome chemistry is known to promote the expression of multiple diseases including type 2 diabetes, cancer, cardiovascular disease, stroke, hypertension, polycystic ovarian syndrome, non-alcoholic fatty liver disease, gallstones, sleep apnea, acne, myopia, male vertex balding, and a reduced age of menarche [138-141]. With such a diverse expression of disease associated with the metabolic syndrome, it is not a surprise that higher postprandial glycemia is considered to be "a universal mechanism for disease progression" [142].

Despite its obvious pervasiveness and associated health risks, it is not uncommon for primary care physicians to fail to identify the presence of the metabolic syndrome [129]. It is important that practitioners of manual therapy avoid this pitfall. As described earlier, the metabolic syndrome and type 2 diabetes are associated with an increased expression of common painful musculoskeletal conditions seen everyday by manual therapists. Additionally, the presence of the metabolic syndrome is directly related to the expression of depression and poor self-rated health [143-147], which are known risk factors for chronic low back pain [6,7].

Knowledge of the metabolic syndrome-pain relationship may be very important, for without it, manual therapists can be led astray to believe that painful conditions not responding to manual care represent "central sensitization syndromes" because it is often assumed that peripheral system is no longer injured or inflamed if manual care is unsuccessful [148]. In contrast, as stated earlier, the emerging impression is that inflammatory chemistry of the metabolic syndrome becomes superimposed over areas of strain or a previous injury and reduces tissue healing and/or leads to ongoing nociception [10,14,35].

As the pro-inflammatory metabolic syndrome is a predecessor of type 2 diabetes, it should not be a surprise that type 2 diabetes is an inflammatory state. At least as early as 2002, review articles outlined how chronic inflammation is the *cause* of insulin resistance and type 2 diabetes [149]. When studies demonstrate that type 2 diabetics have significantly more complications from lumbar fusion surgery [150], the view should not merely be that this is because they have diabetes and do not heal well. While this is true, the correct view is that diabetes is a non-healing state because it is a chronic inflammatory state.

In addition to the pro-inflammatory chemistry outlined in Table 2, patients with type 2 diabetes also have increased circulating painful pro-inflammatory prostaglandins compared to controls [151]. Not surprisingly, these patients are more likely to experience a host of musculoskeletal pain syndromes. Of interest to note is that patients with type II diabetes are known to have altered proteoglycan metabolism in their intervertbral discs, which may promote weakening of the annular fibers and disc herniation [152]. The implication to consider is that the microanatomy of the musculoskeletal system may change in the presence of chronic inflammatory states, such as adiposopathy, the metabolic syndrome, and type 2 diabetes. Recent tendinopathy research supports this contention.

While a waist girth of over 40 inches for men is a risk factor for the metabolic syndrome, it should not be assumed measurements below 40 inches are not associated with inflammation and adiposopathy. A recent study identified that asymptomatic men aged 40 years and older, with a waist girth of more than 33 inches, had the greatest prevalence of Achilles tendinopathy based on ultrasound examination [153]. An earlier study with elite volleyball players also indicated that a waistline measure above 33 inches was associated with an increased risk of tendon pathology; in this case, patella tendinopathy [20]. While a traditional conclusion would be that mechanical loading would be the cause of tendinopathy in such athletes, the authors provided additional insights:

> "Waist girth is a good measure of abdominal adipose tissue, and this tissue releases free fatty acids into the circulation during adipocyte lipolysis, as well as pro-inflammatory cytokines. Free fatty acids and cytokines have been linked to disorders such as heart disease and diabetes. These biochemical substances may also adversely affect tendon function and metabolism and predispose to pathology and abnormal imaging. Therefore, waist girth may have a biochemical as well as a mechanical influence on the development of patellar tendon pathology" [20].

While central accumulation of adipose tissue is known to be harmful to tendons (21), it is unlikely that increased loading adequately explains the development of tendinopathy [19]. It is more likely that tendons are compromised by pro-inflammatory metabolic factors associated with an elevated BMI, such that, "lipid deposition is known to occur in tendons, high cholesterol levels have been observed among individuals with Achilles tendon rupture, and the esterified fraction of cholesterol is elevated in biopsies from Achilles tendinopathy subjects" [19]. In other words, the anatomy, and thus, the integrity of the musculoskeletal system is known to be changed by adiposity, perhaps rendering it more susceptible to injury during mechanical loading. These studies support the suggestion that, "it may be appropriate to redefine our concept of tendinopathy to that of a cardiovascular disease (CVD)," and that "perhaps treating CVD risk factors will improve the treatment of tendinopathy" [19].

Treatment considerations

While the intent of this commentary is not to provide detailed or specific treatments, as this can vary among patients, general management considerations are appropriate to mention. A growing body of evidence clearly implicates pro-inflammatory body chemistry as an initiator and/or perpetuator of musculoskeletal pain syndromes, and thus, the potential for altered chemistry should be considered during patient assessment, especially when an elevated BMI is identified.

While not all patients with an elevated BMI suffer from a chronic inflammatory state, an elevated BMI should be viewed as a potential initiator/promoter of musculoskeletal pain. The risk factors listed in Table 1 can be used to help determine which patients are systemically inflamed. Some are direct markers, including glucose, triglycerides, HDL cholesterol, hsCRP, and vitamin D, while the remainder are surrogate markers of inflammation.

The treatment approach to reduce adiposopathy and the metabolic syndrome can involve multiple anti-inflammatory lifestyle modifications including dietary changes, nutritional supplements, stress management, exercise, and ensuring adequate sleep. Depending on a practitioner's training, practice scope, and the potential need for pharmacologic interventions, co-management of certain patients will be likely.

Conclusion

Historically, an elevated BMI was viewed as a storage depot of excess energy due to overeating and/or a lack of exercise. The systemic pro-inflammatory metabolic consequences of an elevated BMI were unknown until recently, which demands that clinicians modify their views about the influence that weight gain can have on human health.

An elevated BMI may or may not be associated with low back pain and other musculoskeletal pain syndromes. However, as the metabolic syndrome is a universal driver of disease expression, including musculoskeletal pain syndromes, it is incumbent upon the chiropractic profession to identify patients at risk. Identifying adiposopathy and the metabolic syndrome can have a substantial public health impact as patients may only present with musculoskeletal pain and yet have the chronic inflammatory chemistry that promotes heart disease, cancer, and other chronic diseases.

Competing interests
While Dr. Seaman is a paid consultant for Anabolic Laboratories, a manufacturer and distributer of nutritional supplements, no supplements are discussed in this article and he was not financed to write this article.

Author contribution
DRS is the sole author of this manuscript.

References

1. Cordain L, Eaton SB, Sebastian A, Mann N, Lindeberg S, Watkins BA, O'Keefe JH, Brand-Miller J: **Origins and evolution of the Western diet: health implications for the 21st century.** *Am J Clin Nutr* 2005, **81**:341–354.
2. Bays HE, Gonzalez-Campoy M, Henry RR, Bergman DA, Kitabchi AE, Schorr AB, Rodbard HW: **Is adiposopathy (sick fat) an endocrine disease?** *Int J Clin Pract* 2008, **62**:1474–1483.
3. Leboeuf-Yde C: **Body weight and low back pain. A systematic literature review of 56 journal articles reporting on 65 epidemiologic studies.** *Spine* 2000, **25**:226–237.
4. Chou R, Qaseem A, Snow V, Casey D, Cross JT Jr, Shekelle P, Owens DK: **Diagnosis and treatment of low back pain: a joint clinical practice guideline from the American College of Physicians and the American Pain Society.** *Ann Intern Med* 2007, **147**:478–491.
5. Bouwmeester W, van Enst A, van Tulder M: **Quality of low back pain guidelines improved.** *Spine* 2009, **34**:2562–2567.
6. Rubin DI: **Epidemiology and risk factors for spine pain.** *Neurol Clin* 2007, **25**:353–371.
7. Lebovits A, Hainline B, Stone LS, Seminowicz DA, Brunz JT, Rosenquist RW, Cowan P: **Struck from behind: maintaining quality of life with chronic low back pain.** *J Pain* 2009, **10**:927–931.
8. Stone AA, Broderick JE: **Obesity and pain are associated in the United States.** *Obesity* 2012, **20**:1491–1495.
9. Wright LJ, Schur E, Noonan C, Ahumada S, Buchwald D, Afari N: **Chronic pain, overweight, and obesity: findings from a community-based twin registry.** *J Pain* 2010, **11**:628–635.
10. Shiri R, Karppinen J, Leino-Arjas P, Solovieva S, Viikari-Juntura E: **The association between obesity and low back pain: a meta-analysis.** *Am J Epidemiol* 2010, **171**:135–154.
11. Heuch I, Hagen K, Heuch I, Nygaard Ø, Zwart JA: **The impact of body mass index on the prevalence of low back pain: the HUNT study.** *Spine* 2010, **35**:764–768.
12. Heuch I, Heuch I, Hagen K, Zwart JA: **Body mass index as a risk factor for developing chronic low back pain: A Follow-up in the Nord-Trøndelag Health Study.** *Spine* 2012: [Epub ahead of print].
13. Briggs MS, Givens DL, Schmitt LC, Taylor CA: **The relationships of C-reactive protein and obesity to the prevalence and odds of reporting low back pain.** *Arch Phys Med Rehabil* 2012, **S0003-9993**(12):01187–09993. doi:10.1016/j.apmr.2012.11.026. Epub ahead of print].
14. Mantyselka P, Miettola J, Niskanen L, Kumpusalo E: **Persistent pain at multiple sites-connection to glucose derangement.** *Diabetes Res Clin Pract* 2009, **84**(2):e30–e32.
15. Mantyselka P, Miettola J, Niskanen L, Kumpusalo E: **Glucose regulation and chronic pain at multiple sites.** *Rheumatology* 2008, **47**:1235–1238.
16. Mantyselka P, Miettola J, Niskanen L, Kumpusalo E: **Chronic pain, impaired glucose tolerance and diabetes: a community-based study.** *Pain* 2008, **137**:34–40.
17. Mantyselka P, Kautianen H, Vanhala M: **Prevalence of neck pain in subjects with metabolic syndrome - a cross-sectional population-based study.** *BMC Musculoskelet Disord* 2010, **11**:171.
18. Rechardt M, Shiri R, Karppinen J, Jula A, Heliövaara M, Viikari-Juntura E: **Lifestyle and metabolic factors in relation to shoulder pain and rotator**

cuff tendinitis: A population-based study. *BMC Musculoskelet Disord* 2010, **11**:165.
19. Gaida JE, Alfredson L, Kiss ZS, Wilson AM, Alfredson H, Cook JL: **Dyslipidemia in Achilles tendinopathy is characteristic of insulin resistance.** *Med Sci Sports Exerc* 2009, **41**:1194–1197.
20. Malliaras P, Cook JL, Kent PM: **Anthropometric risk factors for patellar tendon injury among volleyball players.** *Br J Sports Med* 2007, **41**:259–263.
21. Shiri R, Viikari-Juntura E, Varonen H, Heliovaara M: **Prevalence and determinants of lateral and medial epicondylitis: a population study.** *Am J Epidemiol* 2006, **164**:1065–1074.
22. Jhawar BS, Fuchs CS, Colditz GA, Stampfer MJ: **Cardiovascular risk factors for physician-diagnosed lumbar disc herniation.** *Spine J* 2006, **6**:684–691.
23. Kauppila LI, McAlindon T, Evans S, Wilson PW, Kiel D, Felson DT: **Disc degeneration/back pain and calcification of the abdominal aorta: a 25-year follow-up study in Framingham.** *Spine* 1997, **22**:1642–1647.
24. Kurunlahti M, Tervonen O, Vanharanta H, Ilkko E, Suramo I: **Association of atherosclerosis with low back pain and the degree of disc degeneration.** *Spine* 1999, **24**:2080–2084.
25. Kauppila LI, Mikkonen R, Mankinen P, Pelto-Vasenius K, Mäenpää I: **MR aortography and serum cholesterol levels in patients with long-term non-specific lower back pain.** *Spine* 2004, **29**:2347–2352.
26. Leino-Arjas P, Kaila-Kangas L, Solovieva S, Riihimäki H, Kirjonen J, Reunanen A: **Serum lipids and low back pain: an association? A follow-up study of a working population sample.** *Spine* 2006, **31**:1032–1037.
27. Leino-Arjas P, Solovieva S, Kirjonen J, Reunanen A, Riihimäki H: **Cardiovascular risk factors and low-back pain in a long-term follow-up of industrial employees.** *Scand J Work Environ Health* 2006, **32**:12–19.
28. Shiri R, Karppinen J, Leino-Arjas P, Solovieva S, Varonen H, Kalso E, Ukkola O, Viikari-Juntura E: **Cardiovascular and lifestyle risk factors in lumbar radicular pain or clinically defined sciatica: a systematic review.** *Eur Spine J* 2007, **16**:2043–2054.
29. Leino-Arjas P, Kauppila L, Kaila-Kangas L, Shiri R, Heistaro S, Heliövaara M: **Serum lipids in relation to sciatica among Finns.** *Atherosclerosis* 2008, **197**:43–49.
30. Kauppila LI: **Atherosclerosis and disc degeneration/low back pain – a systematic review.** *Eur J Vasc Endovasc Surg* 2009, **37**:661–670.
31. Heuch I, Heuch I, Hagen K, Zwart JA: **Associations between serum lipid levels and chronic low back pain.** *Epidemiology* 2010, **21**:837–841.
32. Conaghan PG, Vanharanta H, Dieppe PA: **Is progressive osteoarthritis an atheromatous vascular disease?** *Ann Rheum Dis* 2005, **64**:1539–1541.
33. Masuko K, Murata M, Suematsu N, Okamoto K, Yudoh K, Nakamura H, Kato T: **A metabolic aspect of osteoarthritis: lipid as a possible contributor to the pathogenesis of cartilage degradation.** *Clin Exp Rheumatol* 2009, **27**:347–353.
34. Gkretsi V, Simopoulou T, Tsezou A: **Lipid metabolism and osteoarthritis: lessons from atherosclerosis.** *Prog Lipid Res* 2011, **50**:133–140.
35. Berenbaum F: **Osteoarthritis as an inflammatory disease (osteoarthritis is not osteoarthrosis).** *Osteoarthr Cartil* 2013, **21**:16–21.
36. Abate M, Schiavone C, Pelotti P, Salini V: **Limited joint mobility (LJM) in elderly subjects with type II diabetes mellitus.** *Arch Gerontol Geriatrics* 2011, **53**:135–140.
37. Lotan R, Oron A, Anekstein Y, Shalmon E, Mirovsky Y: **Lumbar stenosis and systemic diseases: is there any relevance.** *J Spinal Disord Tech* 2008, **21**:247–251.
38. Anekstein Y, Smorgick Y, Lotan R, Agar G, Shalmon E, Floman Y, Mirovsky Y: **Diabetes mellitus as a risk factor for the development of lumbar spinal stenosis.** *Isr Med Assoc J* 2010, **12**:16–20.
39. Sakellaridis N: **The influence of diabetes mellitus on lumbar intervertebral disk herniation.** *Surg Neurol* 2006, **66**:152–154.
40. Sakellaridis N, Androulis A: **Influence of diabetes mellitus on cervical intervertebral disc herniation.** *Clin Neurol Neurosurg* 2008, **110**:810–812.
41. Bays HE: **Adiposopathy: is sick fat a cardiovascular disease?** *J Am Coll Cardiol* 2011, **57**:2461–2473.
42. Bays H: **Adiposopathy, diabetes mellitus, and primary prevention of atherosclerotic coronary artery disease: treating "sick fat" through improving fat function with antidiabetes therapies.** *Am J Cardiol* 2012, **110**(suppl):4B–12B.
43. Sommer C, Birklein F: **Resolvins and inflammatory pain.** *F1000 Med Rep* 2011, **3**:19. doi:10.3410/M3-19.
44. Sommer C, Birklein F: **Fighting off pain with resolvins.** *Nat Med* 2010, **16**(5):518–520.
45. Ji RR, Xu ZZ, Strichartz G, Serhan CN: **Emerging roles of resolvins in the resolution of inflammation and pain.** *Trends Neurosci* 2011, **34**:599–609.
46. Xu ZZ, Zhang L, Liu T, Park JY, Berta T, Yang R, Serhan CN, Ji RR: **Resolvins RvE1 and RvD1 attenuate inflammatory pain via central and peripheral actions.** *Nat Med* 2010, **16**:592–597.
47. Nathan C, Ding A: **Nonresolving inflammation.** *Cell* 2010, **140**:871–882.
48. Serhan CN, Brain SD, Buckley CD, Gilroy DW, Haslett C, O'Neill LA, Perretti M, Rossi AG, Wallace JL: **Resolution of inflammation: state of the art, definitions and terms.** *FASEB J* 2007, **21**:325–332.
49. Zhang MJ, Spite M: **Resolvins: anti-inflammatory and proresolving mediators derived from omega-3 polyunsaturated fatty acids.** *Annu Rev Nutr* 2012, **32**:203–227.
50. Campbell EL, Serhan CN, Colgan SP: **Antimicrobial aspects of inflammatory resolution in the mucosa: a role for proresolving mediators.** *J Immunol* 2011, **187**:3475–3481.
51. Das UN: **Is multiple sclerosis a proresolution deficiency disorder?** *Nutrition* 2012, **28**:951–958.
52. Ross R: **Atherosclerosis–an inflammatory disease.** *N Engl J Med* 1999, **340**:115–126.
53. Biasucci LM, Colizzi C, Rizzello V, Vitrella G, Crea F, Liuzzo G: **Role of inflammation in the pathogenesis of unstable coronary artery diseases.** *Scand J Clin Lab Invest Suppl* 1999, **230**:12–22.
54. Das UN: **Is obesity and inflammatory condition?** *Nutrition* 2001, **17**:953–966.
55. Seaman DR: **The diet-induced pro-inflammatory state: a cause of chronic pain and other degenerative diseases?** *J Manip Physiol Ther* 2002, **25**:168–179.
56. Ridker PM: **C-reactive protein: a simple test to help predict risk of heart attack and stroke.** *Circulation* 2003, **108**:81–85.
57. Nicklas BJ, You T, Pahor M: **Behavioural treatments for chronic systemic inflammation: effects of dietary weight loss and exercise training.** *CMAJ* 2005, **172**:1199–1209.
58. Esposito K, Marfella R, Ciotola M, Di Palo C, Giugliano F, Giugliano G, D'Armiento M, D'Andrea F, Giugliano D: **Effect of a mediterranean-style diet on endothelial dysfunction and markers of vascular inflammation in the metabolic syndrome: a randomized trial.** *JAMA* 2004, **292**:1440–1446.
59. Esposito K, Giugliano D: **Diet and inflammation: a link to metabolic and cardiovascular diseases.** *Eur Heart J* 2006, **27**:15–20.
60. Giugliano D, Ceriello A, Esposito K: **The effects of diet on inflammation: emphasis on the metabolic syndrome.** *J Am Coll Cardiol* 2006, **48**:677–685.
61. Basu A, Devaraj S, Jialol I: **Dietary factors that promote or retard inflammation.** *Arterioscler Thromb Vasc Biol* 2006, **26**:995–1001.
62. O'Keefe JH, Bell DS: **Postprandial hyperglycemia/hyperlipidemia (postprandial dysmetabolism) is a cardiovascular risk factor.** *Am J Cardiol* 2007, **100**:899–904.
63. O'Keefe JH, Gheewala NM, O'Keefe JO: **Dietary strategies for improving post-prandial glucose, lipids, inflammation, and cardiovascular health.** *J Am Coll Cardiol* 2008, **51**:249–255.
64. Frassetto LA, Schloetter M, Mietus-Synder M, Morris RC, Sebastian A: **Metabolic and physiologic improvements from consuming a paleolithic, hunter-gatherer type diet.** *Eur J Clin Nutr* 2009, **63**:947–955.
65. Egger G, Dixon J: **Inflammatory effects of nutritional stimuli: further support for the need for a big picture approach to tackling obesity and chronic disease.** *Obes Rev* 2010, **11**:137–149.
66. Guyton AC, Hall JE: *Textbook of medical physiology.* Philadelphia: Saunders; 2011.
67. Kumar V, Abbas AK, Fausto N, Aster J (Eds): *Robbins & Cotran Pathologic Basis of Disease.* 8th edition. Philadelphia: Saunders; 2010.
68. Bonner WM, Jonsson H, Malanos C, Bryant M: **Changes in lipids of human articular cartilage with age.** *Arthritis Rheum* 1975, **18**:461–473.
69. Goldenberg DL, Egan MS, Cohen AS: **Inflammatory synovitis in degenerative joint disease.** *J Rheumatol* 1982, **9**:204–209.
70. Adkisson HD, Risener FS, Zarrinkar PP, Walla MD, Christie WW, Wuthier RE: **Unique fatty acid composition of normal cartilage: discovery of high levels of n-9 eicosatrienoic acid and low levels of n-6 polyunsaturated fatty acids.** *FASEB J* 1991, **5**:344–353.
71. Nakamura H, Yoshino S, Kato T, Tsuruha J, Nishioka K: **T-cell mediated inflammatory pathway in osteoarthritis.** *Osteoarthritis Cart* 1999, **7**:401–402.
72. Nishioka K: **Autoimmune response in cartilage-derived peptides in a patient with osteoarthritis.** *Arth Res Ther* 2003, **6**:6–7.

73. Kato T, Xiang Y, Nakamura H, Nishioka K: **Neoantigens in osteoarthritic cartilage.** *Curr Opin Rheumatol* 2004, **16:**604–608.
74. Lamon BD, Hajjar DP: **Inflammation at the molecular interface of atherogenesis: an anthropological journey.** *Am J Pathol* 2008, **173:**1253–1264.
75. Bonnet CS, Walsh DA: **Osteoarthritis, angiogenesis and inflammation.** *Rheumatology* 2005, **44:**7–16.
76. Tiku ML, Shah R, Allison GT: **Evidence link chondrocyte lipid peroxidation to cartilage matrix protein degradation: possible role in cartilage aging and the pathogenesis of osteoarthritis.** *J Biol Chem* 2000, **275:**20069–20076.
77. Tiku ML, Allison GT, Naik K, Karry SK: **Malondialdehyde oxidation of cartilage collagen by chondrocytes.** *Osteoarthr Cartil* 2003, **11:**159–166.
78. Sturmer T, Sun Y, Sauerland S, Zeissig I, Gunther KP, Puhl W, Brenner H: **Serum cholesterol and osteoarthritis. The baseline examination of the Ulm Osteoarthritis Study.** *J Rheumatol* 1998, **25:**1827–1832.
79. Maes M, Song C, Lin A, Van Gastel A, Kenis G, Bosmans E, De Meester I, Benoy I, Neels H, Demedts P, Janca A, Scharpé S, Smith RS: **The effects of psychological stress on humans: increased production of pro-inflammatory cytokines and TH-1 like response in stress-induced anxiety.** *Cytokine* 1998, **10:**313–318.
80. Bierhaus A, Humpert PM, Nawroth PP: **Linking stress to inflammation.** *Anesthesiol Clin N Am* 2006, **24:**325–340.
81. Simpson N, Dinges DF: **Sleep and inflammation.** *Nutr Rev* 2007, **65:**S244–S252.
82. Irwin MR, Carrillo C, Omstead R: **Sleep loss activates cellular markers of inflammation: sex differences.** *Brain Behav Immunity* 2010, **24:**54–57.
83. Baker RG, Hayden MS, Ghosh S: **NF-κB, inflammation, metabolic disease.** *Cell Metab* 2011, **13:**11–22.
84. Ahn KS, Aggarwal BB: **Transcription factor NF-κB: a sensor for smoke and stress signals.** *Ann NY Acad Sci* 2005, **1056:**218–233.
85. Lekander M, Elofsson S, Neve IM, Hansson LO, Undén AL: **Self-rated health is related to levels of circulating cytokines.** *Psychosom Med* 2004, **66:**559–563.
86. Christian LM, Glaser R, Porter K, Malarkey WB, Beversdorf D, Kiecolt-Glaser JK: **Poorer self-rated health is associated with elevated inflammatory markers among older adults.** *Psychoneuroendocrinology* 2011, **36:**1495–1504.
87. Wium-Andersen MK, Orsted DD, Nielsen SF, Nordestgaard BG: **Elevated C-reactive protein levels, psychological distress, and depression in 73,131 individuals.** *JAMA Psychiatry* 2013, **70:**176–184.
88. Khairova RA, Machado-Vieira R, Du J, Manji HK: **A potential role for pro-inflammatory cytokines in regulating synaptic plasticity in major depressive disorder.** *Int J Neuropsychopharmacol* 2009, **12:**561–578.
89. Miller AH, Maletic V, Raison CL: **Inflammation and its discontents: the role of cytokines in the pathophysiology of major depression.** *Biol Psychiatry* 2009, **65:**732–741.
90. Krishnadas R, Cavanagh J: **Depression: an inflammatory illness?** *J Neurol Neurosurg Psychiatry* 2012, **83:**495–502.
91. Irwin MR: **Inflammation at the intersection of behavior and somatic symptoms.** *Psychiatr Clin N Am* 2011, **34:**605–620.
92. Bonaccorso S, Meltzer HY, Maes M: **Psychological and behavioral effects of interferons.** *Curr Opin Psychiatry* 2000, **13:**673–677.
93. Dantzer R, O'Connor JC, Freund GG, Johnson RW, Kelley KW: **From inflammation to sickness and depression: when the immune system subjugates the brain.** *Nat Rev Neurosci* 2008, **9:**46–56.
94. Spiegel K, Tasali E, Penev P, Van Cauter E: **Sleep curtailment in healthy young men is associated with decreased leptin levels, elevated ghrelin levels and increased hunger and appetite.** *Ann Intern Med* 2004, **141:**846–850.
95. Knutson KL, Spiegel K, Penev P, van Cauter E: **The metabolic consequences of sleep deprivation.** *Sleep Med Rev* 2007, **11:**163–178.
96. Morselli L, Leproult R, Balbo M, Spiegel K: **Role of sleep duration in the regulation of glucose metabolism and appetite.** *Best Prac Res Clin Endocrinol Metab* 2010, **24:**687–702.
97. Lucassen EA, Rother KI, Cizza G: **Interacting epidemics? Sleep curtailment, insulin resistance, and obesity.** *Ann NY Acad Sci* 2012, **1264:**110–134.
98. Dallman MF, Pecoraro NC, la Fleur SE: **Chronic stress and comfort foods: self-medication and abdominal obesity.** *Brain Behav Immun* 2005, **19:**275–280.
99. Adam TC, Epe ES: **Stress, eating and the reward system.** *Physiol Behav* 2007, **91:**449–458.
100. Maniam J, Morris MJ: **The link between stress and feeding behaviour.** *Neuropharmacol* 2012, **63:**97–110.
101. Nedeltcheva AV, Kilkus JM, Imperial J, Schoeller DA, Penev PD: **Insufficient sleep undermines dietary efforts to reduce obesity.** *Ann Int Med* 2010, **153:**435–441.
102. Edwards R, Almeida DM, Klick B, Haythornthwaite JA, Smith MT: **Duration of sleep contributes to next-day pain report in the general population.** *Pain* 2008, **137:**202–207.
103. Mullington JM, Simpson NS, Meier-Ewert HK, Haak M: **Sleep loss and inflammation.** *Best Prac Res Clin Endocrinol Metab* 2010, **24:**775–784.
104. Motivala SJ: **Sleep and inflammation. psychoneuroimmunology in the context of cardiovascular disease.** *Ann Behav Med* 2011, **42:**141–152.
105. Black PH: **The inflammatory consequences of psychologic stress: relationship to insulin resistance, obesity, atherosclerosis and diabetes mellitus, type II.** *Med Hypoth* 2006, **67:**879–891.
106. Petersen AM, Pedersen BK: **The anti-inflammatory effects of exercise.** *J Appl Physiol* 2005, **98:**1154–1162.
107. Mathur N, Pedersen BK: **Exercise as a means to control low-grade systemic inflammation.** *Mediators Inflamm* 2008, **2008:**109502.
108. Rethorst CD, Toups MS, Greer TL, Nakonezny PA, Carmody TJ, Brannermann BD, Huebinger RM, Barber RC, Trivedi MH: **Pro-inflammatory cytokines as predictors of antidepressant effects of exercise in major depressive disorder.** *Mol Psychiatry* 2012. doi:10.1038/mp.2012.125 [Epub ahead of print].
109. Santos RV, Viana VA, Boscolo RA, Marques VG, Santana MG, Lira FS, Tufik S, de Mello MT: **Moderate exercise training modulates cytokine profile and sleep in elderly people.** *Cytokine* 2012: [Epub ahead of print].
110. Teixeira de Lemos E, Oliveira J, Páscoa Pinheiro J, Reis F: **Regular physical exercise as a strategy to improve antioxidant and anti-inflammatory status: benefits in type 2 diabetes mellitus.** *Oxid Med Cell Longev* 2012, **2012:**741545.
111. Lees SJ, Booth FW: **Sedentary death syndrome.** *Can J Appl Physiol* 2004, **29:**447–460.
112. Norman A, Bellocco R, Vaida F, Wolk A: **Total physical activity in relation to age, body mass, health and other factors in a cohort of Swedish men.** *Int J Obesity* 2002, **26:**670–675.
113. Sodergren M, Sundquist J, Johansson SE, Sundquist K: **Physical activity, exercise and self-rated health: a population-based study from Sweden.** *BMC Publ Health* 2008, **8:**352. doi:10.1186/1471-2458-8-352.
114. Darviri C, Fouka G, Gnardellis C, Artemiadis AK, Tigani X, Alexopoulos EC: **Determinants of self-rated health in a representative sample of a rural population: a cross-sectional study in Greece.** *Int J Environ Res Public Health* 2012, **9:**943–954.
115. Babyak M, Blumenthal JA, Herman S, Khatri P, Doraiswamy M, Moore K, Craighead E, Baldewicz TT, Krishnan R: **Exercise treatment for major depression: maintenance of therapeutic benefit at 10 months.** *Psychosom Med* 2000, **62:**633–638.
116. Galic S, Oakhill JS, Steinberg GR: **Adipose tissue as an endocrine organ.** *Mol Cell Endocrinol* 2010, **316:**129–139.
117. Sell H, Eckel J: **Adipose tissue inflammation: novel insight into the role of macrophages and lymphocytes.** *Curr Opin Clin Nutr Metab Care* 2010, **13:**366–370.
118. Chandran M, Phillips SA, Ciaraldi T, Henry RR: **Adiponectin: more than just another fat cell hormone?** *Diabetes Care* 2003, **26:**2442–2450.
119. Lustig Y, Hemi R, Kanety H: **Regulation and function of adiponectin receptors in skeletal muscle.** *Vitam Horm* 2012, **90:**95–123.
120. Uceyler N, Valenza R, Stock M, Schedel R, Sprotte G, Sommer C: **Reduced levels of antiinflammatory cytokines in patients with chronic widespread pain.** *Arthritis Rheum* 2006, **54:**2656–2664.
121. Saraiva M, O'Garra A: **The regulation of IL-10 production by immune cells.** *Nat Rev Immunol* 2010, **10:**170–181.
122. Park HS, Park LY, Yu R: **Relationship of obesity and visceral adiposity with serum concentrations of CRP, TNF-alpha and IL-6.** *Diabetes Res Clin Pract* 2005, **69:**29–35.
123. Harford KA, Reynolds CM, McGillicuddy FC, Roche HM: **Fats, inflammation and insulin resistance: insights to the role of macrophage and T-cell accumulation in adipose tissue.** *Proc Nutr Soc* 2011, **70:**408–417.
124. Schipper HS, Prakken B, Kalkhoven E, Boes M: **Adipose tissue-resident immune cells: key players in immunometabolism.** *Trends Endocrinol Metab* 2012, **23:**407–415.
125. Antuna-Puente B, Feve B, Fellahi S, Bastard AP: **Adipokines: the missing link between insulin resistance and obesity.** *Diabetes Metab* 2008, **34:**2–11.

126. Suganami T, Ogawa Y: **Adipose tissue macrophages: their role in adipose tissue remodeling.** *J Leukoc Biol* 2010, **88**:33–39.
127. Fain JN: **Release of inflammatory mediators by human adipose tissue is enhanced in obesity and primarily by the nonfat cells: a review.** *Mediators Inflamm* 2010: Article ID: 513948.
128. Wilson PW, Grundy SM: **The metabolic syndrome: practical guide to origins and treatment: Part I.** *Circulation* 2003, **108**:1422–1424.
129. Helminen EE, Mäntyselkä P, Nykänen I, Kumpusalo E: **Far from easy and accurate - detection of metabolic syndrome by general practitioners.** *BMC Fam Pract* 2009, **10**:76.
130. Golbidi S, Mesdaghinia A, Laher I: **Exercise in the metabolic syndrome.** *Oxid Med Cell Longev* 2012, **2012**:349710.
131. Pussinen PJ, Havulinna AS, Lehto M, Sundvall J, Salomaa V: **Endotoxemia is associated with an increased risk of incident diabetes.** *Diabetes Care* 2011, **34**:392–397.
132. de la Llera MM, McGillicuddy FC, Hinkle CC, Byrne M, Joshi MR, Nguyen V, Tabita-Martinez J, Wolfe ML, Badellino K, Pruscino L, Mehta NN, Asztalos BF, Reilly MP: **Inflammation modulates human HDL composition and function in vivo.** *Atherosclerosis* 2012, **222**:390–394.
133. Guillot X, Semerano L, Saidenberg-Kermanac'h N, Falgarone G, Boissier MC: **Vitamin D and inflammation.** *Joint Bone Spine* 2010, **77**:552–557.
134. Hypponen E, Boucher BJ, Berry DJ, Power C: **25-hydroxyvitamin D, IGF-1, and the metabolic syndrome at 45 years of age. A cross-sectional study in the 1958 British Birth Cohort.** *Diabetes* 2008, **57**:298–305.
135. Schwalfenberg G: **Improvement of chronic back pain or failed back surgery with vitamin D repletion: a case series.** *J Am Board Fam Med* 2009, **22**:69–74.
136. Ford ES, Giles WH, Dietz WH: **Prevalence of the metabolic syndrome among US adults: findings from the Third National Health and Nutrition Examination Survey.** *JAMA* 2002, **287**:356–359.
137. Dandona P, Aljada A, Chaudhuri A, Mohanty P, Garg R: **Metabolic Syndrome - a comprehensive perspective based on interactions between obesity, diabetes, and inflammation.** *Circulation* 2005, **111**:1448–1454.
138. Blaha M, Elasy TA: **Clinical use of the metabolic syndrome: why the confusion?** *Clin Diabetes* 2006, **24**:125–131.
139. Facchini FS, Hua N, Abbasi F, Reaven GM: **Insulin resistance as a predictor of age-related disease.** *J Clin Endocrinol Metab* 2001, **86**:3574–3578.
140. Cordain L, Eades MR, Eades MD: **Hyperinsulinemic diseases of civilization: more than just syndrome X.** *Compar Biochem Physiol* 2003, **136**:95–112.
141. Cowy S, Hardy RW: **The metabolic syndrome: A high-risk state for cancer?** *Am J Pathol* 2006, **169**:1505–1522.
142. Barclay AW, Petocz P, McMillan-Price J, Flood VM, Prvan T, Mitchell P, Brand-Miller JC: **Glycemic index, glycemic load, and chronic disease risk–a meta-analysis of observational studies.** *Am J Clin Nutr* 2008, **87**:627–637.
143. Heiskanen TH, Niskanen LK, Hintikka JJ, Koivumaa-Honkanen HT, Honkalampi KM, Haatainen KM, Viinamäki HT: **Metabolic syndrome and depression: a cross-sectional analysis.** *J Clin Psychiatry* 2006, **67**:1422–1427.
144. Koponen H, Jokelainen J, Keinänen-Kiukaanniemi S, Kumpusalo E, Vanhala M: **Metabolic syndrome predisposes to depressive symptoms: a population-based 7-year follow-up study.** *J Clin Psychiatry* 2008, **69**:178–182.
145. Miettola J, Niskanen LK, Viinamäki H, Kumpusalo E: **Metabolic syndrome is associated with self-perceived depression.** *Scand J Prim Health Care* 2008, **26**:203–210.
146. Akbaraly TN, Ancelin ML, Jaussent I, Ritchie C, Barberger-Gateau P, Dufouil C, Kivimaki M, Berr C, Ritchie K: **Metabolic syndrome and onset of depressive symptoms in the elderly: findings from the three-city study.** *Diabetes Care* 2011, **34**:904–909.
147. Saudny H, Cao Z, Egeland GM: **Poor self-reported health and its association with biomarkers among Canadian Inuit.** *Int J Circumpolar Health* 2012, **71**:18589. http://dx.doi.org/10.3402/ijch.v71i0.18589.
148. Nijs J, Van Houdenhove B, Oostendorp RA: **Recognition of central sensitization in patients with musculoskeletal pain: Application of pain neurophysiology in manual therapy practice.** *Manual Ther* 2010, **15**:135–141.
149. Grimble RF: **Inflammatory status and insulin resistance.** *Curr Opin Clin Nutr Metab Care* 2002, **5**:551–559.
150. Glassman SD, Alegre G, Carreon L, Dimar JR, Johnson JR: **Perioperative complications of lumbar instrumentation and fusion in patients with diabetes mellitus.** *Spine J* 2003, **3**:496–501.
151. Helmersson J, Vessby B, Larsson A, Basu S: **Association of type 2 diabetes with cylcooxygenase-mediated inflammation and oxidative stress in an elderly population.** *Circulation* 2004, **109**:1729–1734.
152. Robinson D, Mirovsky Y, Halperin N, Evron Z, Nevo Z: **Changes in proteoglycans of intervertebral disc in diabetic patients: a possible cause of increased back pain.** *Spine* 1998, **23**:849–856.
153. Gaida JE, Alfredson H, Kiss ZS, Bass SL, Cook JL: **Asymptomatic Achilles tendon pathology is associated with a central fat distribution in men and a peripheral fat distribution in women: a cross sectional study of 298 individuals.** *BMC Musculoskelet Disord* 2010, **11**:41.

25

Mapping intended spinal site of care from the upright to prone position: an interexaminer reliability study

Robert Cooperstein* and Morgan Young

Abstract

Background: Upright examination procedures like radiology, thermography, manual muscle testing, and spinal motion palpation may lead to spinal interventions with the patient prone. The reliability and accuracy of mapping upright examination findings to the prone position is unknown. This study had 2 primary goals: (1) investigate how erroneous spine-scapular landmark associations may lead to errors in treating and charting spine levels; and (2) study the interexaminer reliability of a novel method for mapping upright spinal sites to the prone position.

Methods: Experiment 1 was a thought experiment exploring the consequences of depending on the erroneous landmark association of the inferior scapular tip with the T7 spinous process upright and T6 spinous process prone (relatively recent studies suggest these levels are T8 and T9, respectively). This allowed deduction of targeting and charting errors. In experiment 2, 10 examiners (2 experienced, 8 novice) used an index finger to maintain contact with a mid-thoracic spinous process as each of 2 participants slowly moved from the upright to the prone position. Interexaminer reliability was assessed by computing Intraclass Correlation Coefficient, standard error of the mean, root mean squared error, and the absolute value of the mean difference for each examiner from the 10 examiner mean for each of the 2 participants.

Results: The thought experiment suggesting that using the (inaccurate) scapular tip landmark rule would result in a 3 level targeting and charting error when radiological findings are mapped to the prone position. Physical upright exam procedures like motion palpation would result in a 2 level targeting error for intervention, and a 3 level error for charting. The reliability experiment showed examiners accurately maintained contact with the same thoracic spinous process as the participant went from upright to prone, ICC (2,1) = 0.83.

Conclusions: As manual therapists, the authors have emphasized how targeting errors may impact upon manual care of the spine. Practitioners in other fields that need to accurately locate spinal levels, such as acupuncture and anesthesiology, would also be expected to draw important conclusions from these findings.

Introduction

Manual therapists use a great variety of physical examination methods to identify the optimal site of care for spinal complaints. Examiners have generally focused on joint malposition and joint hypomobility, or static and dynamic findings of abnormality, respectively. In addition, some contemporary practitioners have emphasized so-called provocation listings, which entail determining the impact of provocative interventions. These include changes in patient body position, orthopedic testing, joint challenges, and contacts with putative reflex points of various kinds [1]. Mnemonics such as P.A.R.T.S. [2,3] in chiropractic and TART [4,5] in osteopathy conveniently categorize the examination methods used by manual therapists. As convenient as such categorizations may be to inventory and assay manual therapy examination methods, they do not capture how the procedures are performed nor what differences may exist among practitioners methods of deployment. (Table 1 lists the components of P.A.R.T.S. and TART). As a case in point, neither P.A.R.T.S. nor TART specifies the *position* in which the patient is assessed. Variations in the patient positioning procedure may lead to very different conclusions about the optimal site of care,

* Correspondence: cooperstein_r@palmer.edu
Palmer West College of Chiropractic, 90 East Tasman Drive, San Jose, CA 95134, USA

Table 1 Acronyms used in manual therapy to summarize examination procedures

PARTS acronym (chiropractic) [2,3]	TART acronym (osteopathy) [4,5]
*P*ain: location, quality, intensity of pain or tenderness	*T*issue texture changes: temperature, tense, flabby, edematous, fibrotic, indurated, hypertonic, hypertrophied
*A*symmetry: of sectional or regional spinal components identified by static palpation of structures	*A*symmetry in joint motion; e.g., compared with contralateral tissues
*R*ange of motion: Decrease or loss of specific active or passive movements identified by motion palpation	*R*estriction of joint motion: degree and quality of pliability, mobility, stability; quality of end-feel
*T*one, *T*exture, *T*emperature: changes in specific soft tissues identified through palpation	*T*enderness (or sensitivity) of soft tissues: unnaturally sensitive, tender, painful, numb with pressure or on active/passive movement
*S*pecial tests: linked to proprietary technique systems, not in general use	

Table 2 Inferior scapular angle and spinal landmark association

	Spinal level, conventional wisdom	Spinal level, evidence-based
Upright IAS	T7	T8
Prone IAS	T6	T9

the vector, and the other force characteristics deployed in spinal manipulation and other interventions. This may impact upon the reliability, validity, and ultimately clinical utility of the examination procedure.

As an example, there is some evidence that supine measurements of cervical rotational range of motion are not correlated with seated measurements [6-9]. Notwithstanding the gross similarity of supine and seated measuring methods, seated weight-bearing and supine non-weight bearing measures of range of motion apparently assess different clinical phenomena. This could lead to different clinical interventions. As another example of patient position-dependent examination findings, the relative position of the posterior superior iliac spines depends on whether the patient is standing or upright. Asymmetry seen in the standing position might be different and even reversed in the seated position [10]. As a final example of how patient position impacts physical examination findings, the position of the inferior angle of the scapula (IAS) in relation to the spine varies between the upright and prone positions; and also depends on the patient's arm position [11-13]. Furthermore, the scapula tends to be relatively inferior on the side of the dominant arm [14]. These scapular anatomic findings and their clinical implications became the impetus for this study.

Although it is widely believed that on average the IAS is at the T7 spinous process (SP) when upright, and the T6 SP when prone, there are data in the manual therapy literature suggesting otherwise [11-13]. Table 2 compares the conventional wisdom ("7 up, 6 down"), with evidence-based findings ("8 up, 9 down") on the location of the IAS in relation to the SPs. The position of the IAS also varies according to the patient's arm positions on the table [12]. The data show a range of T6-T10 for the standing scapular tip, and T7-T11 for the prone scapular tip [11-13].

Three studies by anesthesiologists came to similar conclusions. Using a radiological reference standard, Teoh [15] found the IAS in the standing position to be on average nearest to the T8 SP, as did Arzola [16] using a portable ultrasound system reference standard. Kim [17], using a radiological reference standard, found the scapular tip usually lined up with the T7 rather than T8 SP as in the other 2 anesthesiology studies. The discrepancy is only in appearance, since Kim's data were gathered in the "epidural position" (seated, back arched, neck flexed, arms across the chest), which is known to raise the scapular tip by one level compared to where it lies in the "anatomical position" (thorax fully upright, palms anterior). Thus, Kim's data for the upright position can be easily transformed to upright findings by simply subtracting one vertebral level from each reported data point, rendering this researcher's data consistent the other anesthesiology studies. Ernst [18], using cross-comparison with other manually palpated anatomical landmarks, also reported the IAS to correspond to the T8 SP.

The purpose of the present study was two-fold, resulting in two experiments. In the first, the authors derive conclusions based on scapular landmarks for the practice of manual therapy and other professions (including nursing, surgery, anesthesiology, and acupuncture). In the second experiment, the authors propose and determine the reliability of a novel procedure for mapping spinal sites initially identified upright to the prone position. The overarching goal was to improve upon scapula-based landmark protocols for localizing spinal landmarks that are position-dependent, thus reducing the likelihood of targeting errors.

There has been some assessment of the reliability of static palpation, but these did not explore any issues pertaining to patient-position variations. A systematic review of static palpation of the spine and sacroiliac joints [19] identified 14 studies focused on locating painful or tender points, 10 on the location of landmarks, and 5 on position or alignment of bone structures. Palpation for pain was more reliable than palpation for position, for which examiner concordance was low. A systematic review of the methods used by manual therapists to identify the optimal site for spine care came to the following conclusion for static palpation: "Based on high quality evidence, the validity of palpation for localizing the site of care is unclear" [20]. Neither of these 2 static palpation reviews addressed the complications of using landmarks in the upright position to determine care to be rendered prone.

Experiment 1: Estimating the magnitude of targeting errors

To determine the magnitude of targeting errors attributable to incorrect scapular landmark rules, the authors conducted a *Gedankenexperiment*, or "thought experiment". Thought experiments explore the potential consequences of a principle or hypothesis, sometimes where the outcome is so intuitively obvious that a physical demonstration of this same principle could or would be deemed superfluous.

The magnitude of spinal targeting errors due to using an inaccurate scapular landmark rule may be heuristically calculated by working out two examples, one for radiographic and the other for physical examination procedures. There would be errors in both the site of care and numerated level of care that is charted. In these examples, to simplify the discussion, it is assumed that the IAS is even with a specific vertebral level; even though the IAS lies within a range, as discussed above. Equally discounted is the fact that that the IAS may not lie at the same level on the left and right sides of the body, and would be expected to be relatively inferior on the side of the dominant arm [14].

Example 1: Upright radiographic examination

Suppose a radiograph is being scrutinized to determine a spinal level of interest warranting clinical intervention. (It is acknowledged that the use of radiographic examination for biomechanical analysis is controversial, but that is beyond the scope of this project). Having directly and hypothetically correctly identified T7 on a radiograph, the clinician now attempts to identify the prone T7 SP for the purpose of a manipulative or other manual procedure. If the clinician uses the (inaccurate) landmark rule that the IAS is at the T6 SP while prone, with hands placed on the arm rests, an adjustive contact is made one level lower than the IAS. Since in reality the IAS is at the T9 SP prone, [12] counting down one spinal level results in the clinician contacting T10, not the intended T7 level. Thus, there is a 3-level targeting error. There would also be a 3 level charting error in numerating the site of care, since T7 was the intended but T10 the actual site of care.

Example 2: Upright physical examination

The targeting error for other forms of upright patient assessment is less severe, at least for treatment if not charting. Let us assume that upright (sitting or standing) thermography, manual muscle testing, or motion palpation identifies a vertebral site of care whose SP is at the ISA. Using the traditional benchmark rule, the clinician believes this to be T7, whereas in fact it is more likely closer to T8. If the clinician uses the (inaccurate) landmark rule that the IAS is at the T6 SP while prone, with hands placed on the arm rests, an adjustive contact is made one level lower than the prone IAS. Since the it is actually at T9, counting down one level identify T10. Thus there is a 2-level targeting error: the clinician treats T10 rather than T8, the actual intended site of care. Since the clinician believes this to the T7 level, there would be a 3 level charting error in numerating the site of care, the same degree of charting error made in the case of radiographic examination.

Although these examples assumed findings at either T7 or T8, if the clinician applies the "7 up, 6 down" rule, findings in other thoracic locations would be associated with the same 3 or 2 level targeting error (for radiographic and other physical examination procedures, respectively). In this highly simplified experiment, the authors did not consider the possibility of examiner errors other than those accruing to the use of an erroneous landmark rule; nor did they explore the consequences of variation in scapular positions among between patients, nor within patients between the left and right sides of the body.

Experiment 2: The reliability of an alternative targeting "SP-to-prone" targeting procedure

Since the application of inaccurate scapular benchmark rules likely results in targeting errors for the site and numeration of spine care, it would be useful to devise a more accurate way to identify a prone site of care based on upright examination findings. Experiment 2 was based on the hypothesis that palpators could identify a spinal site of care landmark in the upright patient and then reliably track that site to the prone position. The described procedure requires maintaining contact with a SP as a patient moves from the upright to the prone position; for this reason the authors created the descriptive term "SP-to-prone" to name the procedure.

Methods

There were 2 experienced examiners in this study, with many years of teaching experience and clinical practice and 8 novice student examiners. The first author was experienced in the SP-to-prone method in a private practice setting for several years. The second author has taught palpation at a chiropractic college and practiced for several years. There were no practice or rehearsal sessions for this study. It was approved by the Palmer Chiropractic College Institutional Review Board and the 2 participants provided written consent. They were a convenience sample of asymptomatic young men. A very small mark using an erasable marker was placed on the skin at the SP most closely even with the inferior tip of the right scapula in the standing position. Another mark was placed on the SP that was most closely even with the iliac crest, at either L4 or L5 [21]. Then, standing somewhat behind the participant and to his left, each palpator positioned the distal tip of the left middle digit parallel to the skin mark, trying as closely as possible to align the skin mark with the middle of the nail, as indicated with a penciled line parallel to the length of the line. With the fingernail in position the skin mark was not visible. The palpator kept the palpating finger firmly on the SP underlying the skin mark while the participant carefully and deliberately repositioned himself on the table in the prone position (Figure 1). A study assistant then measured the distance in mm from the lumbar marker to the middle of the nail, which was kept parallel to the participant's mid-thoracic spine (Figure 2). Each of 10 palpators performed this protocol on each of the two participants, in the same order for each participant. Approximately 2 minutes elapsed between observations. The examiners waiting to be tested were at least 5 meters away from the location where the measurements were being recorded and could not have visually ascertained the site localized in the prone position.

Statistical analysis included calculating the absolute value of the mean difference for each examiner from the 10 examiner mean for each of the 2 participants (MAD), the standard error of the mean (SEM), the root mean square error (RMSE, or σ_e), and the intraclass correlation coefficient (ICC). Some of the analyses were performed using Excel® 2013(Microsoft Corporation) and some with SPSS® v.19 (IBM Corporation).

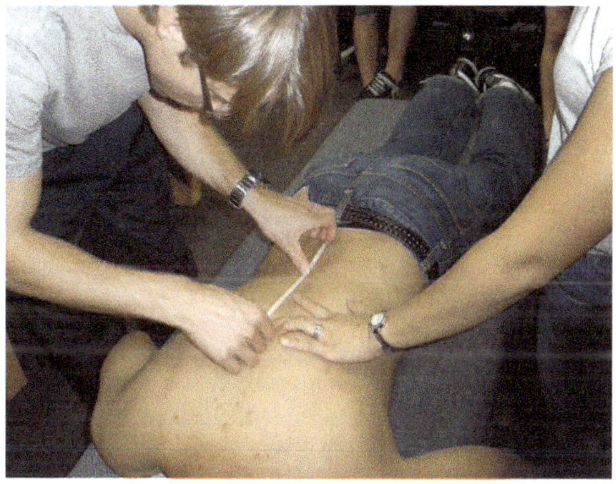

Figure 2 Determining distance of palpatory end-point to lumbar skin mark.

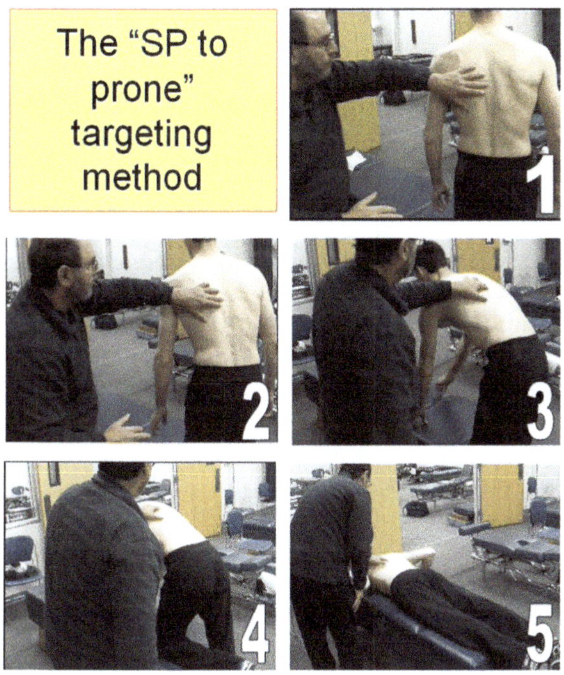

Figure 1 The SP-to-prone targeting procedure.

Results

The data are summarized in Table 3, all distances in millimeters. For participant 1, the average distance from lumbar to thoracic skin marker was 243.4 mm; and for participant 2, was 221.4 mm. The ranges for examiner errors (differences in mm for each measurement from the 10 measure mean) were -8.4 to 11.6, and -6.4 to 10.6, for participants 1 and 2 respectively. The mean examiner error for 20 observations ≈ 0. Stratified by experience and averaged for the two participants, MAD values for the 8 novice examiners and 2 experienced examiners were 4.4 and 6.7 mm, respectively. The 10 examiner MAD for each of the 2 participants = 5.2 mm for participant 1, and

Table 3 Results

(mm)	Participant 1	Participant 2	
Distance IAS-SP to L4 SP	243.4	221.4	
Range, examiner errors	-8.4, 11.6	-6.4, 10.6	Mean
MAD exp (n = 2)	7.4	6.0	6.7
MAD non-exp. (N = 8)	4.7	4.1	4.4
			Participants combined
MAD all, n = 10 95% CI: (lower, upper)	5.2 (2.7, 7.7)	4.5 (2.7, 6.3)	4.8 (3.3, 6.4)
SEM	1.3	0.9	0.8
RMSE (σ_e)	6.5	5.3	5.9
ICC (2,1)		0.83	

MAD = mean absolute difference; *SEM* = standard error mean; *CI* = confidence interval; *ICC* = intraclass correlation coefficient; σ_e = root mean square error (*RMSE*); *SEM* = (MAD SD / √N; 95% *CI* = SD ± SE*1.96; *RMSE* (σ_e) = √MSE.

4.5 mm for participant 2; an average of 4.7 mm. Since the computed t value was less than the t-critical value, the null hypothesis that MAD was not different from zero at a 95% confidence level was not rejected. Standard error of the mean (SEM) for all examiners and participants = 0.8 mm, and root mean square error (RMSE, or σ_e) = 5.9 mm. For all 10 examiners and participants, ICC (2,1) = 0.83, which is judged "excellent" according to the Landis scale [22].

Discussion

Manual therapists often examine the patient in a position different from the one in which the patient will be treated. Thermographic assessment [23], manual muscle testing for spine dysfunction [24], and spinal motion palpation [25] are usually performed with the patient upright, but often lead to spinal interventions, including but not limited to manipulation, that are performed on a prone patient. Since chiropractors usually take or order upright x-rays, radiographic examination is also upright yet may lead to treatment in a prone position. Where is the guarantee that vertebral sites identified as areas of concern in the upright position can be reliably palpated and treated in the prone position? It seems that the ability of manual therapists to accurately proceed from upright examination findings to prone interventions has been simply assumed. Targeting errors could in turn lead to sub-optimal clinical outcomes, depending on the degree to which specificity in identifying sites of spine and sacroiliac care is clinically important. These targeting errors could also lead to charting errors, in that the *intended* sites of care and/or *actual* sites of care could be incorrectly numerated. Byfield and Kissinger, addressing the issue of errors in identifying spinal segmental levels, consider the impact of problems in locating anatomical landmarks due to tissue movement, examiner bias, and recording mistakes. This, they write, could "pose potential problems when palpatory findings are compared from one palpating posture to another" ([26], p.19). These authors also draw a distinction between end play or end feel palpated in the seated position, and joint play or challenge that is palpated prone both assessed at the endpoint of passive spinal motion, at the elastic barrier of the joint ([26], p.10).

The thought experiments suggested that targeting errors using the IAS to locate spinal levels identified in the upright position on a prone patient would be substantial, ranging from 2 to 3 spinal levels. To address that problem, the first author devised a novel method which attained substantially perfect reliability and probably accuracy, among both experienced and novice palpators, in mapping upright levels to the prone position. The authors proposed that the described SP-to-prone targeting method could be utilized in any patient population in which potential spinal sites of care need to be mapped from upright to prone position. Since the reliability experiment was construed to be an IRB-approved full-dress rehearsal for a future larger study, it was not considered important to perform a power analysis to decide upon the numbers of participants and examiners. When it became clear during data analysis that the reliability was extremely high, with very modest variability in examiner errors, it was decided that a larger study was not required. In small studies with relatively few participants, the number of examiners is also commensurately few [27].

Although the length of the thoracic spine varies between individuals, on average it is about 28 cm in length [28], which corresponds to about 23.3 mm per level. Therefore, with a range of −8.4 to 11.6 mm for examiner differences from the 10 measurement mean for each of 2 participants, none of the 20 measurements from the L4 SP to the targeted thoracic skin marker were discrepant by more than half a vertebral level (approximately 11.7 mm). In fact, the 20-measurement MAD = 4.8 mm was less than 1/4 the length of a typical thoracic spinal level. Therefore, the examiners in this study should be considered to have been 100% successful in their effort to maintain contact on the same spinal level as the participants moved from the standing to the prone position. The square root of mean squared error (MSE) yields root-mean-square error (RMSE), yet another measure of examiner accuracy. In this study, combined RMSE = 5.9 mm, while combined (10 observers, 2 participants) MAD = 4.8 mm. MAD = RMSE when all the errors are of the same magnitude. With increasing variance in the errors, RMSE increases in relation to MAD, and thus becomes a more useful (certainly a more conservative) estimate of accuracy. These computations confirm the examiners most likely identified the same spinal level in the prone position in all cases. With ICC (2,1) =0.83, using the Landis scale [22] for classifying ICC values (below 0.40 = poor, 0.40-0.59 = fair, 0.60-0.74 = good, above 0.75 = excellent) interexaminer agreement on the prone spinal level corresponding to the upright thoracic skin marker was judged to be "excellent".

By design, experiment 2 only addressed interexaminer reliability, not the validity (i.e., accuracy) of the attempt to identify the same segment in the upright and prone positions. Since there was no reference standard in this study, the authors thought it reasonable to use the 10 examiner mean for the prone targeted level as a surrogate for such a reference standard. Examiners may highly agree with each other, and yet be inaccurate – that is, they may both be wrong. However, the authors think it highly unlikely that the palpators in this study were subject to systematic measurement error, such as may have resulted in all 10 palpators identifying the same wrong level in the prone position. This is due to the fact that the mean examiner error ≈ 0, ruling out systematic bias. The results using mostly novice examiners most likely represents a worst case scenario, since one would expect more experienced examiners who might use the SP-to-prone procedure in actual clinical situations to achieve even higher accuracy. Therefore, the excellent interexaminer reliability achieved with an examiner pool in which 8/10 (80%) were novice palpators bodes well for clinical relevance.

To the extent clinicians in the manual therapy professions feel that spinal level specificity improves the outcome of interventions, they may find it worthwhile to use the described SP-to-prone method as an alternative to the more usual but suspect scapula landmark when they need to locate spinal levels identified in the upright position on a prone patient. As an alternative, they could use some other landmark to locate a prone spinal level, such as the iliac crest (thought to be in line with the SP of L4 or L5 [21] or the vertebra prominens (VP), thought usually – but not always – to line up with C7 [29]. Due to the variability of the L4 = iliac crest and VP = T1 landmark rules, the authors think the upright-to-prone targeting method herein described would be more reliable. Although it enables reliably mapping upright physical examination finding to the prone position, it does not facilitate accuracy in charting. Indeed, that would have to be accomplished using some other counting method, one that best not involve any scapular landmark rules. Although the SP-to-prone targeting method most directly supplants using landmarks to target a prone spinal level base on upright *physical* examination, it is unlikely to reduce targeting errors accruing to *radiographic* examination.

Beyond the manual therapy professions, these findings may be relevant to other professions that commonly use the IAS as a landmark to target spinal levels. Practitioners of orthopedic medicine, neurology, nursing, and acupuncture should also be interested in this updated information on the anatomical relation of the scapula and spine. For example, anesthesiologists require precise placement of thoracic epidural catheters to optimize postoperative analgesia and minimize adverse effects [15,17,30]. Anatomic landmarks are also used to locate acupuncture points, and specifically the IAS has been cited as a reference point for the T7 spinous process ([31], p.11). Surgeons may decide upon a location to begin their incision based at least in part on the location of the IAS ([32], p18, 26).

In manual therapy, the preponderance of research justifies considerable confidence in treatment success, but not nearly as much in diagnostic acumen. This creates a challenging paradox. It is widely believed that successful treatment requires an accurate diagnosis. If so, it is difficult to explain the apparent success of a great variety of manual treatment procedures, when demonstrated low levels of interexaminer reliability in widely used examination procedures suggests the notion of a specific chiropractic diagnosis (i.e., "listing") remains somewhat hypothetical. As an example, in the derivation of a clinical prediction rule for spinal manipulation, not one of 18 sacroiliac orthopedic tests were retained in the final model that predicted clinical success [33], even though the manipulative procedure used in the study was intended for the sacroiliac joint.

Limitations of experiments 1 and 2

Experiment 1 is a *Gedankenexperiment*. A thought experiment is only capable of attaining face validity, deriving conclusions that seem to make sense. Not all such experiments have good outcomes, such as the one prior to the time of the ancient Greeks (and still widely embraced up to the time of Columbus) by which visual cues led to the conclusion that the earth was flat.

In experiment 2, the investigators did not attempt to numerate the spinal level of the skin marker that was parallel to the IAS, nor how much it changed between the upright and prone levels. Since that had been done in previous studies [11-13], this study was confined to targeting reliability. Since the authors were not aware of what proportion of clinicians actually uses the scapula to localize spinal sites as compared with other landmarks, they did not have an estimate of the magnitude of the problem being addressed. That stated, the authors do believe this proportion is high, certainly for localizing thoracic spine sites.

In principle an examiner could have deceitfully moved the index finger he or she was attempting to keep on a skin mark (concealed under the fingernail) had he or she seen the index finger slip to such a degree that the skin mark could be seen as the participant assumed the prone position. The examiners were asked to look away from their index fingers to preclude that opportunity, and in no cases did the research assistant who recorded the distance of the endpoint from the lumbar skin mark report that the thoracic skin mark was no longer occluded by the distal index finger.

This study did not address the *clinical importance* of targeting specificity for manual therapists. A comprehensive systematic review [20], while it describes the methods that are typically used by chiropractors to target sites of spinal care and rates their validity and reliability, does not address the clinical utility of this information. Although studies in recent years have questioned the ability to deliver forces to intended targets [34-42], it is not known to what extent diagnostic and/or adjustive imprecision in the manual therapy professions leads to suboptimal clinical consequences. The authors would be outside their scope of practice to comment on to what extent targeting errors impact clinical outcomes in the other health care professions that use spinal landmarks.

Experiment 2, the reliability study, was intended to be a pilot study to test the methodology. When the data were analyzed and showed very high levels of examiner concordance, it became clear that a larger study was not necessary. This explains why there were only 10 examiners and 2 participants in this study, resulting in only 20 observations. Caution should be exercised in extrapolating the results to diverse patient populations who might differ significantly from the 2 healthy young male participants in this study. Symptomatic patients, were they to exhibit awkward movements as they change from the upright to the prone position, could make it more difficult to maintain contact on the targeted spinous process, threatening accuracy.

Conclusions

This is a deceptively simple study that addresses a matter that in the authors' opinion is very important, and yet is rarely discussed let alone studied: how does a manual therapist know that a spinal site identified as worthy of treatment with the patient in the upright position has been accurately located when the patient has moved to the prone position? The ability to be accurate in this endeavor using spinal landmarks such as the IAS, crest of ilium, and vertebral prominens has been more or less assumed. It would be presumptuous to assume this in turn has rendered clinical outcomes suboptimal and yet that is clearly possible. Even in the case there had been no deleterious impact on the quality of care, it would then seem that the information supplied by typical spinal examination procedures would have been of little import. That would certainly be worth knowing. As manual therapists, the authors have emphasized how targeting errors might impact upon manual care of the spine. Practitioners in other fields that need to accurately locate spinal levels, such as acupuncture and anesthesiology, would also be expected to draw important conclusions from these findings.

The clinical rationale for insisting on a high degree of diagnostic specificity, the ability of examiners to agree on an optimal site and vector for care, and their ability to direct an intervention accurately at an intended site of care, are far from established. Despite the ample evidence that manipulative and other manual spinal interventions are both safe and effective, the degree to which the results of clinical studies would change were targeting practices more accurate remains speculative. The authors suggest it would be easier research the possibility of optimizing the site of spinal care were there reliable methods to track spinal sites of interest identified in the upright position to the prone and other positions; that is the spirit in which the SP-to-prone targeting procedure has been proposed.

Competing interests

The authors declare they have no competing interests.

Authors' contribution

RC developed the targeting procedure that is the focus of this study, participated in data collection, and drafted the first draft of the manuscript. MY participated in data collection and the production of the final manuscript. Both authors read and approved the final manuscript.

References

1. Cooperstein R: **The limits of traditional chiropractic listings and the advent of provocation testing.** *JACA Online* 2008, **45**:29–31. Online access only.
2. Bergmann T: **P.A.R.T.S. joint assessment procedure.** *Chiropr Tech* 1993, **5**:135–136.
3. Bergmann T: **Toward a reliable, valid method of manual diagnosis. More than the sum of its P.A.R.T.S.** *J Am Chiropr Assoc* 1997, **34**:24–27.
4. Chaitow L: *Muscle Energy Techniques*. 4th edition. London: Churchill Livingstone; 2013.
5. Licciardone JC, Nelson KE, Glonek T, Sleszynski SL, Des Anges C: **Osteopathic manipulative treatment of somatic dysfunction among patients in the family practice clinic setting: a retrospective analysis.** *J Am Osteopath Assoc* 2005, **105**:537–544.
6. Chaves TC, Nagamine HM, Belli JF, De Hannai MC, Bevilaqua-Grossi D, De Oliveira AS: **Reliability of fleximetry and goniometry for assessing cervical range of motion among children.** *Rev Bras Fisioter* 2008, **12**:283–289.
7. Hole DE, Cook JM, Bolton JE: **Reliability and concurrent validity of two instruments for measuring cervical range of motion: effects of age and gender.** *Man Ther* 1995, **1**:36–42.
8. Prushansky T, Deryi O, Jabarreen B: **Reproducibility and validity of digital inclinometry for measuring cervical range of motion in normal subjects.** *Physiother Res Int* 2010, **15**:42–48.
9. Tucci SM, Hicks JE, Gross EG, Campbell W, Danoff J: **Cervical motion assessment: a new, simple and accurate method.** *Arch Phys Med Rehabil* 1986, **67**:225–230.
10. Cooperstein R: **Assessment of sitting-standing pelvic landmarks for anatomical LLI: or Darwin's finches and leg checking.** *J Am Chiropr Assoc* 2006, **43**:12–14.
11. Cooperstein R, Haneline M: **Spinous process palpation using the scapular tip as a landmark vs a radiographic criterion standard.** *J Chiropr Med* 2007, **6**:87–93.
12. Cooperstein R, Haneline MT, Young MD: **The location of the inferior angle of the scapula in relation to the spinal level of prone patients.** *JCCA J Can Chiropr Assoc* 2009, **53**:121–128.
13. Haneline M, Cooperstein R, Young M, Ross J: **Determining spinal level using the inferior angle of the scapula as a reference landmark: a retrospective analysis of 50 radiographs.** *J Can Chiropr Assoc* 2008, **52**:24–29.
14. Kendall FP, McCreary EK, Provance PG, Rodgers MM, Romani WA: *Muscles: Testing and Function, with Posture and Pain*. 5th edition. Baltimore: LippincottWilliams & Wilkins; 2005.
15. Teoh DA, Santosham KL, Lydell CC, Smith DF, Beriault MT: **Surface anatomy as a guide to vertebral level for thoracic epidural placement.** *Anesth Analg* 2009, **108**:1705–1707.
16. Arzola C, Avramescu S, Tharmaratnam U, Chin KJ, Balki M: **Identification of cervicothoracic intervertebral spaces by surface landmarks and ultrasound.** *Can J Anaesth* 2011, **58**:1069–1074.
17. Kim MG, Ok SY, Kim SH, Lee SJ, Park SY, Koh EH, Bae HY, Hur KY: **Is the spinous process of t7 usually at the same level as the inferior tips of the scapulae?** *Soonchunhyang Med Sci* 2012, **18**:9–11.
18. Ernst MJ, Rast FM, Bauer CM, Marcar VL, Kool J: **Determination of thoracic and lumbar spinal processes by their percentage position between C7 and the PSIS level.** *BMC Res Notes* 2013, **6**:58.
19. Haneline MT, Young M: **A review of intraexaminer and interexaminer reliability of static spinal palpation: a literature synthesis.** *J Manipulative Physiol Ther* 2009, **32**:379–386.
20. Triano J, Budgell B, Bagnulo A, Roffey B, Bergmann T, Cooperstein R, Gleberezon B, Good C, Perron J, Iepe R: **Review of methods used by chiropractors to determine the site for applying manipulation.** *Chiropr Man Ther* 2013, **21**(1):36.

21. Chakraverty R, Pynsent P, Isaacs K: **Which spinal levels are identified by palpation of the iliac crests and the posterior superior iliac spines?** *J Anat* 2007, **210**:232–236.
22. Landis JR, Koch GG: **The measurement of observer agreement for categorical data.** *Biometrics* 1977, **33**:159–174.
23. Plaugher G: **Skin temperature assessment for neuromusculoskeletal abnormalities of the spinal column.** *J Manipulative Physiol Ther* 1992, **15**:365–381.
24. Cuthbert SC, Goodheart GJ Jr: **On the reliability and validity of manual muscle testing: a literature review.** *Chiropr Osteopat* 2007, **15**:4.
25. Haneline MT, Cooperstein R, Young M, Birkeland K: **Spinal motion palpation: a comparison of studies that assessed intersegmental end feel vs excursion.** *J Manipulative Physiol Ther* 2008, **31**:616–626.
26. Byfield DC, Kinsigner S: *A Manual Therapists Guide to Surface Anatomy & Palpation Skills.* Oxford: Butterworth Heinemann; 2002.
27. Kottner J, Audige L, Brorson S, Donner A, Gajewski BJ, Hrobjartsson A, Roberts C, Shoukri M, Streiner DL: **Guidelines for Reporting Reliability and Agreement Studies (GRRAS) were proposed.** *Int J Nurs Stud* 2011, **48**:661–671.
28. Campbell RM Jr, Hell-Vocke AK: **Growth of the thoracic spine in congenital scoliosis after expansion thoracoplasty.** *J Bone Joint Surg Am* 2003, **85-A**:409–420.
29. Stonelake PS, Burwell RG, Webb JK: **Variation in vertebral levels of the vertebra prominens and sacral dimples in subjects with scoliosis.** *J Anat* 1988, **159**:165–172.
30. Holmaas G, Frederiksen D, Ulvik A, Vingsnes SO, Ostgaard G, Nordli H: **Identification of thoracic intervertebral spaces by means of surface anatomy: a magnetic resonance imaging study.** *Acta Anaesthesiol Scand* 2006, **50**:368–373.
31. Omi S: *Who Standard Acupuncture Point Locations in the Western Pacific Region.* Manila, Philippines: World Health Organization; 2008. 2008.
32. Little GL, Merrill WH: *Complications in Cardiothoracic Surgery: Avoidance and Treatment.* 2nd edition. Hoboken: Wiley-Blackwell; 2011.
33. Flynn T, Fritz J, Whitman J, Wainner R, Magel J, Rendeiro D, Butler B, Garber M, Allison S: **A clinical prediction rule for classifying patients with low back pain who demonstrate short-term improvement with spinal manipulation.** *Spine* 2002, **27**:2835–2843.
34. Bereznick DE, Ross JK, McGill SM: **The frictional properties at the thoracic skin-fascia interface: implications in spine manipulation.** *Clin Biomech (Bristol, Avon)* 2002, **17**:297–303.
35. Cooperstein R: **Specificity failure and petrified thought.** *Dyn Chiropr* 1999, **17**:20–21. 50-51.
36. Hestbaek L, Leboeuf-Yde C: **Are chiropractic tests for the lumbo-pelvic spine reliable and valid? A systematic critical literature review.** *J Manipulative Physiol Ther* 2000, **23**:258–275.
37. Leboeuf C: **The sensitivity and specificity of seven lumbo-pelvic orthopedic tests and the arm fossa test.** *J Manipulative Physiol Ther* 1990, **13**:138–143.
38. Perle S: **The illusion of specificity.** *J Am Chiropr Assoc* 2002, **39**:30–31.
39. Ross JK, Bereznick DE, McGill SM: **Determining cavitation location during lumbar and thoracic spinal manipulation: is spinal manipulation accurate and specific?** *Spine* 2004, **29**:1452–1457.
40. Perle SM, Kawchuk GN: **Pressures generated during spinal manipulation and their association with hand anatomy.** *J Manipulative Physiol Ther* 2005, **28**:e1–e7.
41. Cooperstein R, Haas M: **The listings continuum: driving a truck through a paradox.** *Dyn Chiropr* 2001, **19**:28–29. 36.
42. Gal J, Herzog W, Kawchuk G, Conway P, Zhang Y-T: **Biomechanical studies of spinal manipulative therapy (SMT): quantifying the movements of vertebral bodies during SMT.** *J Can Chiropr Assoc* 1994, **38**:11–24.

Summary of the findings of the International Collaboration on Mild Traumatic Brain Injury Prognosis

James Donovan[1*], Carol Cancelliere[1,2] and J David Cassidy[1,2,3]

Abstract

In 2004, the WHO Collaborating Centre for Neurotrauma, Prevention, Management and Rehabilitation Task Force published the first large systematic review and best evidence synthesis on the clinical course and prognosis for recovery after MTBI. Ten years later, the International Collaboration on Mild Traumatic Brain Injury Prognosis (ICoMP) formed to update the original WHO Task Force results. This summary review highlights important clinical findings from the full ICoMP results including the current evidence on the course and prognosis of recovery after MTBI in diverse patient populations (e.g., adults, athletes and children) and injury environments (e.g., motor vehicle collisions) as well as on the risk of long-term outcomes after MTBI, such as Parkinson's disease and dementia. Additional clinical areas of interest in MTBI are also discussed including the similarities between MTBI and other traumatic injuries and the risk of Second Impact Syndrome after sport concussion. Clinicians can use this information to help inform patients on the likely course of recovery after MTBI/concussion and guide better decision-making in the care of these patients.

Keywords: Prognosis, Concussion, Mild traumatic brain injury

Introduction

Over the past decade, mild traumatic brain injury (MTBI) or concussion has become a prominent public health concern. The annual incidence likely now exceeds 600 per 100,000 person-years and though popularized by injuries to prominent sports figures, MTBI most commonly occurs after falls and motor vehicle collisions [1]. In 2004, the WHO Collaborating Centre for Neurotrauma, Prevention, Management and Rehabilitation Task Force (WHO Task Force) published the first large systematic review and best evidence synthesis on MTBI course and prognosis. After reviewing the literature from 1980–2000, the WHO Task Force found the prognostic literature to be of poor quality [2]. For instance, inconsistent MTBI definitions, weak study designs and pervasive biases were common problems throughout the literature. In addition, knowledge gaps were found in such areas as prognosis in the elderly, risk of long-term outcomes, and non-surgical intervention studies [2]. The WHO Task Force concluded that more high quality prognostic research was needed to address these evidence gaps and advance the understanding on the course and prognosis after MTBI [3].

In 2011 an international group of 21 research scientists and clinicians, the International Collaboration on MTBI Prognosis (ICoMP), was formed and funded to update the WHO Task Force findings on MTBI prognosis (see Table 1) [4]. ICoMP undertook a systematic review and best-evidence synthesis to identify the clinical course and prognostic factors for recovery after MTBI within diverse patient populations (e.g., children, adults, athletes, and military personnel) as well as to provide insight into the risk of long-term outcomes, such as movement- and dementia-related disorders.

Information on the course and prognosis after MTBI can help clinicians make better informed decisions such as when a patient can safely return to work or play and it can also help clinicians identify those patients who may not be recovering as expected [3]. Further, it is important for clinicians to understand what factors determine prognosis in MTBI, especially those that are potentially modifiable. For

* Correspondence: jamesd@uhnresearch.ca
[1]Division of Health Care and Outcomes Research, Toronto Western Research Institute, University Health Network, University of Toronto, Toronto, Canada
Full list of author information is available at the end of the article

Table 1 The complete list of all 21 ICoMP team members

ICoMP members	Institutional Associations
J. David Cassidy, DC, PhD, DrMedSc	• Senior Scientist, Division of Health Care and Outcomes Research, Toronto Western Research Institute, University Health Network, University of Toronto, Canada.
	• Professor, Institute of Health Policy, Management and Evaluation, University of Toronto, Canada.
	• Professor, Division of Epidemiology, Dalla Lana School of Public Health, University of Toronto, Canada.
	• Globalization Professor, Institute of Sports Science and Clinical Biomechanics, Faculty of Health, University of Southern Denmark, Odense, Denmark
Linda Carroll, PhD	• Professor, Department of Public Health Sciences and Alberta Centre for Injury Control and Research, University of Alberta, Edmonton, Canada
Lena Holm, DrMedSc	• Associate Professor, Division of Epidemiology, Institute of Environmental Medicine, Karolinska Institutet, Stockholm, Sweden
Jörgen Borg MD, PhD	• Department of Clinical Sciences, Rehabilitation Medicine, Karolinska Institutet, Danderyd University Hospital, Stockholm, Sweden
Jan Hartvigsen DC, PhD	• Professor, Institute of Sports Science and Clinical Biomechanics, University of Southern Denmark, Odense, Denmark
	• Nordic Institute of Chiropractic and Clinical Biomechanics, Odense, Denmark
Pierre Côté DC, PhD	• Associate Professor, Faculty of Health Sciences, University of Ontario Institute of Technology, Oshawa, Canada.
	• UOIT-CMCC Centre for the Study of Disability Prevention and Rehabilitation, University of Ontario Institute of Technology, Toronto, Canada.
	• Associate Professor, Division of Epidemiology, Dalla Lana School of Public Health, University of Toronto, Canada.
	• Associate Professor, Institute of Health Policy, Management and Evaluation, University of Toronto, Canada.
Carol Cancelliere, DC, MPH	• Trainee, Division of Health Care and Outcomes Research, Toronto Western Research Institute, University Health Network, University of Toronto, Canada.
	• Doctoral Student, Institute of Health Policy, Management and Evaluation, University of Toronto, Canada.
Cesar Hincapié DC, MHSc	• Trainee, Division of Health Care and Outcomes Research, Toronto Western Research Institute, University Health Network, University of Toronto, Canada.
	• Doctoral student, Division of Epidemiology, Dalla Lana School of Public Health, University of Toronto, Canada
James Donovan DC	• Research Associate, Division of Health Care and Outcomes Research, Toronto Western Research Institute, University Health Network, University of Toronto, Canada
Victor Coronado MD, MPH	• Medical Epidemiologist, National Center for Injury Prevention and Control, Centers for Disease Control and Prevention (CDC), Atlanta, United States
Jean-Luc af Geijerstam MD, PhD	• Section Head, Department of Rehabilitation Medicine, Karolinska Institutet, Danderyd University Hospital, Stockholm, Sweden
Britt-Marie Stålnacke MD, PhD	• Adjunct Professor, Department of Rehabilitation Medicine, Community Medicine and Rehabilitation, Umeå University, Sweden
Connie Marras MD, PhD	• Assistant Professor, Division of Neurology, Faculty of Movement Disorder, University of Toronto
	• Morton and Gloria Shulman Movement Disorders Centre, and the Edmond J. Safra Program in Parkinson's Research, Toronto Western Hospital, University Health Network, University of Toronto, Canada.
Vicki Kristman PhD	• Assistant Professor, Department of Health Sciences, Lakehead University, Thunder Bay, Canada
	• Institute for Work and Health, Toronto, Canada.
	• Division of Epidemiology, Dalla Lana School of Public Health, University of Toronto, Canada.
	• Division of Human Sciences, Northern Ontario School of Medicine, Lakehead University, Thunder Bay, Canada
Eleanor Boyle PhD	• Associate Professor, Institute of Sports Science and Clinical Biomechanics, Faculty of Health, University of Southern Denmark, Odense, Denmark.
	• Division of Epidemiology, Dalla Lana School of Public Health, University of Toronto, Canada

Table 1 The complete list of all 21 ICoMP team members *(Continued)*

Michelle Keightly PhD	• Departments of Occupational Science and Occupational Therapy, Psychology and Graduate Department of Rehabilitation Science, University of Toronto, Canada.
	• Bloorview Research Institute, Holland Bloorview Kids Rehabilitation Hospital, Toronto, Canada.
L. Rachid Salmi MD, PhD	• Professor, University of Bordeaux, ISPED, Centre INSERM U897-Epidemiologie-Biostatistique, F-33000 Bordeaux, France (Salmi); INSERM, ISPED, Centre INSERM U897-Epidemiologie-Biostatistique, F-33000 Bordeaux, France (Salmi); CHU de Bordeaux, Pole de sante publique, Service d'information medicale, F-33000 Bordeaux, France
Ryan Hung, MD MSc	• Department of Rehabilitation and Complex Continuing Care, Holland Bloorview Kids Rehabilitation Hospital, Toronto, Canada.
	• Department of Pediatrics, University of Toronto, Canada
Alison Godbolt MBChB, MD,	• Department of Clinical Sciences, Rehabilitation Medicine, Karolinska Institutet, Danderyd University Hospital, Stockholm, Sweden
Catharina Nygren-de Boussard MD, PhD	• Department of Clinical Sciences, Rehabilitation Medicine, Karolinska Institutet, Danderyd University Hospital, Stockholm, Sweden
Peter Rumney MD	• Department of Rehabilitation and Complex Continuing Care, Holland Bloorview Kids Rehabilitation Hospital, Toronto, Canada

example, the WHO Task Force found the presence of spine and head-related pain to be significant determinants of prognosis after MTBI [3]. Chiropractors as well as other health practitioners may be well positioned to improve care for MTBI patients by reducing pain-related MTBI symptoms and in turn may help play an important role in lessening the burden of this growing public health concern. The main purpose of this review is to present a summary of some of the key clinical findings of the full ICoMP results and to highlight other relevant clinical topics such as the similarities between MTBI and other traumatic injuries and the risk of Second Impact Syndrome after sport concussion.

Review

ICoMP search strategy and critical review process

ICoMP performed a comprehensive literature search from 2001–2012. All 10 included systematic reviews complied with the Preferred Reporting Items of Systematic Reviews and Meta-Analyses (PRISMA) statement [5]. Details of the full systematic search and review procedures are available in Cancelliere et al. [6]. Overall, ICoMP screened 77,914 records, reviewed 299 full-text articles, and deemed 101 (34%) to be scientifically admissible, based on the Scottish Intercollegiate Guidelines Network (SIGN) criteria, and included in the ICoMP synthesis [7]. Key findings from papers found to be of low risk of bias were extracted into evidence tables. ICoMP undertook best-evidence syntheses by linking conclusions and recommendations to the evidence tables. Prognostic factor evidence was prioritized based on the phases of study framework described by Côté et al. [8]: Phase I studies are preliminary, hypothesis-generating investigations that explore crude associations between potential prognostic factors and disease outcomes; Phase II studies are exploratory and test associations between sets of prognostic factors and outcomes using multivariable analyses; Phase III studies are confirmatory analyses, including well-defined pre-stated hypotheses allowing for focused examination of the strength, direction and independence of a prognostic factor to disease outcome taking into account potential confounding factors. Phase III studies are confirmatory and provide the strongest prognostic evidence.

ICoMP results

Sport concussion prognosis and return to play

By understanding sport concussion prognosis, clinicians can help to better educate athletes, coaches, and parents regarding their primary concerns, such as the likely duration of post-concussion symptoms, immediate versus delayed return-to-play (RTP), and potential sequelae of repetitive concussion. Similar to the results of the WHO Task Force, recent literature suggests that most athletes recover quickly (i.e., days to a few weeks) with respect to both cognitive functioning (e.g., attention and memory) and post-concussion symptoms (e.g., headache, fatigue, dizziness, etc.) [9]. While most athletes experience a favourable recovery, factors such as a history of previous concussion, number and duration of post-concussion symptoms and being a younger-aged/high school athlete are associated with delayed recovery. The literature also shows that cognitive functioning is not significantly (if at all) impaired and the mild deficits that do occur resolve quickly in high school, collegiate, and professional athletes [9].

Although RTP guidelines are popular there are no high-quality studies assessing their impact on recovery or prevention of additional injury and most of the research on RTP focuses on contact sports that include male professional American and Australian football players [9]. There is some evidence that the majority of athletes do RTP within the same game or within a few days afterward [9]. Despite the growing concern over RTP after sport concussion, research quality continues to be poor, demonstrating little to no methodological improvement since the WHO Task Force review. Furthermore, RTP decision-making tools, such as the Zurich Consensus guidelines, though widely used, continue to be based on expert opinion and clinical judgement, rather than scientific evidence [10].

In order to develop evidence-based recommendations for the management of sport concussion, ICoMP recommends randomized controlled trials to test the efficacy of existing RTP guidelines [9]. Sport concussion study methodologies remain highly heterogeneous (e.g., different follow-up durations and outcome measures), and include predominantly male American football players 16 years of age and older. Clinicians, however, are responsible for managing male and female athletes of all ages, skill levels, and sporting activities (e.g., hockey, soccer, basketball, etc.) and for these groups, evidence is lacking. Firm conclusions regarding the long-term outcome of repetitive sport concussion cannot be made at this time due to the lack of evidence. Conversely, short-term recovery after sport concussion was found to be delayed in athletes with a history of previous concussion and clinicians need to consider this when making future decisions about RTP or even ending sports participation, especially in younger-aged athletes and those at high risk for repeat concussion such as in contact sports.

One final concern in the sports setting is the potential for Second-Impact Syndrome (SIS) [11]. This very rare condition can occur when a second concussion or head injury happens before the brain has fully healed from a first concussion, resulting in increased intracranial pressure and death [11,12]. Some experts cite this concern when cautioning against early RTP [13]. The WHO Task Force found no scientific evidence on the incidence or risk of SIS, other than a few case reports from North America [1]. The WHO Task Force reviewed these cases and came to the conclusion that the evidence that a second concussion increases the risk for cerebral swelling and death is not well established and another systematic review [14] reached this same conclusion. ICoMP found no studies addressing SIS as an outcome after an initial concussion. While SIS may not be well established in the company of high quality scientific evidence, it nevertheless remains a potentially very serious complication after MTBI and as a result a real concern for clinicians and patients. Accordingly, there is an urgent need for improved research in the area of SIS, including better reporting of fatal outcomes after MTBI and better study designs to address the incidence and risk of SIS.

Adult prognosis after MTBI

Self-reported symptoms

Self-reported symptoms (e.g., headache, fatigue, and dizziness) are the main reason for seeking care after MTBI. Indeed, ICoMP found adult self-reported symptoms to be the most frequently reported of outcomes after MTBI [15]. Recent evidence suggests that these symptoms are common and typically resolve over the course of weeks to several months [15]. Also, ICoMP found adult patients after MTBI may devalue or minimize pre-existing symptoms such as headache and fatigue and therefore misattribute symptoms occurring before the injury to the injury itself [15]. Furthermore, self reported post-concussion symptoms are not unique or specific to head injury per se: injured control groups (i.e., orthopedic injuries) report similar post-traumatic symptoms. Since post-concussion symptoms appear both common and non-specific, the ICoMP recommends possibly dropping the diagnostic label of "post-concussion syndrome" and using the more appropriate "post-traumatic symptoms" as a replacement [15].

Despite post-concussion symptoms being common and resolving in the short-term for the majority, 22 to 36% of MTBI patients continue to report three or more post-traumatic symptoms six months after injury [15]. Interestingly, ICoMP found persistent symptom duration and overall recovery to be more associated with psychosocial factors, such as poor expectations for recovery and negative injury perceptions, rather than biomedical or injury-related factors such as duration of loss of consciousness (LOC) and post-traumatic amnesia (PTA), which are factors commonly used to diagnose and indicate initial head-injury severity.

The above results are in accordance with the WHO Task Force regarding the commonality and lack of specificity of adult self-reported cognitive and somatic symptoms [3]. However, symptoms can persist in a minority of patients and therefore may be challenging for the treating clinician. Clinical importance should be placed on early identification of injury perceptions and other psychosocial factors, as these appear to be strong determinants of recovery. Furthermore, much needed methods such as prognostic prediction rules could help clinicians to triage those at higher risk for poor recovery into early treatment programs, if such programs can be shown to be effective.

One important ICoMP accepted study developed a useful and easy-to-implement prediction rule identifying a favourable recovery six months after MTBI [16]. Prediction rules include combinations of prognostic factors, or markers, strongly associated with a particular outcome, favourable or otherwise. This study examined a range of pre-, peri- and post-injury prognostic factors and results demonstrated a 90% probability for favourable MTBI recovery in those who have no pre-existing physical problems, experience fewer and less severe post-concussion symptoms and suffer lower levels of post-traumatic stress. Absent from these results are the typical peri-injury biomedical factors that are often related to head-injury prognosis (e.g., LOC, PTA, and Glasgow Coma Scale (GCS)). In turn, this suggests the need to shift from a biomedical towards a more biopsychosocial model to understand MTBI recovery. ICoMP recommended that this clinical prediction rule be independently externally validated before being implemented in other settings [15].

Cognitive outcomes

Instead of relying on patient self-report, traditional or computerized neuropsychological testing is often used to more objectively measure deficits and monitor cognitive recovery after MTBI. The WHO Task Force results suggested that early cognitive deficits are common and usually resolve within one to three months after MTBI [3]. Similar to the WHO Task Force, recent evidence suggests adults commonly demonstrate cognitive deficits initially after MTBI, despite variability in the nature of these deficits (e.g., attention, distractibility, learning, etc.) [17]. ICoMP found substantial evidence for the presence of cognitive deficits in the first two weeks after injury, while the timing of recovery of these deficits is less well known. Although the WHO Task Force found good cognitive recovery within three months after MTBI, limited evidence now suggests for some, full recovery may take six months to a year [17].

MTBI after motor vehicle collisions (MVC)

It is important for clinicians to understand the course of recovery after MTBI within the context of different injury environments. For example, an ICoMP original study by Cassidy et al. [18] examined the incidence, course and potential prognostic factors in traffic-related MTBI in the Saskatchewan population. MTBI was found to affect 24% of those with traffic injuries, with a median time to recovery of 100 days; however, 23% of those affected continued to report not being recovered at one year. In those with MTBI, somatic symptoms such as neck pain (90%), headache (84%) and low- and mid-back pain (63%, 58%) were commonly reported. Back pain and headache were also found to be important factors associated with poor recovery in patients with MTBI. Moreover, strong determinants of MTBI recovery, in addition to pain, continue to be factors more psychosocial in nature (e.g., poor expectations of recovery, negative injury perceptions, etc.). This study reflects the reality of multiple injuries after traffic collisions and the fact that head injuries are often accompanied by neck injuries [19].

Another ICoMP original study by Hartvigsen et al. [20] used the same cohort as Cassidy et al. [18] to determine the symptom course and health-care use in MTBI sufferers after motor vehicle collision (MVC). Significant somatic pain complaints (e.g., headache and neck pain) were common, lasting up to one year after MTBI. Though less prevalent at one year, spine-related pain complaints such as neck and low back pain continued to be reported in up to one-quarter of subjects. Medical physicians provided care for the majority of patients (96%); however, many also sought early care from allied health professionals, with 42% seeing a physiotherapist and 20% seeing a chiropractor. For the majority with MTBI, care was provided by multiple health professionals, with non-medical physician care increasing over time. Furthermore, those most likely to report on-going symptoms also sought the most non-physician care. This study underlines the importance of somatic pain (e.g., head and spine pain) in the prognosis of MTBI.

Prognostic research on MTBI is now shedding light on possible similarities between MTBI and other traumatic injuries. For instance, similar post-traumatic symptom patterns can occur after whiplash, or MTBI including headache, neck pain, dizziness, fatigue, and concentration difficulties, to name a few [21]. Further, expectations for recovery appear highly prognostic for actual recovery in both MTBI and whiplash (i.e., those not expecting to get better tend to recover more slowly) [22,23]. In light of these similarities as well as others, it has recently been proposed that those suffering whiplash may also have also suffered a concussion and even more that direct impact to the head is no longer necessary for a diagnosis of concussion [13]. While similarities in post-traumatic symptom patterns and determinants of recovery do exist, care must be taken before blurring the diagnostic lines between MTBI and whiplash. Evidence-based definitions (e.g., WHO Task Force) include trauma to the head as an important diagnostic criteria for defining MTBI. However, it is possible that a coup-contrecoup mechanism of injury during whiplash might also negatively affect the brain. More research in this respect is required to fully delineate the relationship between MTBI and whiplash associated disorder (WAD).

Return to activity after MTBI

Current treatment methods for MTBI bear striking resemblance to historical methods once recommended for low back pain (LBP). For instance, a lengthy course of bed rest was once standard practice for acute LBP. However, this all changed after a randomized controlled trial showed that bed-rest prolongs LBP [24]. At present, the sport-medicine literature recommends full physical and cognitive rest until acute symptoms resolve as the universally accepted treatment after sport concussion, even though there are no trials showing this approach is the best way to manage MTBI [10]. Further, for adult patients, acute post-concussion symptoms such as headache, fatigue and concentration problems can last weeks to several months [15]; thus, recommending continued rest for these patients may not be prudent. Caution is also needed when recommending prolonged rest for patients with a low risk of repeat MTBI/concussion such as athletes not involved in contact sports and those injured after a fall or MVC. In a recent review, Silverberg & Iverson [25] caution against recommending full rest beyond three days for the majority who suffer MTBI, and suggest that management of MTBI be guided by specific patient circumstances and characteristics. Recommending prolonged rest might lead to de-conditioning and withdrawal from activities of daily living that could assist recovery. An ICoMP accepted randomized controlled trial showed that extensive rest was no better at improving recovery after MTBI than a briefer period of rest followed by a prompt return to normal activity [26]. Bear in mind, the current best evidence for LBP now discourages rest, having been replaced by 'remain active' as the new standard of care [27]. The ICoMP, in accordance with the WHO Task Force, also recommends early but careful activation for most MTBI patients [26]. However, the current authors recognize that clinical judgement in this respect is important.

Return to work (RTW)

MTBI can result from accidents occurring in various settings including the workplace and clinicians are often called upon to make a prognosis for return to work (RTW). The ICoMP performed the first systematic review and evidence synthesis on RTW prognosis after MTBI and found four admissible cohort studies [28]. The results indicate that most individuals RTW within three to six months. Predictors of full RTW after MTBI include high levels of education, younger age, absence of severe pain on initial hospital admission, job independence, and high job decision-making latitude [28]. Those factors not predictive however, include duration of LOC and PTA, dizziness, fatigue and headache. Injury-related factors have therefore only a partial impact on predicting RTW after MTBI, and this is consistent with studies of other injuries [29]. More evidence is needed to replicate these findings, and there is a need to investigate return to sustained employment (i.e., follow up beyond two years) in MTBI patients.

Pediatric prognosis after MTBI

Parents and family members can have significant fears and concerns after a child suffers an MTBI. The fear that a child will suffer long-term physical or cognitive symptoms is certainly important, not to mention the eventual concerns over academic performance once the child returns to school. As a result, it can be challenging for clinicians to address parental and family worries while at the same time directing care for the injured child. The WHO Task Force review found the prognosis for children after MTBI to be good, with symptoms resolving within two to three months and little to no evidence of any lasting cognitive or academic deficits [3]. Recent evidence also suggests that for the majority of children, self-reported symptoms resolve over time and there are no MTBI-specific long-term cognitive deficits [30]. However, limited evidence from one Phase III and one Phase II study found that children with lower cognitive ability and a more complicated MTBI (i.e., intracranial MRI abnormalities) reported more post-concussion physical and cognitive symptoms at three months and one year post-injury, respectively [30]. Unfortunately, ICoMP did not find any acceptable studies on return to school after MTBI and highlight this as an area of priority for future research. Clinical practice guidelines on the management of pediatric MTBI including persistent symptoms have recently been published online and clinicians may wish to consult these guidelines when managing young, head-injured patients [31].

Long-term outcomes after MTBI

There is increasing media attention and public concern over the purported risk that repeated MTBI can lead to subsequent chronic cognitive impairment (CCI), dementia, or to other distinct neurodegenerative disorders (e.g., chronic traumatic encephelopathy (CTE), Parkinson's disease (PD)). Nearly a decade removed from the WHO Task Force, evidence addressing the possible latent outcomes after adult MTBI continues to remain insufficient: ICoMP found only one cohort study (Phase III) on dementia in adults after MTBI [32]. Limited evidence from this Phase III study indicates that a history of reported MTBI is not associated with a diagnosis of dementia, five years later [32]. ICoMP concluded that there is a lack of evidence of an increased risk of dementia after MTBI [32].

To scientifically answer the question "What is the risk of developing dementia or other neurodegenerative disorders after suffering repeat MTBI?" for example, requires cohort studies with long-term follow up, or more realistically, case–control studies. Unfortunately, studies to appropriately address these questions are still needed. The present literature is dominated by uncontrolled case reports and case series, such as the highly cited study by McKee et al. [33], which raise interesting hypotheses for example about CTE risk, but cannot infer causality.

ICoMP accepted five studies examining the risk of developing Parkinson's disease (PD) following MTBI [34]. One Phase III study found an association between MTBI and PD, but only if the first PD diagnosis occurred within nine or less years of the initial injury. Further, no association was found when examining longer time delays (i.e., >10 years) between MTBI and PD development. Reverse causality however, likely explains the shorter time interval associated with injury and disease onset; that is to say that early stages of PD when it is not yet diagnosed may cause a fall resulting in MTBI. Collectively, the ICoMP evidence does not suggest an association between PD and MTBI [34].

In children however, there is limited evidence indicating possible long-term neurological sequelae after MTBI [30]. One ICoMP accepted Phase III study found children with MTBI to be twice as likely to develop epilepsy as those without [30]. The risk was highest in the first year after MTBI, but there remained a 50% higher risk of developing epilepsy even 10 years after injury. Although an elevated risk does exist, the absolute number of new cases of epilepsy in children after MTBI (i.e., the absolute risk) is actually quite low and this is important information to consider when addressing the concerns of parents, family members or others about this risk. For example, in children aged 5–10 years, this risk translated into 1.56 compared to 0.87 new cases of epilepsy per 1000 person-years in those with versus without a history of MTBI, respectively [30]. The previous WHO Task Force also found an increased risk of epilepsy in children within the first four years after MTBI [3]. Taken together, these consistent findings substantiate the small yet sustained risk of developing epilepsy after suffering MTBI as a child.

Research recommendations

The ICoMP systematically searched and included 101 (34%) articles within the best-evidence synthesis on MTBI prognosis. This is virtually the same low acceptance rate reported by the WHO Task Force (i.e., 28%). Despite being a decade on from the original review, significant methodological issues persist in the MTBI literature [35]. For example, of those accepted studies, only 10% were Phase III confirmatory studies. In turn, MTBI prognosis research remains highly heterogeneous and primarily exploratory in nature (i.e., consists of mainly Phase I and II studies) [35]. Also, there is no universally accepted definition of MTBI and ICoMP tallied over 50 unique case definitions [35]. Significant knowledge gaps still remain. For instance, quality studies on prognosis after sport concussion fail to include female athletes, male and female athletes between 13–15 years of age, and sports other than American or Australian football. In addition, RTP guidelines have yet to be scientifically tested. Lastly, the current evidence largely comprises short-term studies with only one year of follow-up. As such, pertinent questions surrounding the long-term outcomes after MTBI remain unanswered.

Conclusions

Despite the media's attention, concussion or MTBI is not a problem limited only to professional athletes and those wanting to return-to-play. Children and adults suffer MTBI after motor vehicle collisions and falls and these patients all need to be informed on the likely course and prognosis of recovery after MTBI. In the acute management of MTBI patients, initial importance is placed on identifying the rare, but serious complications that can potentially occur after head injury, such as intracranial bleeding. Clinicians need to promptly identify those with new symptom onset or increasing symptom severity, as immediate neurosurgical attention may be required. While complications can occur, recovery is generally good for the majority after MTBI or concussion. Chiropractors as well as other clinicians can facilitate a path to good recovery for MTBI patients through early education and positive reassurance as well as by providing treatments aimed at reducing associated spine and headache-related pain. Similar to care for whiplash injuries and LBP, MTBI patients may benefit from early, but careful activation, while limiting passive care reliance. For those with persistent post-concussion symptoms, psychosocial factors (e.g., poor expectations of recovery, negative injury perceptions) as well as co-morbidities (e.g., somatic pain) need to be addressed and modified to help direct a patient's course towards a positive recovery. Also for those with persistent symptoms, caution must be exercised before seeking excessive diagnostic testing or applying diagnostic labels (i.e., post-concussion syndrome) as unnecessary diagnoses as well as testing can increase patient anxiety and delay further recovery. Integrating care with a patient's primary medical physician is recommended if additional symptom-specific treatments are required (e.g., pain medication or neurocognitive testing). Forming similar therapeutic partnerships may also be necessary to facilitate a plan for RTW after MTBI. While there is much work to be done to better understand MTBI prognosis, the recent ICoMP review has provided strong preliminary evidence which clinicians can use to help improve and inform clinical decision making and thus promote better recovery and limit disability after MTBI.

Abbreviations

AD: Alzheimer's disease; CCI: Chronic cognitive impairment; CDC: Centers for disease control; CTE: Chronic traumatic encephalopathy; GCS: Glasgow coma scale; ICoMP: International collaboration on MTBI prognosis; LBP: Low back pain; LOC: Loss of consciousness; MTBI: Mild traumatic brain injury; MVC: Motor vehicle collision; PD: Parkinson's disease; PRISMA: Preferred reporting items of systematic reviews and meta-analyses; PTA: Post-traumatic amnesia; RTP: Return to play; RTW: Return to work; SIGN: Scottish intercollegiate guidelines network; SIS: Second impact syndrome; WAD: whiplash associated disorders; WHO: World Health Organization.

Competing interests

The authors declare that they have no competing interests.

Authors' contributions

JD, CC and JDC conceived of the concept and outline of this commentary and JD drafted the manuscript. CC and JDC provided guidance and assistance in the overall development and drafting of this manuscript. All authors read and approved the final manuscript.

Author details

[1]Division of Health Care and Outcomes Research, Toronto Western Research Institute, University Health Network, University of Toronto, Toronto, Canada. [2]Institute of Health Policy, Management and Evaluation, University of Toronto, Toronto, Canada. [3]Institute of Sports Science and Clinical Biomechanics, Faculty of Health, University of Southern Denmark, Odense, Denmark.

References

1. Cassidy JD, Carroll LJ, Peloso PM, Borg J, von Holst H, Holm L, Kraus J, Coronado VG, WHO Collaborating Centre Task Force on MTBI: **Incidence, risk factors and prevention of mild traumatic brain injury: results of the WHO collaborating centre task force on mild traumatic brain injury.** *J Rehabil Med* 2004, **36**(Suppl 43):28–60.
2. Carroll LJ, Cassidy JD, Holm L, Kraus J, Coronado VG, WHO Collaborating Centre Task Force on MTBI: **Methodological issues and research recommendations for mild traumatic brain injury: the WHO collaborating centre task force on mild traumatic brain injury.** *J Rehabil Med* 2004, **36**(Suppl 43):113–125.
3. Carroll LJ, Cassidy JD, Peloso PM, Borg J, von Holst H, Holm L, Paniak C, Pepin M, WHO Collaborating Centre Task Force on MTBI: **Prognosis for mild traumatic brain injury: results of the WHO collaborating centre task force on mild traumatic brain injury.** *J Rehabil Med* 2004, **36**(Suppl 43):84–105.
4. Cancelliere C, Cassidy JD, Côté P, Hincapié CA, Hartvigsen J, Carroll LJ, Marras C, Boyle E, Kristman V, Hung R, Stålnacke BM, Rumney P, Coronado V, Holm LW, Borg J, Nygren-de Boussard C, Af Geijerstam JL, Keightley M: **Protocol for a systematic review of prognosis after mild traumatic brain injury: an update of the WHO collaborating centre task force findings.** *Syst Rev* 2012, **1**:17.
5. Moher D, Liberati A, Tetzlaff J, Altman DG, PRISMA Group: **Preferred reporting items for systematic reviews and meta-analyses: the PRISMA statement.** *PLoS Med* 2009, **6**:e1000097.
6. Cancelliere C, Cassidy JD, Li A, Donovan J, Côté P, Hincapié CA: **Systematic search and review procedures: results of the International Collaboration on Mild Traumatic Brain Injury Prognosis.** *Arch Phys Med Rehabil* 2014, **95**(Suppl 3):S101–S131.
7. **Scottish intercollegiate guidelines network (SIGN).** In [http://www.sign.ac.uk/]
8. Côté P, Cassidy JD, Carroll L, Frank JW, Bombardier C: **A systematic review of the prognosis of acute whiplash and a new conceptual framework to synthesize the literature.** *Spine (Phila Pa 1976)* 2001, **26**:E445–E458.
9. Cancelliere C, Hincapié CA, Keightley M, Godbolt AK, Côté P, Kristman VL, Stålnacke BM, Carroll LJ, Hung R, Borg J, Nygren-de Boussard C, Coronado VG, Donovan J, Cassidy JD: **Systematic review of prognosis and return to play after sport concussion: results of the International Collaboration on Mild Traumatic Brain Injury Prognosis.** *Arch Phys Med Rehabil* 2014, **95**(Suppl 3):S210–S229.
10. McCrory P, Meeuwisse WH, Aubry M, Cantu B, Dvorak J, Echemendia RJ, Engebretsen L, Johnston K, Kutcher JS, Raftery M, Sills A, Benson BW, Davis GA, Ellenbogen RG, Guskiewicz K, Herring SA, Iverson GL, Jordan BD, Kissick J, McCrea M, McIntosh AS, Maddocks D, Makdissi M, Purcell L, Putukian M, Schneider K, Tator CH, Turner M: **Consensus statement on concussion in sport: the 4th international conference on concussion in sport held in Zurich, November 2012.** *Br J Sports Med* 2013, **47**:250–258.
11. Cantu RC: **Second-impact syndrome.** *Clin Sports Med* 1998, **17**:37–44.
12. Saunders RL, Harbaugh RE: **The second impact in catastrophic contact-sports head trauma.** *JAMA* 1984, **252**:538–539.
13. Tator CH: **Concussions and their consequences: current diagnosis, management and prevention.** *CMAJ* 2013, **185**:975–979.
14. McCrory PR, Berkovic SF: **Second impact syndrome.** *Neurology* 1998, **50**:677–683.
15. Cassidy JD, Cancelliere C, Carroll LJ, Côté P, Hincapié CA, Holm LW, Hartvigsen J, Donovan J, Nygren-de Boussard C, Kristman VL, Borg J: **Systematic review of self-reported prognosis in adults after mild traumatic brain injury: results of the International Collaboration on Mild Traumatic Brain Injury Prognosis.** *Arch Phys Med Rehabil* 2014, **95**(Suppl 3):S132–S151.
16. Stulemeijer M, van der Werf S, Borm GF, Vos PE: **Early prediction of favourable recovery 6 months after mild traumatic brain injury.** *J Neurol Neurosurg Psychiatry* 2008, **79**:936–942.
17. Carroll LJ, Cassidy JD, Cancelliere C, Côté P, Hincapié CA, Kristman VL, Holm LW, Borg J, Nygren-de Boussard C, Hartvigsen J: **Systematic review of the prognosis after mild traumatic brain injury in adults: cognitive, psychiatric, and mortality outcomes: results of the International Collaboration on Mild Traumatic Brain Injury Prognosis.** *Arch Phys Med Rehabil* 2014, **95**(Suppl 3):S152–S173.
18. Cassidy JD, Boyle E, Carroll LJ: **Population-based, inception cohort study of the incidence, course, and prognosis of mild traumatic brain injury after motor vehicle collisions.** *Arch Phys Med Rehabil* 2014, **95**(Suppl 3):S278–S285.
19. Cassidy JD, Carroll L, Côté P, Holm L, Nygren A: **Mild traumatic brain injury after traffic collisions: a population-based inception cohort study.** *J Rehabil Med* 2004, **36**(Suppl 43):15–21.
20. Hartvigsen J, Boyle E, Cassidy JD, Carroll LJ: **Mild traumatic brain injury after motor vehicle collisions: what are the symptoms and who treats them? A population-based 1-year inception cohort study.** *Arch Phys Med Rehabil* 2014, **95**(Suppl 3):S286–S294.
21. Ferrari R, Russell AS, Carroll LJ, Cassidy JD: **A re-examination of the whiplash associated disorders (WAD) as a systemic illness.** *Ann Rhem Dis* 2005, **64**:1337–1342.
22. Holm LW, Carroll LJ, Cassidy JD, Skillgate E, Ahlbom A: **Expectations for recovery important in the prognosis of whiplash injuries.** *PLoS Med* 2008, **5**:e105.
23. Carroll LJ, Holm LW, Ferrari R, Ozegovic D, Cassidy JD: **Recovery in whiplash-associated disorders: do you get what you expect?** *J Rheumatol* 2009, **36**:1063–1070.
24. Deyo RA, Diehl AK, Rosenthal M: **How many days of bed rest for acute low back pain? A randomized clinical trial.** *N Engl J Med* 1986, **315**:1064–1070.
25. Silverberg ND, Iverson GL: **Is rest after concussion "the best medicine?" Recommendations for activity resumption following concussion in athletes, civilians, and military service members.** *J Head Trauma Rehabil* 2013, **28**:250–259.
26. Nygren-de Boussard C, Holm LW, Cancelliere C, Godbolt AK, Boyle E, Stålnacke BM, Hincapié CA, Cassidy JD, Borg J: **Nonsurgical interventions after mild traumatic brain injury: a systematic review. Results of the International Collaboration on Mild Traumatic Brain Injury Prognosis.** *Arch Phys Med Rehabil* 2014, **95**(Suppl 3):S257–S264.
27. Chou R, Qaseem A, Snow V, Casey D, Cross JT Jr, Shekelle P, Owens DK, Clinical Efficacy Assessment Subcommittee of the American College of Pain; American College of Physicians, American Pain Society Low Back Pain Guidelines Pain Guidelines Panel: **Diagnosis and treatment of low back pain: a joint clinical practice guideline from the American college of physicians and the American pain society.** *Ann Intern Med* 2007, **147**:478–491.
28. Cancelliere C, Kristman VL, Cassidy JD, Hincapié CA, Côté P, Boyle E, Carroll LJ, Stålnacke BM, Nygren-de Boussard C, Borg J: **Systematic review of return to work after mild traumatic brain injury: results of the International Collaboration on Mild Traumatic Brain Injury Prognosis.** *Arch Phys Med Rehabil* 2014, **95**(Suppl 3):S201–S209.
29. Cancelliere C, Cassidy JD, Colantonio A: **Specific disorder-linked determinants: traumatic brain injury.** In *Handbook of Work Disability: Prevention and Management.* Edited by Loisel P, Anema JR. New York: Springer Publishing Company; 2013:303–314.
30. Hung R, Carroll LJ, Cancelliere C, Côté P, Rumney P, Keightley M, Donovan J, Stålnacke BM, Cassidy JD: **Systematic review of the clinical course, natural history, and prognosis for pediatric mild traumatic brain injury: results of the International Collaboration on Mild Traumatic Brain Injury Prognosis.** *Arch Phys Med Rehabil* 2014, **95**(Suppl 3):S174–S191.
31. Zemek R, Duval S, Dematteo C: *Guidelines for Diagnosing and Managing Pediatric Concussion [Internet].* Toronto, ON: Ontario Neurotrauma Foundation; 2014 [www.onf.org/documents/guidelines-for-pediatric-concussion]
32. Godbolt AK, Cancelliere C, Hincapié CA, Marras C, Boyle E, Kristman VL, Coronado VG, Cassidy JD: **Systematic review of the risk of dementia and chronic cognitive impairment after mild traumatic brain injury: results of the International Collaboration on Mild Traumatic Brain Injury Prognosis.** *Arch Phys Med Rehabil* 2014, **95**(Suppl 3):S245–S256.
33. McKee AC, Cantu RC, Nowinski CJ, Hedley-Whyte ET, Gavett BE, Budson AE, Santini VE, Lee HS, Kubilus CA, Stern RA: **Chronic traumatic encephalopathy in athletes: progressive tauopathy after repetitive head injury.** *J Neuropathol Exp Neurol* 2009, **68**:709–735.
34. Marras C, Hincapié CA, Kristman VL, Cancelliere C, Soklaridis S, Li A, Borg J, Af Geijerstam JL, Cassidy JD: **Systematic review of the risk of Parkinson's disease after mild traumatic brain injury: results of the International Collaboration on Mild Traumatic Brain Injury Prognosis.** *Arch Phys Med Rehabil* 2014, **95**(Suppl 3):S238–S244.

35. Kristman VL, Borg J, Godbolt AK, Salmi LR, Cancelliere C, Carroll LJ, Holm LW, Nygren-de Boussard C, Hartvigsen J, Abara U, Donovan J, Cassidy JD: **Methodological issues and research recommendations for prognosis after mild traumatic brain injury: results of the International Collaboration on Mild Traumatic Brain Injury Prognosis.** *Arch Phys Med Rehabil* 2014, **95**(Suppl 3):S265–S277.

The reliability of a portable clinical force plate used for the assessment of static postural control: repeated measures reliability study

Samira Golriz[1*], Jeffrey J Hebert[2], K Bo Foreman[3] and Bruce F Walker[2]

Abstract

Background: Force plates are frequently used for postural control assessments but they are expensive and not widely available in most clinical settings. Increasingly, clinicians are using this technology to assess patients, however, the psychometric properties of these less sophisticated force plates is frequently unknown. The purposes of the study were to examine the test-retest reliability of a force plate commonly used by clinicians and to explore the effect of using the mean value from multiple repetitions on reliability.

Methods: Thirty healthy volunteer adults were recruited. Postural control measures were obtained using the Midot Posture Scale Analyzer (MPSA). Data were collected in 2 sessions. Five successive repetitions each of 60 seconds duration were obtained from each participant in each session.

Results: The reliability coefficients obtained using single measures were low ($ICC_{3,1}$ = 0.06 to 0.53). The average of two measures allowed for reliable measurements of COP mean velocity and average location of COP. The average of three and five measures was required to obtain acceptable reliability (ICC ≥ 0.70) of relative weight bearing on legs and sway area, respectively. Higher measurement precision values were seen by averaging four or five repetitions for all variables.

Conclusion: Single measures did not provide reliable estimates of postural sway, and the averaging of multiple repetitions was necessary to achieve acceptable levels of measurement error. The number of repetitions required to achieve reliable data ranged from 2 to 5. Clinicians should be wary of using single measures derived from similar equipment when making decisions about patients.

Keywords: Reproducibility, Posture, Stability, Balance, Force plate

Introduction

Postural control organises the orientation and equilibrium of the body during upright stance and is essential to the successful performance of daily movements and activities as well as fall prevention [1]. Postural control depends on visual, vestibular and proprioceptive input and can be disrupted by various perturbations experienced in everyday life [2,3]. Moreover, pathology, medications, alcohol consumption, and the aging process can adversely affect postural control [4,5] .

Postural control can be measured subjectively or objectively. Subjective measures of postural control are obtained through the use of questionnaires. Such questionnaires provide valuable information, however they often have limitations with some special populations such as the elderly or individuals with specific physical or cognitive impairment [6,7]. In addition, subjective methods of measurement may suffer from floor or ceiling effects or lack optimal reliability, validity and the precision to detect small differences [8,9]. It has been suggested that these questionnaires be used in combination with other measures [9].

Objective assessments are the most common method of measuring postural control. Postural control is usually evaluated by interpretation of centre of pressure (COP),

* Correspondence: Samiraa_g@yahoo.com
[1]School of Chiropractic and Sports Science, Murdoch University, 90 South Street, Murdoch, WA 6150, Australia
Full list of author information is available at the end of the article

postural sway and weight bearing distribution measurements [10,11]. COP estimates the position of the ground reaction force vector on the base of support of the body and calculation of the total COP kinematics is frequently used to assess postural sway [12]. Postural sway is an indicator of the displacement and correction of the centre of gravity in relation to the base of support [11]. Relative weight bearing is a gross estimate of postural control. Postural control is influenced by weight bearing distribution and weight bearing distribution asymmetry results in less postural stability [10].

Force plates are frequently used to measure COP and postural sway [11]. This approach requires the individual to stand or walk, while transducers measure ground reaction forces generated by the body. As a clinical tool, force plates are utilised therapeutically [13], and for longitudinal assessment [14]. Force plates can be used to enhance balance training by providing visual feedback to the patient [13]. However, the types of force plates used by clinicians typically lack the sophistication of force plates used in research environments. Moreover, well known force plates used in research have known psychometric properties such as reliability and validity, while the psychometric properties of force plates used in the clinical setting are frequently unknown or poorly defined.

The Midot posture scale analyser (MPSA) is an example of less sophisticated force plate used by clinicians such as physical therapists, chiropractors, and neurologists [15]. The MPSA is relatively inexpensive and includes simple and easy to use software that allows individuals with limited experience to obtain and interpret measures of postural control and weight bearing distribution.

However, when making decisions about patients, it is logical to rely on assessments obtained by instruments shown to be reliable and valid. Reliability is a prerequisite of validity and reflects measurement consistency and the degree to which an instrument is free from errors of measurement [16]. When clinicians obtain measurements to inform clinical decision making, it is necessary that the instruments demonstrate adequate reliability. Therefore, the purpose of this study was to examine the test-retest reliability of a force plate commonly used by clinicians. Additionally, we explored the effect of using the mean value from multiple repetitions on reliability.

Methods

Participants

Participant recruitment was by way of posted advertisements on University bulletin boards. Potential participants were adults between 18 to 60 years of age. A lower age limit of 18 years was chosen to help ensure maturity of the skeletal system [17]. Postural control decreases in the elderly [18], therefore 60 years was considered the upper age limit.

Participants were excluded from the study if they had a history of musculoskeletal injury in the previous three months, a balance deficit stemming from a rheumatologic or neurologic disorder, pregnancy, an ear infection or fever within 72 hours of testing or were currently taking medications that could alter sensory perception. The Human Research Ethics Committee of Murdoch University approved the study protocol (2010/139), and all subjects gave written consent before enrolling in the study. The rights of all subjects were protected.

Instrument

The Midot posture scale analyser (MPSA)- QPS 200 is a portable force plate consisting of 4 electronic weighing plates set in a rectangular position. Analogue signals were sampled and transferred to a laptop computer via a USB-to-serial (RS-232) analogue to digital converter. The MPSA specifications report an acquisition sampling frequency of 200 Hz and cut-off frequency of 0.5 Hz [15].

The MPSA is designed to measure, during quiet standing: (1) the average location of COP with reference to the cross point of the weighing platform (mm), (2) COP mean velocity, which is the average velocity of COP movement (mm/sec), (3) sway area, which is the area of an ellipse enclosing 95% of COP movement (mm^2) and was measured by calculation of the ellipse area, and (4) the relative weight distribution between the subject's right and left sides (%).

Procedure

Calibration of the force plate was conducted each day prior to data collection based on the manufacturer's instructions. We tested all subjects under the same conditions. Participants stood with their feet shoulder width apart on a sheet of paper placed on the top of the platform. The paper remained in place during testing. Both feet were outlined to ensure consistent placement across trials. Participants were asked to remove their shoes, stand upright on the force plate and remain as still as possible in a relaxed posture. We asked participants to put their arms to their sides in a comfortable position and to distribute their body weight evenly on both feet while breathing normally. Finally, the participants were instructed to look straight ahead at an "X" on the opposite wall located 2 meters away at eye level. If the patient usually wore glasses, they continued to do so during this procedure.

Subjects were scheduled for 2 sessions of 5 trials, 5 minutes apart. The second session replicated the first. The duration of each trial was 60 seconds. A 60-second assessment was chosen to mimic constituent periods of standing during typical activities of daily living (e.g., waiting for a bus or elevator). To avoid inconsistencies in the data at transitions, we informed the participants of the data collection start time 5 seconds before the actual start time. Mandatory breaks of 1 minute were allocated between each individual trial during which subjects were allowed to sit. Breaks assured that participants were refreshed for each trial. Five successive trials were recorded during each session. On average, the overall duration of the experiment was approximately 25 minutes.

Statistical analysis

Using the approach of Donner and Eliasziw (1987) [19], considering a minimally acceptable intraclass correlation coefficient (ICC) value of 0.70 [20] and 5 repetitions in each of two sessions, recruitment of 30 participants at an alpha level of 0.05 was estimated to provide 80% power to detect a relationship this strong or stronger.

Data management and statistical analyses were performed using SPSS version 17. Data were entered and inspected to ensure that there were no errors of entry. Descriptive statistics were calculated for all variables.

Values for a single repetition and averages of 2, 3, 4 and 5 repetitions were calculated for all dependant variables. To visually examine for the presence of systematic error (e. g., fatigue or learning effects) average values of COP mean velocity and sway area were plotted against the number of repetitions. Relative reliability of the measures was assessed using $ICC_{3,k}$ [21] and 95% confidence intervals. The standard error of measurement was calculated to assess measurement precision using the formula: Standard error of measurement = pooled standard deviation $\times \sqrt{1 - ICC}$. Additionally, we calculated the minimal detectable difference (MDD) with 95% confidence intervals. The MDD was calculated using the formula: MDD = $1.96 \times$ standard error of measurement $\times \sqrt{2}$. and estimates the smallest difference exceeding measurement error [16]. To explore for systematic differences between the first and second sessions, bias statistics with 95% confidence intervals were calculated by computing the mean difference of measures obtained during the two sessions. Levels of agreement (LOA) were calculated as: LOA = bias $\pm$ 1.96 standard deviation of differences between the 2 sessions. It is expected that 95% of the difference between the first and second sessions would be between these limits [22]. Finally, to compare the effect of the number of repetitions on reliability, all of the above calculations were generated using values from a single repetition as well as the mean of the first 2, 3, 4 and 5 repetitions.

Results

Thirty volunteers aged 20 to 57 years participated in the study. All subjects were able to complete the protocol and all data were included for statistical analysis. The final sample was composed of 16 men and 14 women, with a mean ± SD age of 30.5 ± 7.2 years and BMI of 25.6 ± 5.5.

The profile plots displaying the averages of COP mean velocity and sway area across repetitions were visually inspected and no learning or fatigue effects were identified. Means, standard deviations, reliability coefficients, standard error of measurement, MDD, bias and LOA statistics are presented in Table 1 for each dependant variable.

Each of the five variables measured exhibited unacceptable levels of measurement error when calculated from single measures. For the relative weight distribution on the legs, it was necessary to average 3 or more repetitions to achieve a minimum acceptable reliability value. COP mean velocity required at least 2 trials to obtain an acceptable ICC value. The ICC values of the average COP location are acceptable with 2 measurements; while measures of sway area required 5 repetitions to achieve acceptable reliability.

Bias estimates were small and not significantly different from zero indicating that there were no statistically significant differences between the two sessions. The only exception was the COP mean velocity calculated of two repetitions, which reached the threshold of statistical significance, however the magnitude of this difference was small.

Discussion

The objectives of this study were to examine the test-retest reliability of postural control measurements of a portable force plate commonly used by clinicians and to explore the effect of using the mean value from multiple repetitions on reliability. Our results demonstrated that for measures obtained by the MPSA, single trials do not provide reliable estimates of postural control and that averaging multiple measures is necessary to achieve acceptable levels of measurement error. The number of repetitions necessary to achieve reliable results varied depending of the outcome variable and ranged from two to five. Clinicians should take this into account when measuring postural control on their patients.

ICC values for measures of relative weight bearing appeared lower than ICC values of COP mean velocity and average location of COP. However, inspection of the descriptive statistics (mean and SD) in Table 1 for each of these variables indicates less inter-subject variability in relative weight bearing as compared to the other dependent variables. Low levels of inter-subject variability are known to artificially lower ICC estimates, as this increases the relative magnitude of the error term in the ICC equation [16]. Thus, it can be difficult to interpret

Table 1 Reliability results of single measures and means of 2, 3, 4 and 5 measures for each variable

Variable	Mean ± SD *	ICC (95% CI)	SEM	MDD	Bias (95% CI) ± 95% LOA
Relative weight bearing on right leg (%)					
1 repetition	50.10 ± 2.7	0.44 (−0.18,0.74)	2.0	5.6	0.3(−0.3,0.9) ±6.5
2 repetitions	49.84 ± 2.4	0.65 (0.25,0.83)	1.4	3.9	0.3(−0.2,0.7) ±4.9
3 repetitions	49.69 ± 2.3	**0.75** (0.47,0.88)	1.2	3.2	0.1(−0.3,0.5) ±4.1
4 repetitions	49.69 ± 2.3	**0.82** (0.63,0.92)	1.0	2.7	0.2(−0.2,0.5) ±3.6
5 repetitions	49.64 ± 2.3	**0.83** (0.64,0.92)	0.9	2.6	0.3(−0.1,0.6) ±3.5
Relative weight bearing on left leg (%)					
1 repetition	49.90 ± 2.7	0.44(−0.18,0.75)	2.0	5.6	0.3(−0.3,0.9) ±6.5
2 repetitions	50.16 ± 2.4	0.65 (0.27,0.85)	1.4	3.9	0.3 (−0.2,0.7) ±4.9
3 repetitions	50.31 ± 2.3	**0.75** (0.49,0.89)	1.2	3.2	0.1(−0.3,0.5) ±4.1
4 repetitions	50.31 ± 2.3	**0.81** (0.59-0.91)	1.0	2.7	0.1(−0.2,0.5) ± 3.7
5 repetitions	50.36 ± 2.3	**0.82** (0.63-0.92)	1.0	2.7	0.2(−0.1,0.5) ±3.5
COP mean velocity (mm/sec)					
1 repetition	6.0 ± 4.8	0.19 (−0.75,0.62)	4.4	12.1	−0.6(−1.9,0.7) ±13.50
2 repetitions	5.6 ± 3.4	**0.83** (0.65,0.92)	1.3	3.5	0.2(0.1,0.4)† ±1.81
3 repetitions	5.5 ±3.3	**0.95** (0.90,0.98)	0.7	2	0.2(0.0,0.5) ±2.68
4 repetitions	5.5 ± 3.3	**0.97** (0.94,0.99)	0.6	1.6	0.09(−0.1,0.3) ±2.09
5 repetitions	5.4 ± 3.2	**0.92** (0.84,0.96)	0.9	2.5	0.03(−0.3,0.3) ±3.43
Average location of COP (mm)					
1 repetition	35.0 ± 21	0.53 (−0.01,0.78)	14.4	39.7	−1.8(−6.2,2.6) ±47.2
2 repetitions	38.4 ± 31.1	**0.92** (0.84,0.96)	8.8	24.4	−1.6(−4.7,1.5) ±33.3
3 repetitions	37.3 ± 26.5	**0.91** (0.81,0.96)	8	22.1	−0.4(−3.2,2.4) ±30.2
4 repetitions	38.8 ± 28.9	**0.93** (0.85,0.97)	7.7	21.3	−0.7(−3.4,2.1) ±29.8
5 repetitions	39.0 ± 29.6	**0.94** (0.88,0.97)	7.3	22	−0.6(−3.2,2.0) ±27.9
Sway area (mm^2)					
1 repetition	1549.6 ± 1605.5	0.06(−1.02,0.56)	1556.9	4302.7	−265.6(−686.4,155.1) ± 4517.0
2 repetitions	1442.6 ± 1055.5	0.47 (−0.13,0.75)	763.7	2116.8	−73.2 (−302.3,156.3) ±1399.0
3 repetitions	1456.6 ± 1001.9	0.63 (0.28,0.82)	612.7	1698.3	−159.2 (−350.4,32.1) ±2054.0
4 repetitions	1440.3 ± 889.8	0.68 (0.33,0.85)	504.8	1399.2	−159.2 (−278.9,43.8) ± 1732.7
5 repetitions	1466.9 ± 918.2	**0.83** (0.64,0.92)	380.4	1054.3	−48.6 (−178.7,81.7) ± 1399.0

CI confidence interval, *ICC* intra class correlation coefficient, *LOA* limit of agreement, *MDD* minimal detectable difference, *SEM* standard error of measurement
*Pooled from all repetitions;
† Statistically significant bias (different from zero);
Bold ICCs indicate acceptable reliability values.

ICC values derived from homogenous measures such as relative weight distribution.

We also assessed COP mean velocity, average location of COP, and sway area. Consistent with our results, COP mean velocity has been reported by others to be the most reliable estimate of COP [23-25]. In contrast, others have examined samples of healthy participants and reported low reliability for measures of COP mean velocity [26]. However, it should be noted that in that study, the ICC statistics were calculated by averaging data from 3 10-second repetitions. The longer duration of recording used in our protocol may explain our higher reliability estimates. While longer duration trials of up to 120 seconds are recommended to reduce measurement error [24], sampling duration should be matched to the abilities of participants. For instance, children with cerebral palsy or the elderly may not tolerate standing for an ideal duration of time.

For measures of sway area, it was necessary to average values from five repetitions to achieve an acceptable level of measurement error. Two studies reported similarly low ICC values for sway area [27,28]. Alternatively, others have reported acceptable levels of ICC for this variable; however, these latter studies were conducted under eyes closed.

A potential issue with relying on measures obtained from a suboptimal number of repetitions can arise in clinical practice. For instance, when examining for differences in postural stability over using single measures, a practitioner needs to observe an improvement of at least 12.1 mm/sec in COP mean velocity to be 95% confident that a true change has occurred. However, when using a mean of 3 repetitions, a practitioner can be just as confident that true change has occurred with a change of 2 mm/sec.

The results of this study are limited by several factors. This study was conducted on healthy individuals and the results may or may not generalize to clinical populations. Moreover, the MPSA as an instrument of measurement has several limitations. The MPSA is limited to a fixed duration of data acquisition of between 5 and 60 seconds. It is not possible to set up the recording time to durations longer than 60 seconds, which may be desirable is some circumstances. This technology also has a fixed sampling rate and cut-off frequency and altering these frequencies is not possible. Finally, the MPSA software does not report some variables such as sway area, which we calculated from the raw data.

Future research should examine the validity of the force plates commonly used by clinicians by comparing their measures to those obtained using force plates with known validity. Additionally, it would be useful to assess the reliability of similar force plates in a clinical population, such as those individuals with neurological impairments.

Conclusion

For measures of postural sway obtained by the MPSA, single trials do not provide reliable estimates, and the averaging of multiple repetitions was necessary to achieve acceptable levels of measurement error. Depending on the variable, the number of repetitions required to achieve reliable data ranged from 2 to 5. Clinicians should be wary of using single measures derived from similar equipment when making decisions about patients.

Abbreviations

COP: Centre of pressure; ICC: Intraclass correlation coefficient; LOA: Level of agreement; MDD: Minimal detectable difference; MPSA: Midot posture scale analyser.

Competing interests

The authors declare that they have no competing interests.

Authors' contributions

SG participated in the design of the study, collected data, performed the statistical analysis and drafted the manuscript. JH participated in the design of the study, helped to perform the statistical analysis and drafted the manuscript. BF helped to draft the manuscript. BW participated in the design of the study and helped to draft the manuscript. All authors read and approved the final manuscript.

Author details

[1]School of Chiropractic and Sports Science, Murdoch University, 90 South Street, Murdoch, WA 6150, Australia. [2]School of Chiropractic and Sports Science, Murdoch University, Perth, WA, Australia. [3]Department of Physical Therapy, University of Utah, Salt Lake City, UT, USA.

References

1. Lafond D, Corriveau H, Prince F: **Postural Control Mechanisms during Quiet Standing in Patients with Diabetic Sensory Neuropathy.** *Diabetes Care* 2004, **27**:173–178.
2. Brocklehurst JC, Robertson D, James-Groom P: **Clinical correlates of sway in old age, Sensory modalities.** *Age Ageing* 1982, **11**:1–10.
3. Horak FB, Henry SM, Shumway-Cook A: **Postural perturbations: New insights for treatment of balance disorders.** *Phys Ther* 1997, **77**:517–533.
4. Haas BM, Burden AM: **Validity of weight distribution and sway measurements of the Balance Performance Monitor.** *Physiother res international: j res clinicians therapy* 2000, **5**:19–32.
5. Li X, Aruin AS: **The effect of short-term changes in body mass distribution on feed-forward postural control.** *J Electromyogr Kinesiol* 2009, **19**:931–941.
6. Berg K, Wood-Dauphinee S, Williams JI, Gayton D: **Measuring balance in the elderly: Preliminary development of an instrument.** *Physiother Can* 1989, **41**:304–311.
7. Kairy D, Paquet N, Fung J: **A postural adaptation test for stroke patients.** *Disabil Rehabil* 2003, **25**:127–135.
8. Mercer VS, Hankins CC, Spinks AJ, Tedder DD: **Reliability and validity of a clinical test of reaction time in older adults.** *J Geriatr Phys Ther* 2009, **32**:103–110.
9. Blum L, Korner-Bitensky N: **Usefulness of the Berg Balance Scale in stroke rehabilitation: A systematic review.** *Phys Ther* 2008, **88**:559–566.
10. Anker LC, Weerdesteyn V, van Nes IJW, Nienhuis B, Straatman H, Geurts ACH: **The relation between postural stability and weight distribution in healthy subjects.** *Gait Posture* 2008, **27**:471–477.
11. Prieto TE, Myklebust JB, Myklebust B: **Characterization and modeling of postural steadiness in the elderly: a review.** *IEEE Trans Rehabil Eng* 1993, **1**:26–34.
12. Schiffman JM, Bensel CK, Hasselquist L, Gregorczyk KN, Piscitelle L: **Effects of carried weight on random motion and traditional measures of postural sway.** *Appl Ergon* 2006, **37**:607–614.
13. Geiger RA, Allen JB, O'Keefe J, Hicks RR: **Balance and mobility following stroke: Effects of physical therapy interventions with and without biofeedback/forceplate training.** *Phys Ther* 2001, **81**:995–1005.
14. Lajoie Y: **Effect of computerized feedback postural training on posture and attentional demands in older adults.** *Aging Clin Exp Res* 2004, **16**:363–368.
15. Clark RA, Bryant AL, Pua Y, McCrory P, Bennell K, Hunt M: **Validity and reliability of the Nintendo Wii Balance Board for assessment of standing balance.** *Gait Posture* 2010, **31**:307–310.
16. Portney LG, Watkins MP: *Foundations of clinical research: Application to practice.* 3 ednth edition. Upper Saddle River, NJ: Prentice Hall Health; 2008.
17. Malina RM, Pena Reyes ME, Eisenmann JC, Horta L, Rodrigues J, Miller R: **Height, mass and skeletal maturity of elite Portuguese soccer players aged 11–16 years.** *J Sports Sci* 2000, **18**:685–693.
18. Era P, Sainio P, Koskinen S, Haavisto P, Vaara M, Aromaa A: **Postural balance in a random sample of 7,979 subjects aged 30 years and over.** *Gerontology* 2006, **52**:204–213.
19. Donner A, Eliasziw M: **Sample size requirements for reliability studies.** *Stat Med* 1987, **6**:441–448.
20. Lohr KN, Aaronson NK, Alonso J, Burnam MA, Patrick DL, Perrin EB, Roberts JS: **Evaluating quality-of-life and health status instruments: Development of scientific review criteria.** *Clin Ther* 1996, **18**:979–984.
21. Shrout PE, Fleiss JL: **Intraclass correlations: Uses in assessing rater reliability.** *Psychol Bull* 1979, **86**:420–428.
22. Bland JM, Altman DG: **Statistical methods for assessing agreement between two methods of clinical measurement.** *Lancet* 1986, **1**:307–310.

23. Lin D, Seol H, Nussbaum MA, Madigan ML: **Reliability of COP-based postural sway measures and age-related differences.** *Gait Posture* 2008, **28**:337–342.
24. Lafond D, Corriveau H, Hèlbert R, Prince F: **Intrasession reliability of center of pressure measures of postural steadiness in healthy elderly people.** *Arch Phys Med Rehabil* 2004, **85**:896–901.
25. Hadian MR, Negahban H, Talebian S, Salavati M, Jafari AH, Sanjari MA, Mazaheri M, Parnianpour M: **Reliability of center of pressure measures of postural stability in patients with unilateral anterior cruciate ligament injury.** *J Appl Sci* 2008, **8**:3019–3025.
26. Doyle TL, Newton RU, Burnett AF: **Reliability of traditional and fractal dimension measures of quiet stance center of pressure in young, healthy people.** *Arch Phys Med Rehabil* 2005, **86**:2034–2040.
27. Salavati M, Hadian MR, Mazaheri M, Negahban H, Ebrahimi I, Talebian S, Jafari AH, Sanjari MA, Sohani SM, Parnianpour M: **Test-retest reliabty of center of pressure measures of postural stability during quiet standing in a group with musculoskeletal disorders consisting of low back pain, anterior cruciate ligament injury and functional ankle instability.** *Gait Posture* 2009, **29**:460–464.
28. Takala EP, Korhonen I, Viikari-Juntura E: **Postural sway and stepping response among working population: Reproducibility, long-term stability, and associations with symptoms of the low back.** *Clinical Biomechanics* 1997, **12**:429–437.

The validity of a portable clinical force plate in assessment of static postural control: concurrent validity study

Samira Golriz[1*], Jeffrey J Hebert[2], K Bo Foreman[3] and Bruce F Walker[2]

Abstract

Background: The broad use of force plates in clinical settings for postural control assessment suggests the need for instruments that are easy to use, affordable and readily available. In addition, these instruments of measurement should be reliable and valid as adequate reliability and validity are prerequisites to making correct inferences. The aim of this study was to examine the concurrent validity of postural control measures obtained with a clinical force plate.

Methods: Thirty-one healthy adults were recruited. Participants completed 1 set of 5 trials on each force plate. Postural control measures (centre of pressure [COP] average velocity and sway area) were collected and compared using the Midot Posture Scale Analyzer (clinical force plate) and the Accugait force plate (criterion measure). Intra class correlation coefficient (ICC), standard error of measurement , and paired t-tests were calculated and Bland-Altman plots were constructed to compare the force plates and assess consistency of measurement and agreement between them.

Results: The ICC values (ICC = 0.14-0.60) between the two force plates were lower than the acceptable value for both COP average velocity and sway area. There was significant difference ($p > 0.05$) in COP average velocity and sway area between the force plates. Examination of the plots revealed that there is less difference between the force plates in lower magnitudes of COP for average velocity and sway area however, the greater the average velocity and sway area, the greater the difference between the measures obtained from the two force plates.

Conclusion: Findings of this study showed poor concurrent validity of the clinical force plate. This clinical force plate cannot be a replacement for known reliable and valid force plates and consequently measures obtained from this force plate should be treated with caution especially in a clinical population.

Keywords: Concurrent validity, Force plate, Postural control

Introduction

Postural control is a crucial factor in maintaining balance during standing, walking, task performance and when responding to the unexpected perturbations experienced in everyday life [1]. Postural control assessment can provide useful information when identifying individuals who are susceptible to postural control deficits [2,3]. Furthermore, postural control assessment has been used in sports medicine for selection of talented athletes, identification of athletes at high risk for injury, and for the prevention of sports related injuries [4]. Postural control is usually assessed by interpretation of parameters derived from the centre of pressure (COP) such as velocity and area of COP displacement [5]. COP is defined as the point of application of ground reaction forces under the feet.

In a clinical setting, force plates are regularly used to objectively assess postural control [6]. However, the reliability and validity of these force plates is often unknown. Reliability represents the consistency of measures or the level to which an instrument is free from errors of measurement [7]. Validity represents the extent to which

* Correspondence: Samiraa_g@yahoo.com
[1]School of Chiropractic and Sports Science, Murdoch University, 90 South Street, MurdochWA 6150, Perth, Australia
Full list of author information is available at the end of the article

an instrument measures what it is supposed to measure [7]. Concurrent validity examines the validity of an instrument against a criterion measure to test if the new instrument can be used instead of the criterion [7]. Understanding the reliability and validity of a measurement tool is crucial for making correct inferences from the data collected.

The Midot posture scale analyser (MPSA) is a lower cost portable force plate commonly used in the clinical setting. The MPSA has previously demonstrated acceptable reliability when averaging at least 5 values (ICC > 0.70) [8]. However, the validity of the MPSA has not been previously reported. Therefore, the purpose of this study was to examine the concurrent validity of postural control measures obtained with a clinical force plate when compared to a "gold standard" valid instrument.

Materials and methods

Participants

Participants were recruited through advertisements on University bulletin boards. The inclusion criteria were 18 to 60 years of age. A lower age limit of 18 years was set because the development of the skeletal system reaches its maturity at this age [9]. An upper age limit of 60 years was set because the ability to maintain postural control decreases in the elderly [10]. Potential participants were excluded from the study if they reported having balance deficits stemming from rheumatological or neurological disorders, a recent musculoskeletal injury (within three months), an ear infection or fever within 72 hours of the testing session, current pregnancy or the use of medications that could alter sensory perception. The Human Research Ethics Committee of Murdoch University approved the experimental protocol (2010/220), and all participants gave written consent before enrolment in the study.

Instruments

The MPSA (QPS-200, Midot Medical Technology, Shekel Electronic Scale, Israel) is a portable force plate consisting of four electronic weighing plates set in a rectangular position. The MPSA records data using an internal sampling frequency of 200 Hz and filter frequency of 0.5 Hz. Calibration was conducted in accordance with the manufacturer's recommendations using a 20 kg certified weight.

The Accugait (Advanced Mechanical Technology Inc., Watertown, MA,USA) was used as the criterion measure or reference standard. This force plate is a portable square force plate. There are flat rubber pads in each corner of the force plate to make the force plate less sensitive to vibration from most floor surfaces. The Accugait measures the three dimensional applied forces (Fx, Fy, Fz) and moments (Mx, My, Mz) involved in balance and uses established algorithms to compute the location of the COP and its associated variables from the forces and moments applied to the force plate. Data were acquired, recorded and analyzed using Balance Clinic software (balance software for AMTI's Accusway plus balance platform, version 2.02.01) loaded on a Dell laptop.

The Accugait force plate was initially factory validated prior to its release (personal communication with AMTI). However, to confirm the factory results we validated the Accugait based on the validation manual and validation report provided by AMTI [11]. The validation test represented an absolute COP error (the cumulative effect of noise and drift) of 3.6 mm for the X average, 3.4 mm for the Y average, 33.6 mm/s for average velocity and 2.9 mm^2 for sway area over 40 seconds of data acquisition at a 50 Hz sampling frequency. All of these values were sufficiently close to the values reported in the AMTI validation report and as such the instrument was considered valid. We used data filtration to remove noise [12] and chose a 5Hz cut off frequency as the best level to filter data by performing a residual analysis. Residual analysis computes the differences between filtered and unfiltered signals over a wide range of cut off frequencies. To accomplish this we calculated differences between filtered and unfiltered COP average velocity signals over a wide range of cut off frequencies (1, 2, 3, 5, 10, 20 Hz) and plotted them (Figure 1). The plot was composed of linear and non linear parts. The linear part mostly represented random noise and the non linear part represented true signal. The cut off frequency where the plot turned from linear to non linear was chosen as the best cut off frequency for this experiment [12].

The acquisition sampling frequency of the Accugait was set at 100 Hz with the cut-off frequency of 5 Hz. Data was filtered using a fourth order Butterworth filter [13]. As we considered the Accugait as the criterion measure, the acquisition sampling frequency and cut off frequency of the Accugait was set at the optimal setting regarding the task and environment of our study. The force plate was calibrated with a calibration CD provided by the manufacturer and it was zeroed before each recording.

The COP average velocity (mm/sec) and the sway area, which is the area of an ellipse enclosing 95% of COP movements (mm^2), are the two variables that were assessed and compared.

Procedure

The two force plates were placed on the laboratory floor next to each other. The manufacturer recommends use of the force plate on any flat surface and adds there is no need to install the force plate permanently in the ground [13]. All participants were tested under the same

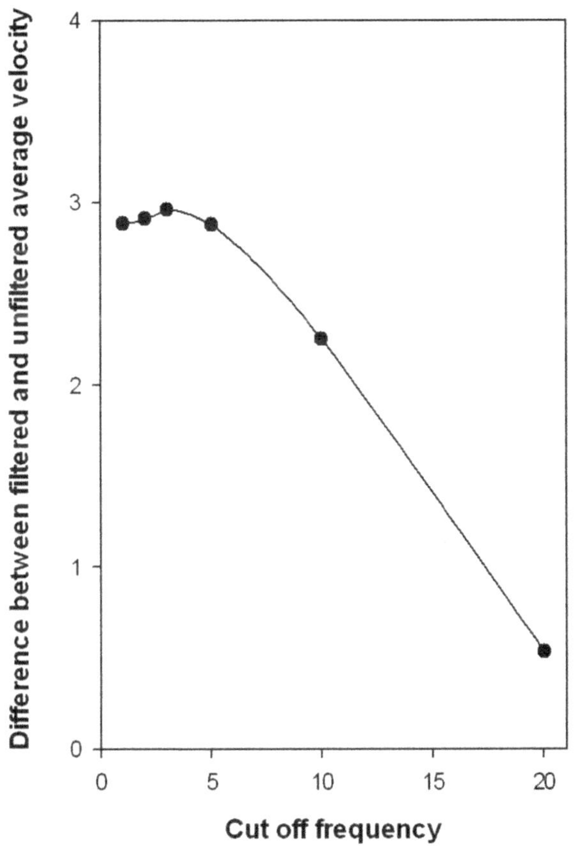

Figure 1 Differences between filtered and unfiltered average velocity vs. cut off frequency to decide the best filter frequency.

conditions. Paper was placed on top of force plates and the force plates were zeroed. Participants were asked to remove their shoes and stand upright on the force plate and remain as still as possible with a relaxed posture. The participants were asked to put their arms to their sides in a comfortable position and distribute their body weight evenly on both feet. Also, they were asked to breathe normally and look straight ahead at an "X" on the opposite wall that was located two meters away at their eye level. Before commencement of data acquisition and after inspection for position symmetry, both feet were outlined on the piece of paper located on top of the force plate to ensure consistent foot placement across trials and between the two force plates. The same procedure was used for testing on the second force plate using the outline of the feet to ensure consistent foot placement.

Participants completed 1 set of 5 trials on each force plate as outlined above. To reduce the potential for bias due to ordering effects, we randomly allocated and counterbalanced the order in which the measurements were obtained on each force plate.

Five successive identical trials of 60 seconds were acquired on each force plate. Mandatory breaks of one minute and 5 minutes were allocated between trials and between force plates, respectively. Data were averaged across five trials, this number of repetitions was informed by a study where we assessed the reliability of the MPSA and found acceptable reliability when averaging at least 5 values [8].

Statistical analysis

We conducted an *a priori* sample size estimation. Using the approach of Donner and Eliasziw (1987), assuming an alpha level of 0.05 and a minimally acceptable ICC value of 0.70 [7], recruitment of 30 participants provided 80% power [14].

Data management and statistical analyses were conducted using SPSS (version 17, Chicago, IL, USA). Data from 31 participants across 2 sets, 5 minutes apart were included for statistical analysis. Averages of 5 trials of COP average velocity and sway area were used for the analyses.

We calculated intraclass correlation coefficients ($ICC_{3,5}$) for comparison between the two force plates. Paired t-tests were also performed to examine for differences in average velocity and sway area between the force plates. We examined the consistency of measurements between the 2 force plates by calculating the standard error of measurement using the formula: Standard error of measurement = pooled standard deviation $\times \sqrt{1 - \text{ICC}}$. Additionally, bias statistics with 95% confidence intervals and limits of agreement (LOA) were calculated and Bland-Altman plots [15] were constructed for COP average velocity and sway area. Bias represents the mean difference between the two force plates, while the LOA examines agreement between the two force plates. LOAs are defined as bias ± 1.96 SD, where SD is the standard deviation of the difference between measures of the two force plates.

Results

Thirty-one healthy participants consisting of 18 males and 13 females, aged 23 to 58 were recruited from the staff and students of Murdoch University. All participants were able to complete all test repetitions and all data were included for statistical analysis. The mean (SD) age of the participants was 32.7 (8.5) years and BMI was 24.7 (5.4). Descriptive statistics, ICC, standard error of measurement, bias and limits of agreement are presented in Table 1 for average velocity and sway area. The ICC values between the two force plates are lower than the acceptable value with wide confidence intervals for both average velocity and sway area. Paired t-tests showed significant differences in average velocity and sway area between the 2 force plates ($p < 0.05$).

Table 1 Criterion validity analysis

	Mean (SD)	t-test (p value)	SEM	ICC $_{(3,5)}$ (CI's)	Bias (95% CI) ± 95% LOA
COP average velocity (mm/s)					
Accugait	8.3 (2.3)				
		0.004*	2	0.60(0.16-0.80)	1.7† (1.1,2.2) ± 5.9
MPSA	6.6 (3.5)				
Sway area (mm^2)					
Accugait	274 (155)				
		0.000*	870	0.14 (−0.24-0.48)	−1660† (−1370,-1950) ± 3134
MPSA	1936 (1720)				

CI, confidence Interval; *$p < 0.05$ indicates a significant difference in values between the 2 force plates; †statistically significant bias (different from zero).

The Bland–Altman plots for the average velocity and sway area are provided in Figures 2 and 3 and demonstrate more variation between the measures obtained from the two force plates when the amount of COP average velocity and sway area were higher.

Discussion

The purpose of this study was to investigate the concurrent validity of the MPSA by measuring COP variables and comparing these with a validated reference standard. The ICCs of the postural control measures were equal to 0.60 for the average velocity and 0.14 for the sway area between the force plates. Results of the reliability study of the MPSA also reported higher agreement for the average velocity and a lower agreement for sway area [8]. The ICC is a ratio estimate and there is no widely agreed upon thresholds for identifying an acceptable level of agreement with ICC reporting. As a result, there are various interpretations of ICC values available in the literature. Landis and Koch [16] suggested the following qualitative approach to ICC interpretation: 0.00-0.20 slight, 0.21-0.40 fair, 0.41-0.60 moderate, 0.61-0.80 substantial and 0.81-1.00 almost perfect. Alternatively, Portney and Watkins [7] suggest that values over 0.75 indicate good agreement, and values below 0.75 are indicative of poor to moderate agreement. The highest level of agreement identified in the current study was ICC = 0.60. Therefore, these results represent evidence that the MPSA does not possess sufficient concurrent validity.

The high standard error of measurement values of both variables especially the sway area, when compared to the mean values obtained by the two force plates, indicates a lack of consistency of measurement between the force plates. Furthermore, our results demonstrated significant differences between the COP measurements obtained from the force plates for the COP average velocity and sway area.

Comparison of standard deviations to means of sway area captured by the two force plates shows that the large standard deviation of MPSA sway area indicates a high degree of random error in the MPSA data. Additionally, the large mean difference between MPSA and Accugait sway area might be a sign of a systematic error in the MPSA when assessing postural control.

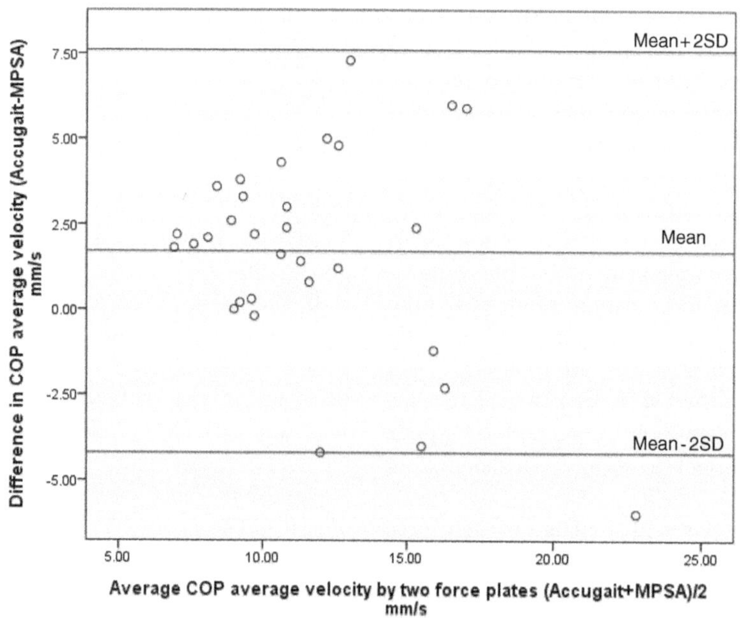

Figure 2 Bland-Altman plot representing comparison of average velocity between the MPSA and the Accugait.

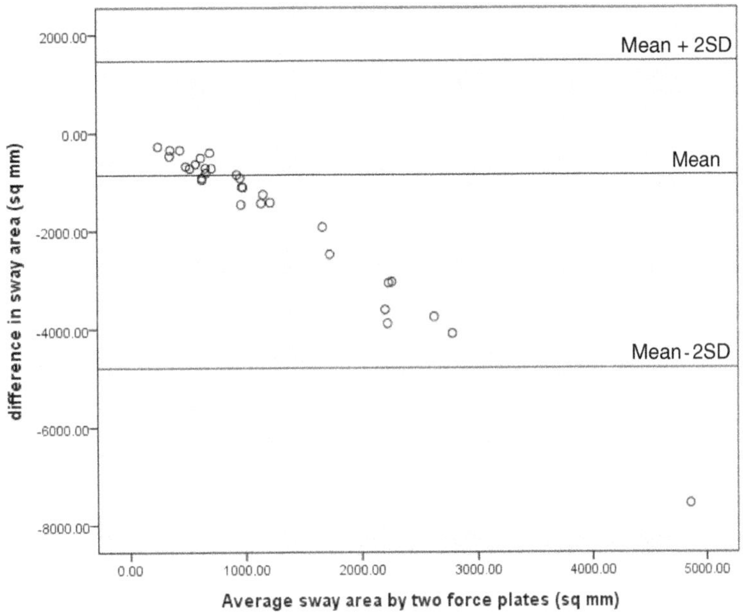

Figure 3 Bland-Altman plot representing comparison of sway area between the MPSA and the Accugait.

Visual inspection of the Bland-Altman plot (Figure 2) of average velocity shows a funnel effect, meaning there is more variability when the magnitude of the average velocity is greater. Our results represent excessive variation between the force plates in higher magnitudes of average velocity and less variation in lower magnitudes of average velocity. Differences between the measures of COP velocity between the force plates depend on the magnitude of the measurement. The excessive variations in higher magnitudes of average velocity indicate that data captured by the MPSA contain errors for measuring higher COP velocities.

The bias estimates for COP velocity were small but statistically different from zero. Statistically significant bias was found for the average velocity variable where the MPSA values underestimate the criterion in most of the cases with an estimate of 1.7 and a 95% confidence interval of 1.1 - 2.2. One possible explanation for this is that data captured by the Accugait was filtered with a 5 Hz cut off frequency whereas data obtained by the MPSA was filtered with a fixed 0.5 Hz cut off frequency. This may have resulted in the MPSA eliminating true signal. The lower cut off frequency causes removing higher proportion of true signals.

The plot of the sway area (Figure 3) shows a systematic trend. With lower magnitudes of sway area the differences between the two force plates are relatively low as compared to higher magnitudes, but the greater the sway area the bigger the difference between the two force plate measures. Moreover, the statistically significant bias of sway area showed that the MPSA overestimated sway area. Overall, larger measures of average velocity and sway area result in increased systematic and random error in MPSA.

While the MPSA previously demonstrated acceptable reliability [8], its validity is not satisfactory; therefore, it cannot be considered a replacement of a known valid force plate for the assessment of postural control. In addition, results obtained by the MPSA on clinical populations should be treated with caution. Clinical populations are potentially less stable and show higher magnitudes of average velocity and sway area [17,18] and the MPSA was incapable of measuring accurate data with higher magnitudes of average velocities and sway areas. Additionally, to reduce measurement error, we used a mean of 5 trials, which is unlikely to be the case with clinical use given the time constraints of clinical practice. Clinicians should consider all the above mentioned issues when assessing postural control using the MPSA.

Although we cannot rely on the MPSA for assessment of postural control, it may possibly be used in obtaining qualitative estimates of postural control, for instance as a biofeedback training tool and to enhance motivation level of patients with balance defects. Having said that, we suggest clinicians intending to use a force plate purchase a reliable and valid instrument.

Limitations exist within this study. The study sample consisted of healthy individuals and the findings may or may not generalize to clinical populations. This study did not attempt to assess the validity of the MPSA in different testing positions such as eyes closed, single limb standing and narrow stance (feet together) although we hypothesis that this would not enhance the MPSA performance.

Future research could be done to assess the validity of the MPSA in different balance testing positions and clinical populations. Estimates of reliability and validity should be known prior to using any type of force plates.

In conclusion, postural control parameters cannot be validly measured in clinical or research settings using the MPSA. The MPSA is a lower cost force plate with a low-technology design and easy to use software but it did not fulfil the criteria to be regarded as a valid force plate for clinical use.

Abbreviations

COP: Centre of pressure; ICC: Intraclass correlation coefficient; LOA: Level of agreement; MPSA: Midot posture scale analyser.

Competing interests

The authors declare that they have no competing interests.

Authors' contributions

SG participated in the design of the study, collected data, performed the statistical analysis and drafted the manuscript. JH participated in the design of the study, helped to perform the statistical analysis and drafted the manuscript. BF helped to draft the manuscript. BW participated in the design of the study and helped to draft the manuscript. All authors read and approved the final manuscript.

Author details

[1]School of Chiropractic and Sports Science, Murdoch University, 90 South Street, MurdochWA 6150, Perth, Australia. [2]School of Chiropractic and Sports Science, Murdoch University, Perth, WA, Australia. [3]Department of Physical Therapy, University of Utah, Salt Lake City, UT, USA.

References

1. Westcott SL, Lowes LP, Richardson PK: **Evaluation of postural stability in children: Current theories and assessment tools.** *Phys Ther* 1997, **77** (6):629–645.
2. McGuine TA, *et al*: **Balance as a predictor of ankle injuries in high school basketball players.** *Clin J Sport Med* 2000, **10**(4):239–244.
3. Lafond D, *et al*: **Postural control during prolonged standing in persons with chronic low back pain.** *Gait Posture* 2009, **29**(3):421–427.
4. Rogind H, *et al*: **Comparison of Kistler 9861A force platform and Chattecx Balance SystemÅ® for measurement of postural sway: Correlation and test-retest reliability.** *Scand J Med Sci Sports* 2003, **13**(2):106–114.
5. Prieto TE, *et al*: **Measures of postural steadiness: Differences between healthy young and elderly adults.** *IEEE Trans Biomed Eng* 1996, **43**(9):956–966.
6. Guskiewicz KM, Perrin DH: **Research and clinical applications of assessing balance.** *J Sport Rehabil* 1996, **5**(1):45–63.
7. Portney LG, Watkins MP: *Foundations of clinical research: Application to practice.* 3rd edition. Upper Saddle River: Prentice Hall Health; 2008.
8. Golriz S, et al.: *Assessment of the reliability of the Midot posture scale analyser for evaluation of the postural stability parameters.* Chiropractic and Manual Therapies, 2012 May, **20**:14 (doi:10.1186/2045-709X-20-14)
9. Malina RM, *et al*: **Height, mass and skeletal maturity of elite Portuguese soccer players aged 11–16 years.** *J Sports Sci* 2000, **18**(9):685–693.
10. Era P, *et al*: **Postural balance in a random sample of 7,979 subjects aged 30 years and over.** *Gerontology* 2006, **52**(4):204–213.
11. AMTI: *Calibration validation manual*, I.A. Advanced Mechanical Technology, Editor: Watertown, MA, USA.
12. Winter DA: *Biomechanics and motor control of human movement.* 4th edition. Hoboken, New Jersey: John Wiley & Sons INC; 2009.
13. AMTI: *Balance software for AMTI's AccuSway plus balance platfrom.* Watertown: I. A. Advanced Medical Technology; 2006.
14. Donner A, Eliasziw M: **Sample size requirements for reliability studies.** *Stat Med* 1987, **6**(4):441–448.
15. Bland JM, Altman DG: **Statistical methods for assessing agreement between two methods of clinical measurement.** *Lancet* 1986, **1**(8476):307–310.
16. Landis JR, Koch GG: **The measurement of observer agreement for categorical data.** *Biometrics* 1977, **33**(1):159–174.
17. Blaszczyk JW, *et al*: **Assessment of postural instability in patients with Parkinson's disease.** *Exp Brain Res* 2007, **183**(1):107–114.
18. Ruhe A, Fejer R, Walker B: **Center of pressure excursion as a measure of balance performance in patients with non-specific low back pain compared to healthy controls: a systematic review of the literature.** *Eur Spine J* 2011, **20**(3):358–368.

The location of the inferior angle of the scapula in relation to the spine in the upright position: a systematic review of the literature and meta-analysis

Robert Cooperstein[1*], Michael Haneline[2] and Morgan Young[1]

Abstract

Practitioners in several of the health care professions use anatomical landmarks to identify spinal levels, both in order to enhance diagnostic accuracy and to specifically target the site of intervention. Authoritative sources usually state the upright inferior scapular angle (IAS) aligns with the spinous process (SP) of T7, but some specify the T7-8 interspace or the T8 SP. The primary goals of this study were to systematically review the relevant literature; and conduct a meta-analysis of the pooled data from retrieved studies to increase their statistical power. Electronic searching retrieved primary studies relating the IAS to a spinal level, as determined by an imaging reference standard, using combinations of these search terms: scapula, location, landmark, spinous process, thoracic vertebrae, vertebral level, palpation, and spine. Only primary studies were included; review articles and reliability studies related to scapular position but lacking spinal correlations were excluded. Eight-hundred and eighty (880) articles of interest were identified, 43 abstracts were read, 22 full text articles were inspected, and 5 survived the final cut. Each article (with one exception) was rated for quality using the QUADAS instrument. Pooling data from 5 studies resulted in normal distribution in which the upright IAS on average aligns closely with the T8 SP, range T4-T11. Since on average the IAS most closely identifies the T8 SP in the upright position, it is very likely that health professionals, both manual therapists and others, who have been diagnosing and treating patients based on the IAS = T7 SP rule (the conventional wisdom), have not been as segmentally accurate as they may have supposed. They either addressed non-intended levels, or made numeration errors in their charting. There is evidence that using the IAS is less preferred than using the vertebra prominens, and may be less preferred than using the iliac crest for identifying spinal levels Manual therapists, acupuncturists, anesthesiologists, nurses, and surgeons should reconsider their procedures for identifying spinal sites in light of this modified information. Inaccurate landmark benchmark rules will add to patient variation and examiner errors in producing spine care targeting errors, and confound research on the importance of specificity in treating spinal levels.

Introduction

Practitioners in several of the health care professions use anatomical landmarks to identify spinal levels, both in order to enhance diagnostic accuracy and to specifically target the site of intervention. Manual therapists palpate spinal and pelvic structures to determine both their position and their movement capacities. Anesthesiologists require precise placement of thoracic epidural catheters to optimize postoperative analgesia and minimize adverse effects [1-6]. Anatomic landmarks are also used to locate acupuncture points [7]; surgeons may decide upon a location to begin their incision based at least in part on the location of the IAS ([8] p.18).

Manual therapists use static palpation to identify asymmetry of bilateral structures, such as the posterior superior iliac spines [9,10]; as well as to identify malposition of contiguous structures, such as that of a spinal motion segment. Motion palpation is used to identify quantitative limitation

* Correspondence: cooperstein_r@palmer.edu
[1]Palmer West College of Chiropractic, 90 East Tasman Drive, San Jose, CA 94577, USA
Full list of author information is available at the end of the article

in the excursion of contiguous structures, or changes in the qualitative properties of an osseous structure that has its movement taken to endrange [11]. Manual therapists generally believe that the confluence of both static and motion findings of abnormality establishes criteria for clinical intervention [12]. Indices of interexaminer agreement were generally found to be low in systematic reviews of both motion palpation [13,14] and static palpation [13], although more recent studies in which examiners determined the "most fixated level" rather than rating specific levels as fixated or not have shown high reliability in both the thoracic [15] and cervical [16] spinal regions.

The various health professions that make use of spinal palpation deploy a litany of spinal and pelvic landmarks to target potential sites of care, as well as chart levels that have been identified or treated. Since these anatomical landmarks are thought to identify corresponding spinal levels, other spinal levels may be located by counting up or down. Some of the most commonly used landmarks used in this way are C7, usually regarded to be the vertebra prominens (but not always) [17]), with the longest cervical spinous process; L4, whose SP is generally thought level with the iliac crest [18]; and S2, thought level with the posterior superior iliac spines [19]. Investigators have reported frequent mistakes in numerating spinal levels [20,21]. Some of these no doubt result from examiner palpatory errors [13,22], while others may result from variations in patient anatomy [17-19,23]. However, errors may also result from anatomical benchmark rules that are inherently inaccurate [24].

In chiropractic education it is commonly taught that the inferior angle of the scapula (IAS) can be located using the rule "7 up, 6 down," referring to the position of the IAS in relation to the thoracic SPs in the upright and prone positions, respectively [25-27]. Spot checking, the T7 SP = IAS benchmark can also be found in other professions: anesthesiology [4,28], physiatry [29], orthopedic medicine [30,31], kinesiology [32], acupuncture [7], and nursing [33]. Other sources state the IAS line up with the T7-8 interspace [34,35], T8 SP, [36,37], or with the T9 SP [38]. The primary goal of this study was to conduct a systematic review of primary studies that addressed the location of the IAS in relation to the upright spine. The secondary goal was to perform meta-analysis using the combined data to increase the level of confidence that could be attached to the individual study findings.

Methods

Table 1 uses the STARLITE mnemonic [39] to summary our search strategy. The titles, abstracts, and (as required) full publications of retrieved citations were independently screened by two reviewers. Any possible discrepancies were resolved by consensus. To be included, a study had to provide data on the location of the IAS in relation to the spine in the upright position, as determined by an imaging reference standard. A study could report the location of the IAS in relation to an SP, an intervertebral space, or a vertebral body. The investigators excluded review articles, reliability studies related to scapular position but not correlated with spinal levels; and studies that involved fractures, dislocations or congenital abnormalities of the scapula (e.g., Klippel-Feil syndrome and Sprengel deformity). Cadeveric and intraoperative studies were also excluded. Once a relevant citation was found, the "related citations" (or equivalent, depending on the website or database) function was deployed to find additional articles. A secondary search was also conducted using the included articles' references. Each of the included articles, except Haneline [40] (which was an anatomy study and did not include a palpation arm) was rated for quality using the QUADAS index [41,42]. Scoring differences were discussed and, where necessary, resolved by a third reviewer. Meta-analysis was conducted on the combined data from the included studies and analysis, and presented

Table 1 STARLITE search strategy summary

Sampling strategy	Electronic databases searched for articles satisfying inclusion criteria
Type of studies	Anatomical studies investigating the spinal level corresponding to the scapula
Approaches	"Related articles" function used following successful retrieval. Secondary search to reach point of data saturation. Google searching.
Range of years	No restrictions.
Limits	Only English-language articles were included.
Inclusions/Exclusions	Included only primary studies where the spinal level corresponding to the scapula was identified through comparison with an imaging reference standard. Reliability studies and reviews of the literature were excluded. Intraoperative and cadaveric studies were excluded.
Terms used	Combinations of Non-MesH terms (Spinous Process, Thoracic Vertebrae, Vertebral Level, Validity) and MeSH terms (Scapula, Spine, Palpation, Diagnostic Techniques and Procedures, Diagnostic Imaging, Physical Examination, Anatomic Landmarks, Thorax, Reproducibility of Results).
Electronic sources	PubMed, MANTIS, ICL, CINAHL, AMED, Osteopathic Research Web, OstMed, Google.

as a forest plot in Figure three (Open Meta-Analyst, available from http://www.cebm.brown.edu/open_meta). Due to differences in how the included studies were done, pooling the data in some cases required transforming their findings, which may have related the scapula to an intervertebral space or a vertebral body, to correspond with a spinous process (SP) level. These transformations are described in the results section.

Results

The initial search retrieved 880 studies. After the authors had scrutinized the titles, 43 abstracts were deemed potentially relevant and were read, which in turn prompted the retrieval of 22 full-text articles which were more carefully inspected. Of these, 5 articles published between 2007 and 2013 survived the final cut and were entered into this review. The procedures involved in the screening and exclusion of studies is shown in the Flow Diagram in Figure 1. Three of these 5 studies required data transformation to allow data pooling. Since Arzola et al [1] reported intervertebral spaces rather than SP levels corresponding to the IAS, the number of participants with the IAS at this intervertebral space was divided equally among the vertebral levels above and below. Although Haneline et al [40] reported the IAS to correspond to the upper vertebral body, lower vertebral body, or intervertebral space; enough methodological detail was supplied to heuristically map the data to corresponding SPs. Although Kim et al [3] examined the participants in the "epidural position" (seated, back arched, neck flexed, arms across the chest), the authors were able to convert their findings to what would have been obtained in "anatomical position" (i.e., thorax fully upright, palms anterior) simply by subtracting one vertebral level from each reported data point, since trunk flexion has been found to raise the scapula by about one level [4]. This 1-level cephalad shift of the scapular position in flexion was also reflected in the data of Arzola et al [1], who reported data for both the epidural and anatomical positions.

Three of the studies [1,3,4] drew a line connecting the left and right IASs, defining the closest SP to this line as corresponding to the IAS. One study [43] did not specify which IAS was used and apparently used either, while another study [40] separately reported the location of both the left and right IASs relative to the spine. In tabulating the data for this latter study, the authors used an average of the left and right IAS positions, resulting in some non-integral values for the SP level. When this was the case, the number was rounded to the nearest integer for the purpose of data pooling. Since rounding protocols would on average distribute the errors in both directions, the authors are confident this loss of accuracy did not significantly alter the estimated spinal levels. Table 2 summarizes the data (transformed as necessary) from the 5 retrieved studies, and Table 3 their quality ratings [41,42]. The quality ratings for all of the included studies were 11 or higher and were considered acceptable.

Following data conversions, the data from all 5 studies were combined to construct a pool of 343 participants. As seen in Figure 2, the data comprise an almost perfect bell curve centered on the T8 SP, the vertebral level whose SP most closely corresponds on average to the IAS. Normality was confirmed using the Shapiro-Wilk

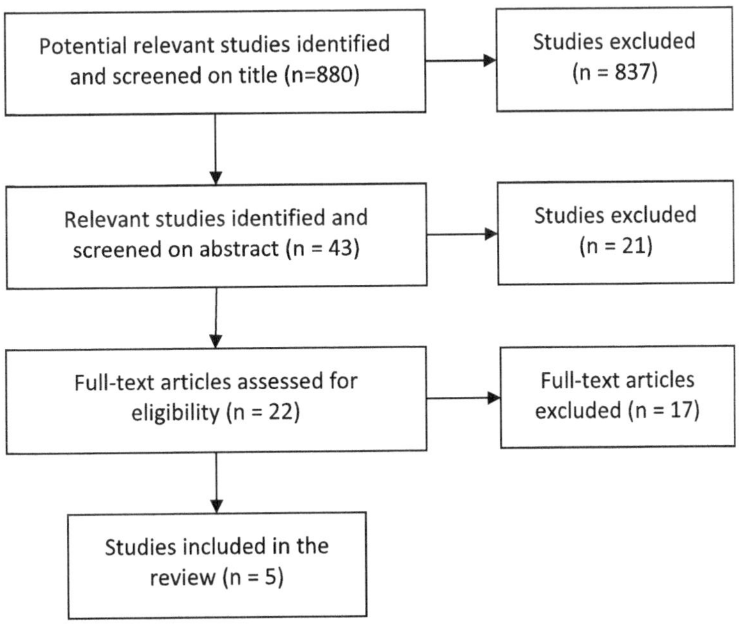

Figure 1 Flow diagram for literature retrieval.

Table 2 Studies mapping the IAS to a spinal landmark in the upright position

Study	Sample size, participant demographics	Reference standard and method	Location IAS relative to thoracic SP*	Method of transforming data, if any	ModifiedQUADAS score (n/14)
Cooperstein, 2007 [43]	n = 34, 59% male; mean Y/O = 26; all healthy	Radio-opaque marker placed on ISA, compared with spinal radiography	T6: 5.9% T7: 17.6% T8: 47.1% T9: 26.5% T10: 2.9	n/a	11
Haneline, 2008 [40]	n = 50, 50% male; mean Y/O = 47.5; health status unknown	Radiographic mensuration of scapula and spine	T6: 8.0% T7: 26.0% T8: 56.0 T9: 10.0%	Left and right scapular positions averaged	n/a
Teoh, 2009 [4]	n = 104, 54.8% male; mean Y/O; receiving chest radiography	Radio-opaque marker placed on ISA, compared with spinal radiography	T6: 1.0% T7: 9.6% T8: 30.8% T9: 36.5% T10: 16.3% T11: 5.8%	n/a	14
Arzola, 2011 [1]	n = 55, 41.8% male; mean Y/O 30.7; all healthy	Ultrasonography	T6: 3.6% T7: 12.7% T8: 29.1% T9: 29.1% T10: 16.4% T11: 9.1%	Intervertebral space findings apportioned equally to segments above and below	13
Kim, 2012 [3]	n = 100, 33% male; mean Y/O = 49.3; all symptomatic, variety of conditions	Epidural insertion level as seen on radiography	T5: 1% T6: 1% T7: 25% T8: 62% T9: 10% T10: 1%	Subtracted 1 spinal level to account for use of epidural position	14

*Spinal levels corresponding to IAS reported following data transformation for uniform reporting and data pooling.

statistic. Two-hundred and ninety-three (85.4%) of measurements were at or within one level of the T8 SP, range T4-T11. Figure 3 is a forest plot that provides the vertebral level point estimate and 95% confidence level for each of the included studies. The areas of the tick marks denoting the point estimates are proportional to the participant size. The confidence intervals for each study overlap each other as well as the grand mean of 8.01, which almost exactly corresponds to the T8 SP. This confirms there are no statistical differences at the 95% confidence interval in the spinal level of the ISA as identified in each of the 5 studies. The very low I-squared summary statistic ($I^2 = 0\%$, $p = 0.93$) suggests very low heterogeneity among the included studies.

Discussion

Among the 5 included articles, in all but that of Haneline et al [40] manual palpation served as an index test to identify the position of the IAS, as compared with either a radiographic or ultrasonographic reference standard. The Haneline study performed a secondary analysis of radiographs taken for reasons unrelated to that of the current study, that permitted visualization of the IAS and the SP that most closely approximated its level. Arzola [1], Teoh [4], and Kim [3] each studied the accuracy of using the IAS to locate the T7 SP, only to find that this landmark rule was not accurate. Although the failure of the benchmark rule is important to note, the purpose of our systematic review was not to assess the degree of landmark failure but rather conduct a purely anatomical secondary analysis to determine the spinal level of the IAS.

In Cooperstein et al [43], a palpator affixed a lead marker to the SP judged closest to the level of the IAS; later radiographically identified most often as the T8 SP. In Teoh et al [4] the palpator used the IAS as a landmark to locate what was expected to be the T7 SP but was later

Table 3 QUADAS ratings

QUADAS ITEM Abbreviations: Y = yes, N = no, U = unclear	Cooperstein, 2009 [47]	Teoh, 2009 [4]	Arzola, 2011 [1]	Kim, 2012 [3]
1. Was the spectrum of patients representative of the patients who will receive the test in practice?	N	Y	N	Y
2. Were selection criteria clearly described?	Y	Y	Y	Y
3. Is the reference standard likely to correctly classify the target condition?	Y	Y	Y	Y
4. Is the time period between reference standard and index test short enough to be reasonably sure that the target condition did not change between the 2 tests?	Y	Y	Y	Y
5. Did the whole sample or a random selection of the sample receive verification using a reference standard of diagnosis?	Y	Y	Y	Y
6. Did patients receive the same reference standard regardless of the index text result?	Y	Y	Y	Y
7. Was the reference standard independent of the index test (ie, the index test did not form part of the reference standard)?	Y	Y	Y	Y
8. Was the execution of the index test described in sufficient detail to permit replication of the test?	Y	Y	Y	Y
9. Was the execution of the reference standard described in sufficient detail to permit its replication?	Y	Y	Y	Y
10. Were the index test results interpreted without knowledge of the results of the reference standard?	N	Y	Y	Y
11. Were the reference standard results interpreted without knowledge of the results of the index test?	N	Y	N	Y
12. Were the same clinical data available when test results were interpreted as would be available when the test is used in practice?	Y	Y	Y	Y
13. Were interpretable/intermediate test results reported?	Y	Y	Y	Y
14. Were withdrawals from the study explained?	Y	Y	Y	Y
Total quality score	**11**	**14**	**12**	**14**

The Haneline study, one of the 5 articles included in this review, was not amenable to QUADAS rating and thus is not included in Table 3.

radiographically determined to correspond closest to the T8 SP. Arzola et al [1] also used the IAS to locate what was expected to be the T7 SP, using a skin marking to identify that location; ultrasononographic examination determined that location to usually lie closer to the T8 SP. Kim et al [3] inserted a catheter at spinal levels identified based on their anatomic relation to the IAS, with the patients in the flexed epidural position. After data transformation, the level of insertion most often corresponded to the T8 SP.

Accuracy in using spinal landmarks to identify segmental levels should be supported by anatomical studies. Some studies suggest that anatomical variability among patients

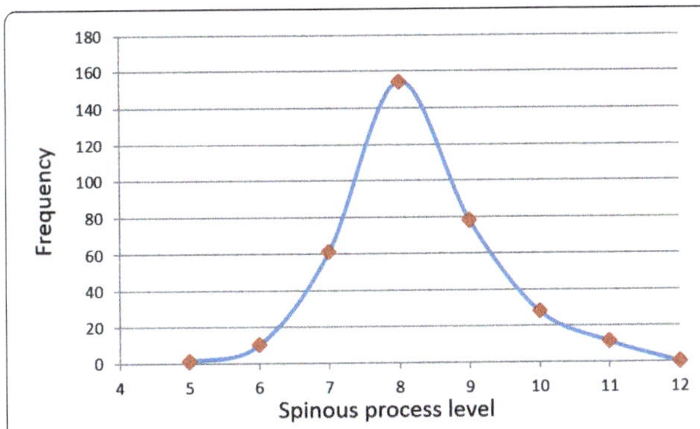

Figure 2 Distribution of pooled data.

can lead to errors in treating and charting sites of care. For example, the vertebra prominens is not always C7 [17], the L4 SP is not always at the same level as the iliac crest [18], and the IAS is not always at the T7 SP standing nor T6 SP prone [44]. The present study endeavored to both systematically review the literature on the location of the IAS in relation to the spine; and transform/pool the data from 5 individual studies to increase the precision and accuracy of their combined results. Since on average the IAS most closely identifies the T8 SP in the upright position, it is very likely that health professionals, both manual therapists and others, who have been diagnosing and treating patients based on the IAS = T7 SP rule (the conventional wisdom), have not been as segmentally accurate as they may have supposed. They either addressed non-intended levels, or made numeration errors in their charting. Arzola [1] Kim [3] and Teoh [4] reported accuracy rates of 18%, 62%, and 41% respectively in using the IAS for identifying T7. Since the IAS lies within a range spanning T4 to T11, the accuracy depends on the anatomy of the individual who is being examined. Teoh [4], comparing the accuracy of two different surface landmarks for locating the T7 SP, found the vertebra prominens (C7) to be more accurate than the tip of the scapula.

Apart from issues related to the between-individuals accuracy of the landmark rule, variability within individuals further compounds its use. The scapula on the side of the dominant arm tends to lie approximately 0.5 cm

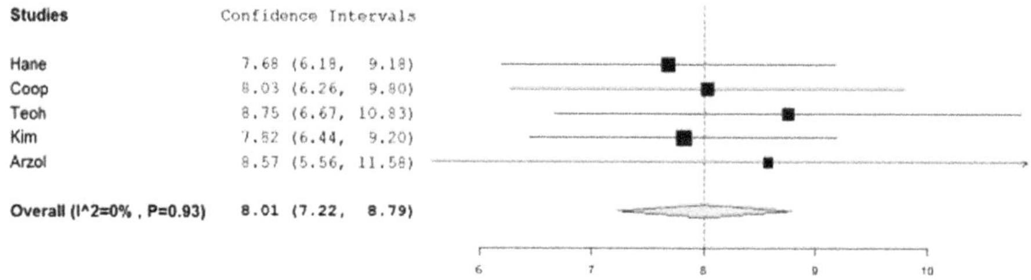

Figure 3 Forest plot summarizing results of included studies.

lower than the scapula on the side of the non-dominant arm [37,45], corresponding to about 0.2 vertebral levels lower [46]. Therefore the accuracy of using the IAS as a benchmark is arm-dependent.

Although a one-level error in the scapular landmark rule may not seem very clinically significant, the error may be compounded by a two-level error related to yet another inaccurate scapular landmark rule, by which the scapula supposedly rises one level in the prone compared with standing positions. Since in fact the scapula tends to move *inferiorly* about one level when the patient is prone (depending on arm position) [47], the potential exists for a three-level error when a clinician applies an intervention in the prone position based on an examination procedure performed in the upright position [24]. Clinicians who intend to treat spinal levels identified by upright examination procedures (including thermography, manual muscle testing, static/motion palpation, and x-ray) in the prone position may miss their target by 2-3 spinal level. Although we do not *assume* that the outcome of chiropractic or other types of manual care for spinal complaints is made better by identifying misalignments accurately, manual therapists and other health professionals who do believe such information improves the outcome of care are now faced with an interesting paradox. They must either consider their clinical outcomes to have been suboptimal due to targeting errors, or derive an alternative explanation for their presumed good clinical outcomes, at least in relation to spinal segments that were identified by using the IAS as a landmark.

Irrespective of whether misdiagnosing the level of a misaligned or dysfunctional segment results in a suboptimal clinical outcome, issues may arise if or when another or the same clinician attempts to intervene on the incorrectly charted level on another day [23]. Level misidentification may also be problematic in attempting to track clinical changes over time. Accurate palpation is crucial when the practitioner is attempting to correlate physical examination findings with the results of an imaging study, in order to decide upon the clinical relevance of manual examination findings [23].

Limitations of the study

The QUADAS instrument was used to rate the quality of 4 of the included studies, each of which compared palpatory results with a reference standard. However, it could not be used to rate Haneline [40], since this purely anatomical study did not include a palpation arm. QUADAS can only be used to assess the comparative validity of an examination method to a reference standard. Using QUADAS as we did to assess the quality of articles used in a secondary analysis is not common.

The need to transform the data in 3 of the studies may have introduced some loss of accuracy. The process of synthesizing data from studies that use different methods is error-prone; the authors did their best to make the necessary transformations with fidelity. When a study reported the location of the IAS in relation to a spinal structure other than the SP, the authors either assigned it to the nearest SP or apportioned it equally to the levels above and below, reducing the risk of systematic bias. The individual studies enrolled participants who were rather different in their demographic characteristics, thus warranting caution in drawing comparisons between studies. Conversely, the conclusions to be drawn from the pooled data are made more credible because data pooling created a rather heterogeneous participant mix, with both healthy and symptomatic, younger and older, participants.

Although the authors are aware of no data on how commonly the IAS is used to identify spinal sites in the manual therapy professions, the existence of abundant examples in the literature [43] suggests this practice is common. The existence of several studies by anesthetists determining the relation of the scapula to the spine lends to this impression. It remains to be seen whether counting up from pelvic landmarks leads to more accurate identification of thoracic spinal levels than using the scapular location as a landmark. Palpating the posterior superior iliac spines (PSISs) has been shown to be more useful than palpating the iliac crests to locate lumbar spinal levels [19], presumably because crest levels show more anatomical variation than PSIS levels [18].

Conclusion

Manual therapists (and other health professionals) use spinal landmarks for a variety of different purposes: corroborating a specific nerve root or other segmental pathology, accurate identification of an intended site of care, accurate positioning of the clinician's contact hand during spinal manipulation and other spinal therapies, and documentation as to the spinal level found subluxated/dysfunctional and/or treated. Although the clinical importance of attaining specificity in the identifying and treating spinal sites of care remains controversial in the manual therapy setting [48], the capacity to attain specificity is a prerequisite for accomplishing the clinical studies that would confirm or refute its importance. Based especially on Teoh's findings [4] using the IAS may be less preferred than using the location of vertebra prominens to identify thoracic spine locations. As a non-fixed structure that may be said to "float" over the rib cage, considering the anatomical variability that follows from that, the scapula does not constitute an acceptable landmark for identifying spinal levels.

Practitioners of manual therapy, orthopedic medicine, primary medical care, neurology, anesthesiology, nursing, and acupuncture should be interested in this updated information on the anatomical relation of the scapula and spine. Anatomically incorrect landmark benchmarks will hinder the accurate identification of spinal sites of clinical interest, beyond what is to be expected due to examiner error and variation among patients. It may be of some value to systematically review the literature addressing other commonly used spinal landmark rules.

Competing interests

The authors declare that they have no competing interests.

Authors' contributions

RC conceived of the study, initiated the literature search, performed the computations, and wrote the first draft of the manuscript. RC and MH reviewed the selected abstracts and determined those articles that were to be included. RC, MH, and MY rated the articles using the QUADAS instrument, and participated in editing the manuscript. All authors read and approved the final manuscript.

Author details

[1]Palmer West College of Chiropractic, 90 East Tasman Drive, San Jose, CA 94577, USA. [2]University of Western States, 2900 NE 132nd Avenue, Portland, OR 97230, USA.

References

1. Arzola C, Avramescu S, Tharmaratnam U, Chin KJ, Balki M. Identification of cervicothoracic intervertebral spaces by surface landmarks and ultrasound. Can J Anaesth. 2011;58:1069–74.
2. Holmaas G, Frederiksen D, Ulvik A, Vingsnes SO, Ostgaard G, Nordli H. Identification of thoracic intervertebral spaces by means of surface anatomy: a magnetic resonance imaging study. Acta Anaesthesiol Scand. 2006;50:368–73.
3. Kim MG, Ok SY, Kim SH, Lee SJ, Park SY, Koh EH, et al. Is the Spinous Process of T7 Usually at the Same Level as the Inferior Tips of the Scapulae? Soonchunhyang Med Sci. 2012;18:9–11.
4. Teoh DA, Santosham KL, Lydell CC, Smith DF, Beriault MT. Surface anatomy as a guide to vertebral level for thoracic epidural placement. Anesth Analg. 2009;108:1705–7.
5. Broadbent CR, Maxwell WB, Ferrie R, Wilson DJ, Gawne-Cain M, Russell R. Ability of anaesthetists to identify a marked lumbar interspace. Anaesthesia. 2000;55:1122–6.
6. Furness G, Reilly MP, Kuchi S. An evaluation of ultrasound imaging for identification of lumbar intervertebral level. Anaesthesia. 2002;57:277–80.
7. Omi S, editor. WHO standard acupuncture point locations in the Western Pacific Region. Manila, Phillippines: World Health Organization; 2008.
8. Little GL, Merrill WH, editors. Complications in Cardiothoracic Surgery: Avoidance and Treatment. 2nd ed. Hoboken: Wiley-Blackwell, 2011.
9. Cooperstein R, Crum E, Morschhauser E, Lisi A. Sitting PSIS positions and prone blocking preferences: a preliminary report. J Chirop Educ. 2004;18:44–5.
10. Levangie PK. The association between static pelvic asymmetry and low back pain [In Process Citation]. Spine. 1999;24:1234–42.
11. Cooperstein R. Two types of motion palpation: The excursion and tne end-feel methods. JACA Online. 2008;45:25-6. Online access only.
12. Kmita A, Lucas N. Reliability of physical examination to assess asymmetry of anatomical landmarks indicative of pelvic somatic dysfunction in subjects with and without low back pain. Int J Osteopath Med. 2008;11:16–25.
13. Haneline MT, Young M. A review of intraexaminer and interexaminer reliability of static spinal palpation: a literature synthesis. J Manipulative Physiol Ther. 2009;32:379–86.
14. Seffinger MA, Najm WI, Mishra SI, Adams A, Dickerson VM, Murphy LS, et al. Reliability of spinal palpation for diagnosis of back and neck pain: a systematic review of the literature. Spine. 2004;29:E413–425.
15. Cooperstein R, Haneline M, Young M. Interexaminer reliability of thoracic motion palpation using confidence ratings and continuous analysis. J Chiropr Med. 2010;9:99–106.
16. Cooperstein R, Young M, Haneline M. Interexaminer reliability of cervical motion palpation using continuous measures and rater confidence levels. J Can Chiropr Assoc. 2013;57:156–64.
17. Stonelake PS, Burwell RG, Webb JK. Variation in vertebral levels of the vertebra prominens and sacral dimples in subjects with scoliosis. J Anat. 1988;159:165–72.
18. Chakraverty R, Pynsent P, Isaacs K. Which spinal levels are identified by palpation of the iliac crests and the posterior superior iliac spines? J Anat. 2007;210:232–6
19. Kim HW, Ko YJ, Rhee WI, Lee JS, Lim JE, Lee SJ, et al. Interexaminer reliability and accuracy of posterior superior iliac spine and iliac crest palpation for spinal level estimations. J Manipulative Physiol Ther. 2007;30:386–9.
20. Billis EV, Foster NE, Wright CC. Reproducibility and repeatability: errors of three groups of physiotherapists in locating spinal levels by palpation. Man Ther. 2003;8:223–32.
21. Huijbregts PA. Spinal motion palpation: a review of reliability studies. J Man Manip Ther. 2002;10:24–39.
22. Hart J, Neely C. Allowing a possible margin of error when assessing student skills in spinous process location. J Chiropr Educ. 2011;25:182–5.
23. Snider KT, Snider EJ, Degenhardt BF, Johnson JC, Kribs JW. Palpatory accuracy of lumbar spinous processes using multiple bony landmarks. J Manipulative Physiol Ther. 2011;34:306–13.
24. Cooperstein R, Young M. Mapping intended spinal site of care from the upright to prone position: an interexaminer reliability study. Chiropr Man Therap. 2014;22:20.
25. Peterson JD, ed. Palmer College of Chiropractic Adjusting Technique Manual. Davenport, Il: PCC; 1998. Bovee M, Burns R, Gindl P, et al., eds
26. Downes JW. Life College School of Chiropractic Technique Manual. 2nd ed. Marietta, GA: Life College School of Chriropractic
27. Walker RA, Lovejoy O, Bedford E, Yee W. Skeletal and Developmental Anatomy for Students of Chiropractic. Philadelphia, PA: F. A. Davis Company; 2007.
28. Anatomy relevant to epidural and subarachnoid blockade [http://www.frca.co.uk/article.aspx?articleid=100361
29. PASSOR Musculoskeletal Physical Examination Competencies List [http://zone.medschool.pitt.edu/ENRICHMENT/rehab/Documents/Advanced%20Clinical%20Skills%20Course/2010/PASSOR%20PE%20Guidelines.pdf]
30. The Five-Minute Shoulder Exam [http://www.usask.ca/cme/learning_resources/CPL_resources/orthopedics/fmse.php]
31. Part 7: The Back [http://www.dartmouth.edu/~humananatomy/part_7/]
32. Oatis CA. Kinesiology: The Mechanics & Pathomechanics of Human Movement. 1st ed. Philadelphia: Lippincott Williams & Wilkins; 2004.

33. Weber J, Kelley J. Health assessment in nursing. New York: Lippincott Williams & Wilkins; 2009.
34. Lewis J, Green A, Reichard Z, Wright C. Scapular position: the validity of skin surface palpation. Man Ther. 2002;7:26–30.
35. Cheek B. The back. http://www.gp-training.net/rheum/backpain/index.htm. Accessed August 13, 2013
36. Shoulder anatomy and function 1 [http://moon.ouhsc.edu/dthompso/NAMICS/labs/shldr1.htm]
37. Gibson MH, Goebel GV, Jordan TM, Kegerreis S, Worrell TW. A reliability study of measurement techniques to determine static scapular position. J Orthop Sports Phys Ther. 1995;21:100–6.
38. Ernst MJ, Rast FM, Bauer CM, Marcar VL, Kool J. Determination of thoracic and lumbar spinal processes by their percentage position between C7 and the PSIS level. BMC Res Notes. 2013;6:58.
39. Booth A. "Brimful of STARLITE": toward standards for reporting literature searches. J Med Libr Assoc. 2006;94:421–9. e205.
40. Haneline M, Cooperstein R, Young M, Ross J. Determining spinal level using the inferior angle of the scapula as a reference landmark: a retrospective analysis of 50 radiographs. J Can Chiropr Assoc. 2008;52:24–9.
41. Whiting P, Rutjes AW, Reitsma JB, Bossuyt PM, Kleijnen J. The development of QUADAS: a tool for the quality assessment of studies of diagnostic accuracy included in systematic reviews. BMC Med Res Methodol. 2003;3:25.
42. Whiting PF, Weswood ME, Rutjes AW, Reitsma JB, Bossuyt PN, Kleijnen J. Evaluation of QUADAS, a tool for the quality assessment of diagnostic accuracy studies. BMC Med Res Methodol. 2006;6:9.
43. Cooperstein R, Haneline M. Spinous process palpation using the scapular tip as a landmark vs a radiographic criterion standard. J Chiropr Med. 2007;6:87–93.
44. Cooperstein R, Haneline M: Where Is the Inferior angle of the scapula? Dynamic Chiropractic 2008, 26(8). http://www.dynamicchiropractic.com/mpacms/dc/article.php?id=53152. Accessed Jan. 18, 2015..
45. Sobush DC, Simoneau GG, Dietz KE, Levene JA, Grossman RE, Smith WB. The lennie test for measuring scapular position in healthy young adult females: a reliability and validity study. J Orthop Sports Phys Ther. 1996;23:39–50.
46. The vertebral column as a whole [http://www.theodora.com/anatomy/the_vertebral_column_as_a_whole.html]
47. Cooperstein R, Haneline MT, Young MD. The location of the inferior angle of the scapula in relation to the spinal level of prone patients. JCCA J Can Chiropr Assoc. 2009;53:121–8.
48. Triano JJ, Budgell B, Bagnulo A, Roffey B, Bergmann T, Cooperstein R, et al. Review of methods used by chiropractors to determine the site for applying manipulation. Chiropr Man Therap. 2013;21:36.

Permissions

All chapters in this book were first published in CMT, by BioMed Central; hereby published with permission under the Creative Commons Attribution License or equivalent. Every chapter published in this book has been scrutinized by our experts. Their significance has been extensively debated. The topics covered herein carry significant findings which will fuel the growth of the discipline. They may even be implemented as practical applications or may be referred to as a beginning point for another development.

The contributors of this book come from diverse backgrounds, making this book a truly international effort. This book will bring forth new frontiers with its revolutionizing research information and detailed analysis of the nascent developments around the world.

We would like to thank all the contributing authors for lending their expertise to make the book truly unique. They have played a crucial role in the development of this book. Without their invaluable contributions this book wouldn't have been possible. They have made vital efforts to compile up to date information on the varied aspects of this subject to make this book a valuable addition to the collection of many professionals and students.

This book was conceptualized with the vision of imparting up-to-date information and advanced data in this field. To ensure the same, a matchless editorial board was set up. Every individual on the board went through rigorous rounds of assessment to prove their worth. After which they invested a large part of their time researching and compiling the most relevant data for our readers.

The editorial board has been involved in producing this book since its inception. They have spent rigorous hours researching and exploring the diverse topics which have resulted in the successful publishing of this book. They have passed on their knowledge of decades through this book. To expedite this challenging task, the publisher supported the team at every step. A small team of assistant editors was also appointed to further simplify the editing procedure and attain best results for the readers.

Apart from the editorial board, the designing team has also invested a significant amount of their time in understanding the subject and creating the most relevant covers. They scrutinized every image to scout for the most suitable representation of the subject and create an appropriate cover for the book.

The publishing team has been an ardent support to the editorial, designing and production team. Their endless efforts to recruit the best for this project, has resulted in the accomplishment of this book. They are a veteran in the field of academics and their pool of knowledge is as vast as their experience in printing. Their expertise and guidance has proved useful at every step. Their uncompromising quality standards have made this book an exceptional effort. Their encouragement from time to time has been an inspiration for everyone.

The publisher and the editorial board hope that this book will prove to be a valuable piece of knowledge for researchers, students, practitioners and scholars across the globe.

List of Contributors

Marion Willard Evans Jr
Texas Chiropractic College, Pasadena, TX, USA

Stephen M Perle
University of Bridgeport, Bridgeport, CT USA

Harrison Ndetan
Parker Research Institute, Dallas, TX, USA

Paul E Dougherty
Research Department, New York Chiropractic College, 2360 State Route 89, Seneca Falls, NY 13148, USA
School of Medicine and Dentistry, University of Rochester, Rochester, NY 14620, USA

Cheryl Hawk
Logan College of Chiropractic, Chesterfield, MO 63017, USA

Debra K Weiner
Anesthesiology & Psychiatry, VA Pittsburgh, Pittsburgh 15261, USA
U. of Pittsburgh, 3550 Terrace Street Pittsburgh, PA 1526, USA

Brian Gleberzon
Canadian Memorial Chiropractic College, 6100 Leslie Street, Toronto, ON M2H 3J1, Canada

Kari Andrew
Palmer College of Chiropractic, 1000 Brady St, Davenport, IA 52803, USA

Lisa Killinger
Palmer College of Chiropractic, 1000 Brady St, Davenport, IA 52803, USA

Richard Brown
The Lansdown Clinic, 1, High Street, Stroud, Gloucestershire GL5 1AU, United Kingdom

Jennifer E Bolton
Anglo-European College of Chiropractic, Parkwood Road, Bournemouth BH5 DF, UK

Hugh C Hurst
Clifton Chiropractic Clinic, 123 Pembroke Road, Clifton BS8 3EU, UK

Andrée-Anne Marchand
Canadian Memorial Chiropractic College (CMCC), Toronto, Ontario and Université du Québec à Trois-Rivieres (UQTR), Trois-Rivieres, Québec, Canada

Julie O'Shaughnessy
Département de chiropratique, Université du Québec à Trois-Rivières (UQTR), Trois-Rivières, Québec, Canada

Kent Stuber
6100 Leslie Street, Toronto, ON M2H 3J1, Canada

Paul Bruno
3737 Wascana Parkway, Regina, Saskatchewan S4S 0A2, Canada

Kevyn Kristmanson
102 - 12 Cheadle St. West Swift Current, Saskatchewan S9H 0A9, Canada

Zara Ali
6100 Leslie Street, Toronto, ON M2H 3J1, Canada

Richard P Saporito
Assistant Professor of Clinical Sciences, University of Bridgeport College of Chiropractic, 75 Linden Avenue, Bridgeport, CT 06604, USA

Farah M Shroff
Department of Family Practice and School of Population and Public Health, University of British Columbia, Third Floor David Strangway Bldg, 5950 University Blvd, Vancouver, BC V6T 1Z3, Canada

Inderjeet S Sahota
Department of Biomedical Physiology and Kinesiology, Simon Fraser University, Simon Fraser, Canada

Rainer Wieser
C3 Chiropractic Clinic, 223-225 Pantbach Road, Rhiwbina, Cardiff, Wales CF14 6AE, UK

Haymo Thiel
Anglo-European College of Chiropractic, 13-15 Parkwood Road, Bournemouth, Dorset BH5 2DF, UK

Diane E Grondin
Canadian Memorial Chiropractic College, 6100 Leslie Street, Toronto, ON M2H 3J1, Canada

John J Triano
Canadian Memorial Chiropractic College, 6100 Leslie Street, Toronto, ON M2H 3J1, Canada

Steve Tran
Canadian Memorial Chiropractic College, 6100 Leslie Street, Toronto, ON M2H 3J1, Canada

David Soave
Canadian Memorial Chiropractic College, 6100 Leslie Street, Toronto, ON M2H 3J1, Canada

Caroline D Peterson
Private Practice, Portland, OR, USA

Mitchell Haas
Division of Research, University of Western States, Portland, OR, USA

W Thomas Gregory
Department of Obstetrics & Gynecology, Oregon Health & Science University, Portland, OR, USA

Benjamin T. Brown
Department of Chiropractic, Macquarie University, Balaclava Road, North Ryde 2109NSW, Australia

Petra L. Graham
Department of Statistics, Macquarie University, Balaclava Road, North Ryde 2109NSW, Australia

Rod Bonello
School of Health Professions - Murdoch University, 90 South Street, Murdoch 6150WA, Australia

Henry Pollard
Private Practice, 84 Kingsway, Cronulla 2230NSW, Australia

Patricia E Fikar
Private Practice, Vienna, Austria

Kent A Edlund
AECC-Anglo-European College of Chiropractic, 13-15 Parkwood Road, Bournemouth, Dorset BH5 2DF, UK

Dave Newell
AECC-Anglo-European College of Chiropractic, 13-15 Parkwood Road, Bournemouth, Dorset BH5 2DF, UK

Hugh MacPherson
Department of Health Sciences, University of York, York, UK

Elizabeth Newbronner
Firefly Research & Evaluation and Visiting Fellow, Department of Health Sciences, University of York, York, UK

Ruth Chamberlain
Firefly Research & Evaluation, North Yorkshire, UK

Ann Hopton
Department of Health Sciences, University of York, York, UK

Jon Adams
Australian Research Centre in Complementary and Integrative Medicine, Faculty of Health, University of Technology Sydney, Australia

Amie Steel
Australian Research Centre in Complementary and Integrative Medicine, Faculty of Health, University of Technology Sydney, Australia
Office of Research, Endeavour College of Natural Health, Brisbane, Australia

Sungwon Chang
Australian Research Centre in Complementary and Integrative Medicine, Faculty of Health, University of Technology Sydney, Australia

David Sibbritt
Australian Research Centre in Complementary and Integrative Medicine, Faculty of Health, University of Technology Sydney, Australia

Alexander Ruhe
Murdoch University. Praxis fuer Chiropraktik Wolfsburg, Porschestrasse 1, 38440 Wolfsburg, Germany

René Fejer
Research Department, Spine Centre of Southern Denmark, Hospital Lillebaelt and University of Southern Denmark, Middelfart, Denmark

Bruce Walker
School of Chiropractic and Sports Science, Murdoch University, Murdoch, 6150, Western Australia, Australia

Francesco Ferrarello
Functional Rehabilitation Unit, Azienda USL 4, Via Cavour 118/120, 59100 Prato, Italy

Gabriella Deluca
Fondazione Don Carlo Gnocchi ONLUS-IRCCS, Florence, Italy

Assunta Pizzi
Fondazione Don Carlo Gnocchi ONLUS-IRCCS, Florence, Italy

Carlo Baldini
Fondazione Don Carlo Gnocchi ONLUS-IRCCS, Florence, Italy

Francesca Iori
Fondazione Don Carlo Gnocchi ONLUS-IRCCS, Florence, Italy

Niccolò Marchionni
Research Unit of Medicine of Aging, Department of Experimental and Clinical Medicine, University of Florence, and Azienda Ospedaliero-Universitaria Careggi, Florence, Italy

Mauro Di Bari
Research Unit of Medicine of Aging, Department of Experimental and Clinical Medicine, University of Florence, and Azienda Ospedaliero-Universitaria Careggi, Florence, Italy

Dayna Pool
Department of Physiotherapy and Paediatric Rehabilitation, Princess Margaret Hospital for Children, Roberts Road, Subiaco, 6008 Perth, Australia

Jane Valentine
Department of Paediatric Rehabilitation, Princess Margaret Hospital for Children, Perth, Australia

A. Marie Blackmore
The Centre for Cerebral Palsy, Perth, Australia

Jennifer Colegate
Department of Occupational Therapy and Paediatric Rehabilitation, Princess Margaret Hospital for Children, Perth, Australia

Natasha Bear
Department of Physiotherapy and Paediatric Rehabilitation, Princess Margaret Hospital for Children, Roberts Road, Subiaco, 6008 Perth, Australia

Katherine Stannage
Department of Orthopaedics, Princess Margaret Hospital for Children, Perth, Australia

Catherine Elliott
Faculty of Health Science, Curtin University of Technology, Perth, Australia

Nichola J. Hatton
Tameside General Hospital, Ashton-u-Lyne, Greater Manchester OL6 9RW, UK

Rachel C. Stockley
Department of Health Professions, Birley Campus, Manchester Metropolitan University, Manchester M15 6GX, UK

Chad E Cook
Department of Orthopaedics, Duke University, 2200 Main Street, 27705 Durham, NC, USA

Thomas J Moore
Department of Physical and Occupational Therapy, Duke University Medical Center, Clinic 1E, Trent Drive and Erwin Road, 27710 Durham, NC, USA

Kenneth Learman
Department of Physical Therapy, One University Plaza, 44555 Youngstown, Ohio, USA

Christopher Showalter
Maitland-Australian, Physiotherapy Seminars, PO Box 1244, 11935 Cutchogue, NY, USA

Suzanne J Snodgrass
Department of Physiotherapy, University Drive, 2308 Callaghan, NSW, Australia

Pawel Kiper
Laboratory of Kinematics and Robotics, IRCCS San Camillo Hospital Foundation, via Alberoni 70, Venice 30126, Italy

Alfonc Baba
Laboratory of Kinematics and Robotics, IRCCS San Camillo Hospital Foundation, via Alberoni 70, Venice 30126, Italy

Michela Agostini
Laboratory of Kinematics and Robotics, IRCCS San Camillo Hospital Foundation, via Alberoni 70, Venice 30126, Italy

Andrea Turolla
Laboratory of Kinematics and Robotics, IRCCS San Camillo Hospital Foundation, via Alberoni 70, Venice 30126, Italy
Department of Neuroscience, University of Sheffield, Glossop Road, Sheffield S10 2JF, UK

Sylvana S Asche, Marjolein Krul and Sita MA Bierma-Zeinstra
Department of General Practice, Erasmus MC-University Medical Centre
Rotterdam, PO Box 2040, 3000 CA, Rotterdam, The Netherlands

Rogier M van Rijn
Department of General Practice, Erasmus MC-University Medical Centre Rotterdam, PO Box 2040, 3000 CA, Rotterdam, The Netherlands
Department of Public Health, Erasmus MC-University Medical Centre Rotterdam, PO Box 2040, 3000 CA, Rotterdam, The Netherlands

Johannes HJM Bessems
Department of Orthopedic Surgery, Erasmus MC-Sophia Children's Hospital Rotterdam, Dr. Molewaterplein 60, 3015 GJ, Rotterdam, The Netherlands

Nadège Lemeunier
Complexité, Innovation et Activités Motrices et Sportives, Bâtiment 335, UFR
STAPS, Université Paris Sud-11, Orsay Cedex 91405, France

Institut Franco- Européen de Chiropratique, 72 Chemin de la Flambère, Toulouse 31300, France

Charlotte Leboeuf-Yde
Complexité, Innovation et Activités Motrices et Sportives, Bâtiment 335, UFR
STAPS, Université Paris Sud-11, Orsay Cedex 91405, France
Research Department, Spine Center of Southern Denmark, Hospital Lillebaelt and Institute of Regional Health Services Research, University of Southern Denmark, Ostre Hougvej 55, Middelfart, Denmark

Olivier Gagey
Complexité, Innovation et Activités Motrices et Sportives, Bâtiment 335, UFR STAPS, Université Paris Sud-11, Orsay Cedex 91405, France

David R Seaman
National University of Health Sciences, SPC-Health Education Center, 7200 66th St, Pinellas Park, FL 33781, USA

Robert Cooperstein and Morgan Young
Palmer West College of Chiropractic, 90 East Tasman Drive, San Jose, CA 95134, USA

James Donovan
Division of Health Care and Outcomes Research, Toronto Western Research Institute, University Health Network, University of Toronto, Toronto, Canada

Carol Cancelliere
Division of Health Care and Outcomes Research, Toronto Western Research Institute, University Health Network, University of Toronto, Toronto, Canada
Institute of Health Policy, Management and Evaluation, University of Toronto, Toronto, Canada

J David Cassidy
Division of Health Care and Outcomes Research, Toronto Western Research Institute, University Health Network, University of Toronto, Toronto, Canada
Institute of Health Policy, Management and Evaluation, University of Toronto, Toronto, Canada
Institute of Sports Science and Clinical Biomechanics, Faculty of Health, University of Southern Denmark, Odense, Denmark

Samira Golriz
School of Chiropractic and Sports Science, Murdoch University, 90 South Street, Murdoch, WA 6150, Australia

Jeffrey J Hebert and Bruce F Walker
School of Chiropractic and Sports Science, Murdoch University, Perth, WA, Australia

K Bo Foreman
Department of Physical Therapy, University of Utah, Salt Lake City, UT, USA

Samira Golriz
School of Chiropractic and Sports Science, Murdoch University, 90 South Street, MurdochWA 6150, Perth, Australia

Jeffrey J Hebert and Bruce F Walker
School of Chiropractic and Sports Science, Murdoch University, Perth, WA, Australia

K Bo Foreman
Department of Physical Therapy, University of Utah, Salt Lake City, UT, USA

Robert Cooperstein and Morgan Young
Palmer West College of Chiropractic, 90 East Tasman Drive, San Jose, CA 94577, USA

Michael Haneline
University of Western States, 2900 NE 132nd Avenue, Portland, OR 97230, USA